COMBATING ONLINE HEALTH MISINFORMATION

Medical Library Association Books

The Medical Library Association (MLA) publishes state-of-the-art books that enhance health care, support professional development, improve library services and promote research throughout the world.

MLA books are dynamic resources for librarians in hospitals, medical research practice, corporate libraries, and other settings. These invaluable publications provide medical librarians, health care professionals and patients with accurate information that can improve outcomes and save lives.

Medical Library Association Books Panel

The MLA Books Panel is responsible for (1) monitoring publishing trends within the industry; (2) exploring new concepts in publications by actively soliciting and proposing ideas for new publications; and (3) coordinating publishing efforts to achieve the best utilization of MLA resources. Each MLA book is directly administered from its inception by the MLA Books Panel, composed of MLA members with expertise spanning the breadth of health sciences librarianship.

About the Medical Library Association

The Medical Library Association (MLA) is a global, nonprofit educational organization, with a membership of more than 400 institutions and 3,000 professionals in the health information field. Since 1898, MLA has fostered excellence in the professional practice and leadership of health sciences library and information professionals to enhance health care, education, and research throughout the world. MLA educates health information professionals, supports health information research, promotes access to the world's health sciences information, and works to ensure that the best health information is available to all.

Recently Published MLA Books

3D Printing in Medical Libraries: A Crash Course in Supporting Innovation in Healthcare by Jennifer Herron
Diversity and Inclusion in Libraries: A Call to Action and Strategies for Success Edited by Shannon D. Jones and Beverly Murphy
Framing Health Care Instruction: An Information Literacy Handbook for the Health Sciences by Lauren M. Young and Elizabeth G. Hinton
The Clinical Medical Librarian's Handbook Edited by Judy C. Stribling
The Engaged Health Sciences Library Liaison Edited by Lindsay Alcock and Kelly Thormodson
A History of Medical Libraries and Medical Librarianship: From John Shaw Billings to the Digital Era by Michael R. Kronenfeld and Jennie Jacobs Kronenfeld
Planning and Promoting Events in Health Sciences Libraries: Success Stories and Best Practices Edited by Shalu Gillum and Natasha Williams
Great Library Events: From Planning to Promotion to Evaluation by Mary Grace Flaherty
Assessing Academic Library Performance: A Handbook by Holt Zaugg
Finding Your Seat at the Table: Roles for Librarians on Institutional Regulatory Boards and Committees Edited by Susan M. Harnett and Laureen P. Cantwell
Virtual Services in the Health Sciences Library: A Handbook Edited by Amanda R. Scull
Combating Online Health Misinformation: A Professional's Guide to Helping the Public Edited by Alla Keselman, Catherine Arnott Smith, and Amanda J. Wilson

COMBATING ONLINE HEALTH MISINFORMATION

A Professional's Guide to Helping the Public

Edited by
Alla Keselman, Catherine Arnott Smith, and Amanda J. Wilson

ROWMAN & LITTLEFIELD
Lanham • Boulder • New York • London

Published by Rowman & Littlefield
An imprint of The Rowman & Littlefield Publishing Group, Inc.
4501 Forbes Boulevard, Suite 200, Lanham, Maryland 20706
www.rowman.com

86-90 Paul Street, London EC2A 4NE

British Library Cataloguing in Publication Information Available

Library of Congress Cataloging-in-Publication Data

Names: Keselman, Alla, editor. | Smith, Catherine Arnott, editor. | Wilson, Amanda J., editor.
Title: Combating online health misinformation : a professional's guide to helping the public / edited by Alla Keselman, Catherine Arnott Smith, and Amanda J. Wilson.
Description: Lanham : Rowman & Littlefield Publishers, [2022] | Series: Medical library association books series | Includes bibliographical references and index.
Identifiers: LCCN 2022014978 (print) | LCCN 2022014979 (ebook) | ISBN 9781538162194 (cloth) | ISBN 9781538162200 (paperback) | ISBN 9781538162217 (ebook)
Subjects: LCSH: Health—Information services. | Medicine—Information services. | Communication in medicine. | Electronic information resource literacy.
Classification: LCC R118.2 .C645 2022 (print) | LCC R118.2 (ebook) | DDC 610.1/4—dc23/eng/20220706
LC record available at https://lccn.loc.gov/2022014978
LC ebook record available at https://lccn.loc.gov/2022014979

Contents

Preface vii

Part I: The Ecology of Online Health Information

1 Defining Health Misinformation 3
Yuan Wang, Kathryn Thier, and Xiaoli Nan

2 The Ecology of Online Health Information and COVID-19 Misinformation 17
David R. Kaufman, Adiebonye E. Jumbo, and Tonya N. Taylor

3 The Health Misinformation Ecosystem on Social Media: Emerging Evidence and Research Gaps 31
Wen-Ying Sylvia Chou, Anna Gaysynsky, and Yuki Lama

4 Flies in the Ointment: Vaccine Hesitancy and Bad Medical Advice during the Russian COVID-19 Pandemic 45
Alexandra Arkhipova and Ian Brodie

Part II: Susceptibility to Misinformation; Literacies as Safeguards

5 Let the Reader and Viewer Beware: Quality Markers for Health Information 61
Catherine Arnott Smith

6 Preventing Health Number Confusion through Clear Communication Design 77
Brian J. Zikmund-Fisher and Jessica S. Ancker

7 The Case of Everyday Science: Science Literacy and Resilience against Health Misinformation 91
Alla Keselman

8 An Examination of the Multiple Dimensions of Public Trust in Science as Health Misinformation Roadblocks 105
Alla Keselman and Amanda J. Wilson

9 Critical Cultural Literacy Education as a Bridge to Improving Health Disparities in BIPOC Communities 121
Jason Alston and Nicole A. Cooke

Part III: Practice

10 When Medical Practice Meets Medical Myth: Confronting Misinformation in the Clinical Encounter 137
Jamie L. Wood, Erin Eckert, Megan von Isenburg, Joseph Jackson, and Brian G. Southwell

11 Teaching Young People to Think Critically about Health Claims and Choices 149
Sarah Rosenbaum, Allen Nsangi, and Daniel Semakula

12 Medical Professionals Using Social Media to Combat Misinformation 167
Lisa Mordell, Eve Bloomgarden, Shikha Jain, and Vineet Arora

13 Participation, Empowerment, and Equity: Addressing eHealth Misinformation with Community Engagement in Libraries 187
Amanda J. Wilson and Laura Bartlett

14 Addressing Health Misinformation in the Infodemic Era: The Alaska Public Health Information Response Team 207
Jennifer Meyer, Joy Chavez Mapaye, Alexandra Edwards, Thomas Hennessy, Tim Hinterberger, and Mary Ryan

Index 221

About the Editors 231

About the Contributors 233

Preface

THE IDEA FOR THIS BOOK was conceived in the summer of 2020. The COVID-19 pandemic and the accompanying infodemic presented us with a particularly urgent example, in a long line of examples, of the critical need to support the public in distinguishing good information from potentially harmful information.

Misinformation has been defined as "objectively incorrect information that is not supported by scientific evidence and expert opinion" (Kim et al. 2020, 588). While the 2016 US presidential election brought intense attention to the phenomenon in politics, Molina et al. (2019) analogize it to a much older problem—"yellow journalism"—dating from the Spanish-American War of 1896. Misinformation differs from disinformation in that disinformation connotes "an intentional, deliberate, or purposeful effort to mislead, deceive, or confuse" (194). Misinformation, conversely, is content that is "explicitly false" (Tan 2015). Regardless of the originator's motives in producing it, the inaccurate content exists on a spectrum from completely false to simply misleading. In the health domain, misinformation manifests itself in a proliferation of promotions of nonevidence-based health advice, treatment recommendations, and outright denialism of medical realities ranging from HIV to COVID-19.

The purpose of this book is to help librarians, journalists, health care professionals, community organizers, health communicators, teachers, and community health workers combat the proliferation of online health misinformation. In order to support the public in dealing with health misinformation, professionals themselves need support. The book will also help researchers who investigate the spread of health misinformation and the contexts and characteristics that make individuals susceptible. While much is written about information literacy, professionals and future professionals need a comprehensive picture of the foundations of ehealth literacy, an in-depth picture of different types of misinformation, and a broad range of solutions. These solutions involve different nonclinical settings, a broad range of professionals and contexts, and a combination of expert-led community and machine approaches to misinformation. This book represents a diversity of perspectives reflective of the authors' geography and disciplines.

This book aims to assist professionals with all phases of information provision and support, from understanding users' information needs, to building relationships, to helping users verify and evaluate sources. The book can be used as a textbook in library and information science programs, as well as nursing, communication, journalism, psychology, and informatics programs.

The content is organized into three parts. Part I: The Ecology of Online Health Information provides the context for the reader to understand health misinformation online. In chapter 1, "Defining Health Misinformation, authors Wang, Thier, and Nan provide a critical review of current definitions of health misinformation, discuss key challenges in defining the concept, propose a unifying definition for future research, and discuss directions for refining that definition. In chapter 2, "The Ecology of Online Health Information and COVID-19 Misinformation," Kaufman, Jumbo, and Taylor provide an overview of the ecology of COVID-19 misinformation, disinformation, and conspiracy theories, focusing on historical accounts, psychological factors, and social media dynamics and strategies that make individuals vulnerable. Chapter 3 in this section, by Chou, Gaysynsky, and Lama, is "The Health Misinformation Ecosystem on Social Media: Emerging Evidence and Research Gaps." This chapter reviews existing research in the spread of misinformation on social media, focusing on user characteristics that increase vulnerability and presenting impact studies of mitigation methods. The authors point out gaps in our current understanding of the subject and suggest directions for future research. In the final chapter of this part, "Flies in the Ointment: Vaccine Hesitancy and Bad Medical Advice during the Russian COVID-19 Pandemic," Arkhipova and Brodie analyze recurrent conspicuous themes of COVID-19-related rumors and other infodemic narratives in the Russian social media. The authors show how these narratives, many of which parallel those in the cyber universe worldwide, are deeply embedded in culture, history, and attitudes toward institutions of power.

Part II: Susceptibility to Misinformation; Literacies as Safeguards explains key competencies that citizens need to acquire in order to benefit from online health information, rather than be harmed by it. This part opens with chapter 5, "Let the Reader and Viewer Beware: Quality Markers for Health Information," by Arnott Smith. This chapter examines the evolution of health information quality criteria, showing that while the strategies for applying these criteria have changed with the emergence of new technologies, their basic principles and objectives remain the same. Chapter 6 is "Preventing Health Number Confusion through Clear Communication Design" by Zikmund-Fisher and Ancker. This chapter discusses reasons why people often have difficulty with numbers that convey health information and outlines strategies for making number communication meaningful and useful. In chapter 7, "The Case of Everyday Science: Science Literacy and Resilience against Health Misinformation," Keselman introduces the multidimensional concept of science literacy and reviews the role that each component has in fostering resilience against misinformation, as well as the place of science literacy among other factors that influence information behaviors. Chapter 8, "An Examination of the Multiple Dimensions of Public Trust in Science as Health Misinformation Roadblocks," by Keselman and Wilson shows how individuals' views of science and scientists, trust in the government, political ideology, religious beliefs, education, and social context affect their trust in science and reactions to health misinformation. The last chapter of this part by Alston and Cooke, "Critical Cultural Literacy Education as a Bridge to Improving Health Disparities in BIPOC Communities," discusses how online health misinformation affects BIPOC communities whose vulnerability to misinformation is furthered by mistrust of authorities, health disparities, racism, and implicit biases among health care providers. The authors propose education grounded in critical cultural literacy as an antidote to health misinformation.

Part III: Practice presents a range of interventions, both human-led and computer-assisted, from the education of patients, students, and consumers to AI technologies. In chapter 10, "When Medical Practice Meets Medical Myth: Confronting Misinformation in the Clinical Encounter," Wood, Eckert, von Isenburg, Jackson, and Southwell discuss physicians' experiences with medical misinformation brought to them by their patients and describe the Duke University Medical Center Program on Medical Misinformation that trains physicians to address misinformation in a clinical encounter. Chapter 11, "Teaching Young People to Think Critically about Health Claims and Choices," by Rosenbaum, Nsangi, and Semakula describes the development and evaluation of primary school learning resources for children ages ten to twelve who support young people's capacity to evaluate health information critically. The project is international in scope, funded by the Norwegian Research Council, pilot-tested in East Africa, and adapted for use in many other countries. In chapter 12, "Medical Professionals Using Social Media to Combat Misinformation," Mordell, Bloomgarden, Jain, and Arora describe their models of combating misinformation and its application by a collaborative team of health care professionals in the state of Illinois in the context of the COVID-19 pandemic. Chapter 13 by Wilson and Bartlett, titled "Participation, Empowerment, and Equity: Addressing eHealth Misinformation with Community Engagement in Libraries," discusses how library-led community engagement, grounded in the framework of critical health literacy (CHL) and principles of community-based participatory research (CBPR), can address ehealth misinformation. The authors also recommend practical strategies for immediate implementation. The final chapter, "Addressing Health Misinformation in the Infodemic Era: The Alaska Public Health Information Response Team," by Meyer, Chavez Mapaye, Edwards, Hennessy, Hinterberger, and Ryan presents another social media intervention by health experts aiming to counter the impact of misinformation, "potentially influencing community norms, and individual health behaviors."

We hope that by publishing this book we not only draw readers' attention to an important issue but also provide them with tools for addressing it.

References

Kim, H. K., J. Ahn, L. Atkinson, and L. A. Kahlor. (2020). Effects of COVID-19 misinformation on information seeking, avoidance, and processing: A multicountry comparative study. *Science Communication*, 42(5), 586-615. doi:10.1177/1075547020959670.

Molina, Maria D., S. Shyam Sundar, Thai Le, and Dongwon Lee. (2019). "Fake news" is not simply false information: A concept explication and taxonomy of online content. *American Behavioral Scientist*, 65(2), 180–212.

Tan, Andy S. L., Chul⊠joo Lee, and Jiyoung Chae. (2015). Exposure to health (mis)information: Lagged effects on young adults' health behaviors and potential pathways. *Journal of Communication* 65, 674–698.

I

THE ECOLOGY OF ONLINE HEALTH INFORMATION

1

Defining Health Misinformation

Yuan Wang, Kathryn Thier, and Xiaoli Nan

According to the World Health Organization (WHO), we are entering an age of "infodemics," with misinformation leading to mistrust in health authorities, increasing risk-taking behaviors, and undermining public health responses (WHO 2020). While concerns are rapidly growing about the prevalence and harmful impact of health misinformation (Nan, Wang, and Thier 2021), scholars have not clearly defined health misinformation or its components. Without a clear definition and shared agreement on what constitutes health misinformation, comparisons across studies purportedly about health misinformation will remain challenging, hampering our efforts to understand this phenomenon, assess its effects, and design effective interventions. However, defining misinformation in the first place is exceedingly difficult, partly because the benchmarks we often use to diagnose misinformation (e.g., scientific evidence and expert consensus) are sometimes moving targets (Vraga and Bode 2020). In light of the ongoing debate about the nature of misinformation and the urgent need for a clear definition of health misinformation, this chapter aims to critically review current definitions of health misinformation, identify key challenges in defining health misinformation, and finally propose a tentative, unifying definition of health misinformation to guide future research. We conclude by discussing directions for future efforts in refining the definition of health misinformation.

Current Definitions of Health Misinformation

To identify current definitions of health misinformation, we conducted a comprehensive review of the literature on health misinformation, including both scholarly and government publications. Scholarly articles were located from nine research databases (Communication & Mass Media Complete, Health Source, Psychology & Behavioral Sciences Collection, APA PsycInfo, Academic Search Ultimate, Medline, Education Source, PubMed, and JSTOR). We found that although some articles on health misinformation provide an explicit definition of health misinformation or misinformation, most do not. Among the peer-reviewed empirical articles we reviewed ($N = 286$), only a small subset (about 15 percent) provided or cited a definition of health misinformation or misinformation. Moreover, publications that do offer a definition often define misinformation generally, not health misinformation specifically. In fact, it appears only two definitions offered so far are specifically tailored to health misinformation. Chou, Oh, and Klein (2018) defined health misinformation as "a health-related claim of fact that is currently false due to a lack of scientific evidence" (2417). Swire-Thompson and Lazer (2020) defined science and health misinformation as "information that is contrary to the epistemic consensus of the scientific community regarding a phenomenon" (434).

Table 1.1 lists all definitions of misinformation or health misinformation identified through our review of the health misinformation literature. Table 1.2 is a collection of definitions for related concepts concurrently studied in health misinformation research, such as disinformation, conspiracy theories, rumors, and medical folk wisdom. As both tables show, there is no shortage of definitions for misinformation and related constructs, which is indicative of a lack of consensus among researchers about what misinformation is generally and what constitutes health misinformation specifically.

Through our review of the current literature on health misinformation, we identified two key challenges for defining health misinformation: (1) a lack of consistent terminology for misinformation and (2) a lack of agreement on the defining features of misinformation.

TABLE 1.1
Conceptual Definitions of Misinformation/Health Misinformation in Current Health Misinformation Literature

Authors	*Definition*
	General context
Al Khaja, AlKhaja, and Sequeira (2018)	"Unintentionally false information" (345).
Bode and Vraga (2015)	"Misinformation, or factual misperception, refers to the presence of or belief in objectively incorrect information" (621).
Bode, Vraga, and Tully (2020)	"Objectively incorrect information, as determined by the best available evidence and expertise on the subject" (227).
CDC (2020)	"False information shared by people who do not intend to mislead others" (n.p.).
Chen, Wang, and Peng (2018)	"False and inaccurate information that is spread intentionally or unintentionally" (2).
Chou, Oh, and Klein (2018)	"A health-related claim of fact that is currently false due to lack of scientific evidence" (2417).
Cook, Lewandowsky, and Ecker (2017)	"Information that people accept as true despite it being false" (1).
Deshpande, Deshpande, and O'Brien (2018)	"Information that is known to be untrue or uninvestigated" (562).
Duplaga (2020)	"False or misleading information" (2).
Featherstone and Zhang (2020)	"Information that has received a consensus of rejection from either the public or experts" (693).
Ferrand et al. (2020)	"Either deliberate or accidental promotion of previously disproved or unproven beliefs, attitudes, and behaviors" (4).
Fode et al. (2020)	"Contradictions of established literature and/or guidelines" (409).
Gesser-Edelsburg et al. (2018)	"Deficient information" (2).
Ghezzi et al. (2020)	"Incorrect information that stems from human error (e.g., a lack of fact checking), whereas disinformation is purposefully and deliberately incorrect" (2).
Hornik et al. (2021)	"False and misleading information" (6).

Authors	Definition
Kim et al. (2020)	"Objectively incorrect information that is not supported by scientific evidence and expert opinion" (588).
Krishna and Thompson (2019)	"Acceptance of false or (scientifically) inaccurate data as useful (a) despite exposure to (scientifically) accurate data, (b) in the absence of accurate data or messages to the contrary, or/and (c) within historical or contextual legacies" (325).
Nyhan and Reifler (2010)	"Cases in which people's beliefs about factual matters are not supported by clear evidence and expert opinion" (305).
Sallam, Dababseh, Yaseen, Al-Haidar, Taim, et al. (2020)	"Inaccurate or false information that are communicated regardless of the deception intent" (2).
Sangalang, Ophir, and Cappella (2019)	"Misinformation can encompass both factually incorrect information and misleading information that leads the public to form incorrect perceptions" (299).
Shah et al. (2019)	"Communications that are not a fair representation of available evidence or communicate that evidence poorly" (2).
Southwell, Thorson, and Sheble (2018)	"Claims to which mass audiences are exposed that do not actually enjoy universal or near-universal consensus as being true at a particular moment in time" (4).
Southwell et al. (2019)	"False or inaccurate information regardless of intentional authorship" (282).
Sullivan (2019)	"Incorrect information" (2).
Swire-Thompson and Lazer (2020)	"Information that is contrary to the epistemic consensus of the scientific community regarding a phenomenon" (434).
S. Zhang et al. (2021)	"A claim that is not supported by scientific evidence and expert opinion" (2).
Tan, Lee, and Chae (2015)	"We define facts or misinformation to be based on what is considered to be correct or incorrect by expert consensus contemporaneous with the time period of this study" (675).
Tran et al. (2020)	"Incorrect information which can seem to be legitimate initially but can mislead and create harmful effects to the individual and the community" (2).
Wang et al. (2019)	"Misinformation involves information that is inadvertently false and is shared without intent to cause harm" (2).
Xiao, Borah, and Su (2021)	"The false information that is circulated without the disseminators' knowledge" (981).
Xu, Chen, and Safarnejad (2020)	"False or inaccurate information that could mislead people regardless of intention" (1561).
Yang et al. (2018)	"Information currently considered to be incorrect by expert consensus" (362).
	Specific context
Badell-Grau et al. (2020) (The Covid-19 context)	"Misinformation is defined as no empirical evidence, nor active published peer reviewed research, regarding their relevance to COVID-19 and their media coverage indicative of their potential for controversy" (8).
van der Meer and Jin (2020) (Crisis context)	"We define crisis misinformation as false information about a crisis, initially assumed to be valid but can be later corrected or retracted, that can lead to factual misperception held by people" (561).

TABLE 1.2
Conceptual Definitions of Misinformation-Related Concepts in Current Health Misinformation Literature

Concepts	*Authors*	*Definition*
Conspiracy beliefs	Sallam, Dababseh, Yaseen, Al-Haidar, Ababneh, et al. (2020)	"Unsubstantiated and implausible beliefs that involve the role of a malevolent force in plotting major events when other explanations are more probable" (2).
Conspiracy theories	Wood (2018)	"Suspicions that powerful people or organizations are secretly carrying out sinister plans by deceiving the public at large" (485).
Conspiracy theories	Y. Zhang et al. (2021)	"Claims that are generally unsubstantiated and thus referred as misinformation to some extent" (585).
Disinformation	Al Khaja et al. (2018)	"Intentionally false or inaccurate information that is spread deliberately" (345).
Disinformation	CDC (2020)	"False information deliberately created and disseminated with malicious intent" (n.p.).
Disinformation	Yoon et al. (2020)	"False information to mislead the public" (5).
Fake news	Sommariva et al. (2018)	"Misinformation that has the trappings of traditional news media, with the presumed associated editorial processes" (246).
Fake news	Waszak, Kasprzycka-Waszak, and Kubanek (2018)	"News that is intentionally false and could mislead readers" (115).
Infodemic	WHO (2020)	"An infodemic is too much information including false or misleading information in digital and physical environments during a disease outbreak" (n.p.).
Medical folk wisdom (MFW)	Motta and Callaghan (2020)	"Popular, yet inaccurate, information about a wide range of medically relevant topics, which are thought to have ancient origins and spread via word of mouth from parents to children" (10722).
Misleading information	Pathak et al. (2015)	"Videos containing at least one scientifically unproven information" (307).
Misleading information	Russo, Metcalf, and Stephens (1981)	"An advertisement is misleading if it creates, increases, or exploits a false belief about expected product performance" (119).
Misperception	van Stekelenburg et al. (2020)	"Factual beliefs that are false or contradict the best available evidence in the public domain" (32).
Rumor	DeClerque et al. (1986)	"An unconfirmed message passed from one person to another in face-to-face interaction that refers to an object" (84).
Rumor	Ozturk, Li, and Sakamoto (2015)	"A rumor is commonly defined as a statement whose informational truthfulness is unverified" (2406).

Key Challenges in Defining Health Misinformation

Lack of Consistent Terminology

The first challenge in defining health misinformation is a lack of consistency in terminology. The term "misinformation" and related concepts such as rumors, misleading advertising, fake news, and conspiracy theories are often used interchangeably. Early research on health misinformation mainly focused on face-to-face settings, and rumors constituted the main subject of study (e.g., DeClerque et al. 1986; Kroeger 2003). A rumor is "an unconfirmed message passed from one person to another" (DeClerque et al. 1986, 84). Rumors are not necessarily false but are unsubstantiated claims. The difference between a false claim and an unsubstantiated claim is that the former is in direct contradiction to available evidence, whereas the latter is unsupported due to lack of evidence. For example, the claim that "vape devices would increase humidity in the lungs and thereby prevent COVID-19 infection" is unsubstantiated because the scientific evidence regarding the relationship between vaping and COVID-19 outcomes is still limited, and no consistent conclusion has been drawn (Majmundar et al. 2020, 1667). In contrast, "COVID-19 vaccines contain microchips" is a false claim because it contradicts established scientific facts (Centers for Disease Control and Prevention 2021a).

Misleading advertising is another type of misinformation frequently studied (e.g., Al Khaja, AlKhaja, and Sequeira 2018; Russo, Metcalf, and Stephens 1981). Misleading advertising "creates, increases, or exploits a false belief about expected product performance" (Russo, Metcalf, and Stephens 1981, 128). Claims in misleading advertising are often inaccurate, rather than false or unsubstantiated. Inaccurate claims have some evidentiary support and are often not in direct contradiction to available evidence, but they are based on incomplete evidence through cherry-picking, namely selecting information that supports a particular position while ignoring relevant contradictory evidence (Fooks et al. 2019). Inaccurate claims, therefore, are often misleading. For example, a drug advertisement which claimed that "Annona muricata is useful for treating different types of cancers and other health disorders" is inaccurate because it omits the important fact that it is not generally recognized as safe (GRAS) by the FDA (Al Khaja, AlKhaja, and Sequeira 2018, 351). Another drug advertisement claiming that "AstraZeneca excretes all ingested sugars by kidney" is also inaccurate because it ignores the clinical evidence that the drug removes some blood sugar but not all as claimed (Al Khaja, AlKhaja, and Sequeira 2018, 347).

More recent research has addressed the phenomenon of fake news. Fake news is "misinformation that has the trappings of traditional news media, with the presumed associated editorial processes" (Sommariva et al. 2018, 246). Unlike advertising, which can be intentionally or unintentionally misleading, fake news is "intentionally false" (Waszak, Kasprzycka-Waszak, and Kubanek 2018, 115). Fake medical news, specifically, is intentionally false medical information, which takes the form of fabricated news that contains fictitious medical facts, manipulated news that includes false recommendations based on evidence with exaggerated clinical usefulness, or advertisement news that promote unsubstantiated alternative treatments (Waszak, Kasprzycka-Waszak, and Kubanek 2018; McGrath et al. 2017).

Finally, there is long-standing research on conspiracy theories. Conspiracy theories are "suspicions that powerful people or organizations are secretly carrying out sinister plans by deceiving the public at large" (Wood 2018, 485). In times of crisis, conspiracy theories become prevalent, as they often fulfill the needs for certainty and a sense of control (Douglas, Sutton, and Cichocka 2017, 538). Conspiracy theories are not necessarily false; instead, they are considered unsubstantiated due to their lack of verifiability (Zhang et al. 2021, 3).

Using the term misinformation and other related concepts interchangeably partly reflects a lack of understanding of the differences among false, unsubstantiated, and inaccurate claims. As tables 1.1 and 1.2 show, current definitions of health misinformation or misinformation diverge substantially in the type of claims that is considered misinformation. For example, Chen, Wang, and Peng (2018) focused on false claims and inaccurate claims; they defined misinformation as "false and inaccurate information that is spread intentionally or unintentionally" (2). In contrast, Deshpande, Deshpande, and O'Brien (2018) considered unsubstantiated claims as misinformation and defined misinformation as "information that is known to be untrue or uninvestigated" (562). Inconsistent terminology emerged partly due to a lack of agreement on misinformation's defining features.

Lack of Agreement on the Defining Features of Misinformation

A lack of agreement on the defining features of misinformation is the second challenge in defining health misinformation. Here we outline four points of disagreement. The first concerns the source's intent to deceive. The second relates to the recipients' perceptions of the information. The third pertains to the criteria or benchmarks for distinguishing misinformation from facts. And the fourth concerns the scope of misinformation and whether it should encompass all forms of misinformation including false claims, unsubstantiated claims, and inaccurate claims.

Intent. Some definitions differentiate misinformation from disinformation on the basis of the source's intent to deceive and consider the two types of information as mutually exclusive. With this approach, disinformation refers to "false information knowingly being created and shared to cause harm," whereas misinformation is false information that is "shared without intent to cause harm" (Wang et al. 2019, 2). Disinformation is intentionally produced and disseminated "for social influence or profit," whereas misinformation is unintentionally circulated, often as a result of "honest mistakes, negligence, or unconscious biases" (Fallis 2015, 402). Although the distinction between misinformation and disinformation is clearly valid, it is generally difficult to determine whether a piece of false information is deliberately created or not, and false information can mislead people regardless of the source's intention (Wu et al. 2019, 81). Therefore, we may consider disinformation as a subtype of misinformation and defining health misinformation as an umbrella term to include all misinformation related to health, which can be "both deliberately promoted and accidentally shared" (Southwell, Thorson, and Sheble 2018, 1).

Perceptions. Some definitions of misinformation rely on recipients' perceptions of misinformation. For example, Krishna and Thompson (2019) proposed that recipients' perceived usefulness of misinformation is a prerequisite for labeling certain content as misinformation. They argued that "simply inaccurate and false messages do not constitute misinformation; in order for such data to be called misinformation, they must be accepted as being useful in an individual's problem-solving information search" (9). Similarly, other definitions conceptualize misinformation based on its potential effects on recipients. For example, Fallis (2015) defined misinformation as "information that is likely to create false beliefs" (406). However, definitions that rely on recipients' perceptions or the effects of misinformation are not as useful as ones that are based on the intrinsic features of the misinformation. Whether or not people accept or are misled by misinformation does not change the false nature of the information itself. Further, defining misinformation as information that misleads is tautological, which impedes our understanding of the objective features that characterize misinformation.

Benchmarks. What distinguishes misinformation from facts? This is perhaps the most challenging part of defining misinformation or health misinformation. Some argue that the key distinction between facts and misinformation lies in whether the information is consistent with expert consensus (e.g., Swire-Thompson and Lazer 2020; Tan, Lee, and Chae 2015; Yang et al. 2018). As mentioned earlier, Swire-Thompson and Lazer (2020) defined science and health misinformation as "information that is contrary to the epistemic consensus of the scientific community regarding a phenomenon" (434). Although expert consensus provides a reasonable standard against which we can evaluate the veracity of information in the health domain, relying on expert consensus alone to define health misinformation can be problematic. This is because expert consensus is not always available, especially for emerging or contentious health issues. A second criterion—best available evidence—should be enlisted to distinguish misinformation from facts (Vraga and Bode 2020). Using the best available evidence as an additional criterion also suggests that what is considered as misinformation can change as new evidence comes to light. Defining misinformation as "information considered incorrect based on the best available evidence from relevant experts at the time" takes into account both expert input and best available evidence as the benchmarks for assessing the truthfulness of a claim (Vraga and Bode 2020, 138). Still, there is ambiguity as to what constitutes the best available evidence. In empirical studies, the criteria used to determine misinformation often include diverse sources of evidence, such as peer-reviewed journal articles (Deshpande, Deshpande, and O'Brien 2018, 562), fact-checking websites (Safarnejad et al. 2020, 341), and the latest guidelines from health agencies such as WHO and CDC (Obiała et al. 2020, 2). To foster evidence-based practices in health settings, researchers proposed the hierarchy of evidence pyramid (Brownson, Fielding, and Maylahn 2009; Evans 2003; Murad et al. 2016; Yetley et al. 2017), suggesting that systematic reviews and meta-analyses of randomized controlled trials (RCTs) rank as the highest quality of evidence, followed by RCTs, cohort studies, case-control studies, cross-sectional studies, case reports, and expert opinions. Depending on the highest level of evidence available, there will be a degree of confidence in categorizing a claim of fact as false. Confidence should increase as the highest level of evidence available approaches the top of the hierarchy of evidence pyramid.

Scope. Finally, there is disagreement on whether unsubstantiated and inaccurate information, along with false information, should be subsumed under misinformation. Some suggest that misinformation is explicitly false (Vraga and Bode 2020). Similarly, others argue that health misinformation should be clearly in contradiction to expert consensus or best available evidence and therefore should not include "information that is currently unverified, speculative, vague, exaggerated, contradictory, or contested" (Tan, Lee, and Chae 2015, 675). As such, a claim like "vaccines cause autism" is clearly health misinformation because it is in conflict with expert consensus and scientific evidence (Centers for Disease Control and Prevention 2021b), whereas a claim like "vaping prevents COVID-19 infection" may not be classified as misinformation because the claim is unsubstantiated. Other scholars support a broader definition of health misinformation that includes both false information and unsubstantiated claims (e.g., Chou, Oh, and Klein 2018, 2417). Moreover, some definitions include inaccurate claims, defining health misinformation as "false or inaccurate information regardless of intentional authorship" (Southwell et al. 2019, 282).

Although most researchers agree that false claims are in contradiction to expert consensus or available evidence and are therefore clear cases of misinformation, whether misinformation should encompass unsubstantiated and/or inaccurate claims is more controversial. Including unsubstantiated and inaccurate claims in the definition of health misinformation may be important, however. First, health claims that are unsubstantiated due to lack of evidence could be equally harmful as those that are explicitly verified as false. For example, during the COVID-19 pandemic, several companies claimed that products such as colloidal silver can cure or prevent coronavirus infections (US Food and Drug Administration 2020). Unsubstantiated (but not explicitly false) claims like this posed severe threats to public health as they might prompt consumers to stop or delay appropriate medical treatment (Majmundar et al. 2020). In addition, inaccurate claims that provide incomplete evidence are also problematic. As Ecker et al. (2014) argued, although laboratory research on misinformation tends to focus on information that is unequivocally false, misinformation in the real world is often more subtly misleading—perhaps technically true but misleading in substance (324). For example, in a content analysis of drug-related messages on social media, Al Khaja, AlKhaja, and Sequeira (2018) found the majority of messages (59.1 percent) consisted of misleading claims that omit important facts about the drug or relied on exaggerated clinical evidence, more than twice the rate of false claims (27.3 percent) that directly contradict scientific evidence (345). Therefore, focusing solely on explicitly false content may not meet the core challenges that public health and medical professionals face in the communication and dissemination of accurate information (Southwell et al. 2019, 282).

Proposing a New Definition of Health Misinformation

Based on our review of prior literature and definitions, we suggest that the definition of health misinformation should be guided by at least three principles: (1) health misinformation should be defined as a message's intrinsic features rather than source intent, recipient perceptions, or message effects; (2) a definition of health misinformation should incorporate both expert consensus and best available evidence as the benchmarks for assessing misinformation with a degree of confidence; and (3) a definition of health misinformation should encompass the types of misinformation consumers typically encounter in their information environment, including false claims, unsubstantiated claims, and inaccurate claims. Relatedly, health misinformation should be understood as an umbrella term comprising health-related rumors, misleading advertising, fake news, and conspiracy theories. Building on Chou, Oh, and Klein's (2018) definition, we propose a tentative, unifying definition for health misinformation in accordance with these principles:

> *Health misinformation is a health-related claim of fact that is currently false due to its contradiction to expert consensus and/or best available evidence at the time, inaccurate due to its use of incomplete evidence, or unsubstantiated due to a lack of evidence.*

Conclusions

Tackling the problem of health misinformation requires a clear definition of the problem. The working definition for health misinformation proposed here addressed some limitations in current definitions by incorporating both expert consensus and best available evidence as benchmarks, including various common forms of misinformation claims, and defining misinformation in terms of its features, rather than intent or effects. However, as noted earlier, the benchmarks for assessing misinformation (e.g., expert consensus and best available evidence) can change over time and therefore applying this definition (or any other definition using similar benchmarks) at different times may result in different categorization of misinformation. Additionally, there does not appear to be general agreement about what constitutes expert consensus and best available evidence. Who qualifies as an expert on a particular subject and what level of agreement among the experts indicates a consensus? Furthermore, what level of evidence in the hierarchy of evidence pyramid meets the minimum threshold as best available evidence? Finally, does health misinformation have any defining features that distinguish it from other types of misinformation (e.g., political misinformation)? These are some of the questions that future research needs to address in order to refine the proposed definition of health misinformation.

References

Al Khaja, Khalid A. J., Alwaleed K. AlKhaja, and Reginald P. Sequeira. 2018. "Drug Information, Misinformation, and Disinformation on Social Media: A Content Analysis Study." *Journal of Public Health Policy* 39, no. 3 (May): 343–57. doi:10.1057/s41271-018-0131-2.

Badell-Grau, Rafael A., Jordan Patrick Cuff, Brendan P. Kelly, Helen Waller-Evans, and Emyr Lloyd-Evans. 2020. "Investigating the Prevalence of Reactive Online Searching in the COVID-19 Pandemic." *Journal of Medical Internet Research* 22, no. 10 (August): 1–17. doi:10.2196/19791.

Bode, Leticia, and Emily K. Vraga. 2015. "In Related News, That Was Wrong: The Correction of Misinformation Through Related Stories Functionality in Social Media." *Journal of Communication* 65, no. 4 (August): 619–38. doi:10.1111/jcom.12166.

Bode, Leticia, Emily K. Vraga, and Melissa Tully. 2020. "Correcting Misperceptions About Genetically Modified Food on Social Media: Examining the Impact of Experts, Social Media Heuristics, and the Gateway Belief Model." *Science Communication* 43, no. 2 (December): 225–51. doi:10.1177/1075547020981375.

Brownson, Ross C., Jonathan E. Fielding, and Christopher M. Maylahn. 2009. "Evidence-Based Public Health: A Fundamental Concept for Public Health Practice." *Annual Review of Public Health* 30, no. 1 (April): 175–201. doi:10.1146/annurev.publhealth.031308.100134.

Centers for Disease Control and Prevention. 2020. "How to Address COVID-19 Vaccine Misinformation." Accessed January 13, 2022. https://www.cdc.gov/vaccines/covid-19/health-departments/addressing-vaccine-misinformation.html.

Centers for Disease Control and Prevention. 2021a. "Myths and Facts about COVID-19 Vaccines." Last modified December 15, 2021. https://www.cdc.gov/coronavirus/2019-ncov/vaccines/facts.html.

Centers for Disease Control and Prevention. 2021b. "Autism and Vaccines." Accessed January 13, 2022. https://www.cdc.gov/vaccinesafety/concerns/autism.html.

Chen, Liang, Xiaohui Wang, and Tai-Quan Peng. 2018. "Nature and Diffusion of Gynecologic Cancer-Related Misinformation on Social Media: Analysis of Tweets." *Journal of Medical Internet Research* 20, no. 10 (October): e11515. doi:10.2196/11515.

Chou, Wen-Ying Sylvia, April Oh, and William M. P. Klein. 2018. "Addressing Health-Related Misinformation on Social Media." *JAMA* 320, no. 23 (December): 2417–18. doi:10.1001/jama.2018.16865.

Cook, John, Stephan Lewandowsky, and Ullrich K. H. Ecker. 2017. "Neutralizing Misinformation through Inoculation: Exposing Misleading Argumentation Techniques Reduces Their Influence." *PLOS ONE* 12, no. 5 (May): e0175799. doi:10.1371/journal.pone.0175799.

DeClerque, J., A. O. Tsui, M. F. Abul-Ata, and D. Barcelona. 1986. "Rumor, Misinformation and Oral Contraceptive Use in Egypt." *Social Science & Medicine* 23, no. 1: 83–92. doi:10.1016/0277-9536(86)90327-8.

Deshpande, Aniruddha K., Shruti Balvalli Deshpande, and Colleen O'Brien. 2018. "A Study of Social Media Utilization by Individuals with Tinnitus." *American Journal of Audiology* 27, no. 4 (December): 559–69. doi:10.1044/2018_AJA-18-0033.

Douglas, Karen M., Robbie M. Sutton, and Aleksandra Cichocka. 2017. "The Psychology of Conspiracy Theories." *Current Directions in Psychological Science* 26, no. 6 (December): 538–42. doi:10.1177/0963721417718261.

Duplaga, Mariusz. 2020. "The Determinants of Conspiracy Beliefs Related to the COVID-19 Pandemic in a Nationally Representative Sample of Internet Users." *International Journal of Environmental Research and Public Health* 17, no. 21 (October): 1–15. doi:10.3390/ijerph17217818.

Ecker, Ullrich K. H., Stephan Lewandowsky, Ee Pin Chang, and Rekha Pillai. 2014. "The Effects of Subtle Misinformation in News Headlines." *Journal of Experimental Psychology: Applied* 20, no. 4 (October): 323–35. doi:10.1037/xap0000028.

Evans, David. 2003. "Hierarchy of Evidence: A Framework for Ranking Evidence Evaluating Healthcare Interventions." *Journal of Clinical Nursing* 12, no. 1 (January): 77–84. doi:10.1046/j.1365-2702.2003.00662.x.

Fallis, Don. 2015. "What Is Disinformation?" *Library Trends* 63, no. 3 (November): 401–26. doi:10.1353/lib.2015.0014.

Featherstone, Jieyu, and Jingwen Zhang. 2020. "Feeling Angry: The Effects of Vaccine Misinformation and Refutational Messages on Negative Emotions and Vaccination Attitude." *Journal of Health Communication* 25, no. 9 (October): 692–702. doi:10.1080/10810730.2020.1838671.

Ferrand, John, Ryli Hockensmith, Rebecca Fagen Houghton, and Eric R. Walsh-Buhi. 2020. "Evaluating Smart Assistant Responses for Accuracy and Misinformation Regarding Human Papillomavirus Vaccination: Content Analysis Study." *Journal of Medical Internet Research* 22, no. 8 (April): e19018. doi:10.2196/19018.

Fode, Mikkel, Alexander B. Nolsøe, Frederik M. Jacobsen, Giorgio Ivan Russo, Peter B. Østergren, Christian Fuglesang S. Jensen, Maarten Albersen, Paolo Capogrosso, Jens Sønksen, and EAU YAU Men's Health Working Group. 2020. "Quality of Information in YouTube Videos on Erectile Dysfunction." *Sexual Medicine* 8, no. 3 (September): 408–13. doi:10.1016/j.esxm.2020.05.007.

Fooks, Gary Jonas, Simon Williams, Graham Box, and Gary Sacks. 2019. "Corporations' Use and Misuse of Evidence to Influence Health Policy: A Case Study of Sugar-Sweetened Beverage Taxation." *Globalization and Health* 15, no. 1 (September): 1–20. doi:10.1186/s12992-019-0495-5.

Gesser-Edelsburg, Anat, Alon Diamant, Rana Hijazi, and Gustavo S. Mesch. 2018. "Correcting Misinformation by Health Organizations during Measles Outbreaks: A Controlled Experiment." *PloS One* 13, no. 12 (December): e0209505. doi:10.1371/journal.pone.0209505.

Ghezzi, Pietro, Peter G. Bannister, Gonzalo Casino, Alessia Catalani, Michel Goldman, Jessica Morley, Marie Neunez et al. 2020. "Online Information of Vaccines: Information Quality, Not Only Privacy, Is an Ethical Responsibility of Search Engines." *Frontiers in Medicine* 7, no. 400 (August): 1–7. doi:10.3389/fmed.2020.00400.

Hornik, Robert, Ava Kikut, Emma Jesch, Chioma Woko, Leeann Siegel, and Kwanho Kim. 2021. "Association of COVID-19 Misinformation with Face Mask Wearing and Social Distancing in a Nationally Representative US Sample." *Health Communication* 36, no.1 (January): 6–14. doi:10.1080/10410236.2020.1847437.

Kim, Hye Kyung, Jisoo Ahn, Lucy Atkinson, and Lee Ann Kahlor. 2020. "Effects of COVID-19 Misinformation on Information Seeking, Avoidance, and Processing: A Multicountry Comparative Study": *Science Communication* 42, no. 5 (September): 586–615. doi:10.1177/1075547020959670.

Krishna, Arunima, and Teresa L. Thompson. 2019. "Misinformation About Health: A Review of Health Communication and Misinformation Scholarship." *American Behavioral Scientist* 65, no. 2 (September): 316–32. doi:10.1177/0002764219878223.

Kroeger, Karen A. 2003. "AIDS Rumors, Imaginary Enemies, and The Body Politic in Indonesia." *American Ethnologist* 30, no. 2 (May): 243–57. http://www.jstor.org/stable/3805375.

Majmundar, Anuja, Jon-Patrick Allem, Tess Boley Cruz, and Jennifer B Unger. 2020. "Public Health Concerns and Unsubstantiated Claims at the Intersection of Vaping and COVID-19." *Nicotine & Tobacco Research* 22, no. 9 (August): 1667–68. doi:10.1093/ntr/ntaa064.

McGrath, Trevor A., Matthew D. F. McInnes, Nick van Es, Mariska M. G. Leeflang, Daniël A. Korevaar, and Patrick M. M. Bossuyt. 2017. "Overinterpretation of Research Findings: Evidence of 'Spin' in Systematic Reviews of Diagnostic Accuracy Studies." *Clinical Chemistry* 63, no. 8 (August): 1353–62. doi:10.1373/clinchem.2017.271544.

Motta, Matthew, and Timothy Callaghan. 2020. "The Pervasiveness and Policy Consequences of Medical Folk Wisdom in the U.S." *Scientific Reports* 10, no. 1 (July): 10722. doi:10.1038/s41598-020-67744-6.

Murad, M. Hassan, Noor Asi, Mouaz Alsawas, and Fares Alahdab. 2016. "New Evidence Pyramid." *BMJ Evidence-Based Medicine* 21, no. 4 (August): 125–27. doi:10.1136/ebmed-2016-110401.

Nan, Xiaoli, Yuan Wang, and Kathryn Thier. 2021. "Health Misinformation." In *The Routledge Handbook of Health Communication* (3rd), edited by Teresa L. Thompson and Nancy Grant Harrington, pp. 318–32. Routledge.

Nyhan, Brendan, and Jason Reifler. 2010. "When Corrections Fail: The Persistence of Political Misperceptions." *Political Behavior* 32, no. 2 (March): 303-30. doi:10.1007/s11109-010-9112-2.

Obiała, Justyna, Karolina Obiała, Małgorzata Mańczak, Jakub Owoc, and Robert Olszewski. 2020. "COVID-19 Misinformation: Accuracy of Articles about Coronavirus Prevention Mostly Shared on Social Media." *Health Policy and Technology* 10, no. 1 (November): 182–86. doi:10.1016/j.hlpt.2020.10.007.

Ozturk, Pinar, Huaye Li, and Yasuaki Sakamoto. 2015. "Combating Rumor Spread on Social Media: The Effectiveness of Refutation and Warning." In *2015 48th Hawaii International Conference on System Sciences*, 2406–14. https://www.computer.org/csdl/proceedings/hicss/2015/12OmNyr8Yts.

Pathak, Ranjan, Dilli Ram Poudel, Paras Karmacharya, Amrit Pathak, Madan Raj Aryal, Maryam Mahmood, and Anthony A. Donato. 2015. "YouTube as a Source of Information on Ebola Virus Disease." *North American Journal of Medical Sciences* 7, no. 7 (July): 306–9. doi:10.4103/1947-2714.161244.

Russo, J. Edward, Barbara L. Metcalf, and Debra Stephens. 1981. "Identifying Misleading Advertising." *Journal of Consumer Research* 8, no. 2 (September): 119–31. doi:10.1086/208848.

Safarnejad, Lida, Qian Xu, Yaorong Ge, Siddharth Krishnan, Arunkumar Bagarvathi, and Shi Chen. 2020. "Contrasting Misinformation and Real-Information Dissemination Network Structures on Social Media During a Health Emergency." *American Journal of Public Health* 110, no. 3 (October): S340–47. doi:10.2105/AJPH.2020.305854.

Sallam, Malik, Deema Dababseh, Alaa' Yaseen, Ayat Al-Haidar, Nidaa A. Ababneh, Faris G. Bakri, and Azmi Mahafzah. 2020. "Conspiracy Beliefs are Associated with Lower Knowledge and Higher Anxiety Levels Regarding COVID-19 among Students at the University of Jordan." *International Journal of Environmental Research and Public Health* 17, no. 14 (July): e0243264. doi:10.3390/ijerph17144915.

Sallam, Malik, Deema Dababseh, Alaa Yaseen, Ayat Al-Haidar, Duaa Taim, Huda Eid, Nidaa A. Ababneh, Faris G. Bakri, and Azmi Mahafzah. 2020. "COVID-19 Misinformation: Mere Harmless Delusions or Much More? A Knowledge and Attitude Cross-Sectional Study among the General Public Residing in Jordan." *PLoS ONE* 15, no. 12 (December): 1–18. doi:10.1371/journal.pone.0243264.

Sangalang, Angeline, Yotam Ophir, and Joseph N Cappella. 2019. "The Potential for Narrative Correctives to Combat Misinformation†." *Journal of Communication* 69, no. 3 (June): 298–319. doi:10.1093/joc/jqz014.

Shah, Zubair, Didi Surian, Amalie Dyda, Enrico Coiera, Kenneth D. Mandl, and Adam G. Dunn. 2019. "Automatically Appraising the Credibility of Vaccine-Related Web Pages Shared on Social Media: A Twitter Surveillance Study." *Journal of Medical Internet Research* 21, no. 11 (March): e14007. doi:10.2196/14007.

Sommariva, Silvia, Cheryl Vamos, Alexios Mantzarlis, Lillie Uyên-Loan Đào, and Dinorah Martinez Tyson. 2018. "Spreading the (Fake) News: Exploring Health Messages on Social Media and the Implications for Health Professionals Using a Case Study." *American Journal of Health Education* 49, no. 4 (June): 246–55. doi:10.1080/19325037.2018.1473178.

Southwell, Brian G., Emily A. Thorson, and Laura Sheble. 2018. *Misinformation and Mass Audiences*. Austin: University of Texas Press.

Southwell, Brian G., Jeff Niederdeppe, Joseph N. Cappella, Anna Gaysynsky, Dannielle E. Kelley, April Oh, Emily B. Peterson, and Wen-Ying Sylvia Chou. 2019. "Misinformation as a Misunderstood

Challenge to Public Health." *American Journal of Preventive Medicine* 57, no. 2 (August): 282–85. doi:10.1016/j.amepre.2019.03.009.

Sullivan, M. Connor. 2019. "Leveraging Library Trust to Combat Misinformation on Social Media." *Library & Information Science Research* 41, no. 1 (January): 2–10. doi:10.1016/j.lisr.2019.02.004.

Swire-Thompson, Briony, and David Lazer. 2020. "Public Health and Online Misinformation: Challenges and Recommendations." *Annual Review of Public Health* 41, no. 1 (April): 433–51. doi:10.1146/annurev-publhealth-040119-094127.

Tan, Andy S. L., Chul-joo Lee, and Jiyoung Chae. 2015. "Exposure to Health (Mis)Information: Lagged Effects on Young Adults' Health Behaviors and Potential Pathways." *Journal of Communication* 65, no. 4 (July): 674–98. doi:10.1111/jcom.12163.

Tran, Thi, Rohit Valecha, Paul Rad, and H. Raghav Rao. 2020. "An Investigation of Misinformation Harms Related to Social Media during Two Humanitarian Crises." *Information Systems Frontiers: A Journal of Research and Innovation* 23, no. 4 (November), 1–9. doi:10.1007/s10796-020-10088-3.

US Food and Drug Administration. 2020. "Coronavirus (COVID-19) Update: November 3, 2020." Accessed January 13, 2022. https://www.fda.gov/news-events/press-announcements/coronavirus-covid-19-update-november-3-2020.

van der Meer, Toni G. L. A., and Yan Jin. 2020. "Seeking Formula for Misinformation Treatment in Public Health Crises: The Effects of Corrective Information Type and Source." *Health Communication* 35, no. 5 (February): 560–75. doi:10.1080/10410236.2019.1573295.

van Stekelenburg, Aart, Gabi Schaap, Harm Veling, and Moniek Buijzen. 2020. "Correcting Misperceptions: The Causal Role of Motivation in Corrective Science Communication About Vaccine and Food Safety." *Science Communication* 42, no. 1 (January): 31–60. doi:10.1177/1075547019898256.

Vraga, Emily K., and Leticia Bode. 2020. "Defining Misinformation and Understanding Its Bounded Nature: Using Expertise and Evidence for Describing Misinformation." *Political Communication* 37, no. 1 (February): 136–44. doi:10.1080/10584609.2020.1716500.

Wang, Yuxi, Martin McKee, Aleksandra Torbica, and David Stuckler. 2019. "Systematic Literature Review on the Spread of Health-Related Misinformation on Social Media." *Social Science & Medicine* 240 (September): 1–12. doi:10.1016/j.socscimed.2019.112552.

Waszak, Przemyslaw M., Wioleta Kasprzycka-Waszak, and Alicja Kubanek. 2018. "The Spread of Medical Fake News in Social Media—The Pilot Quantitative Study." *Health Policy and Technology* 7, no. 2 (June): 115–18. doi:10.1016/j.hlpt.2018.03.002.

Wood, Michael J. 2018. "Propagating and Debunking Conspiracy Theories on Twitter During the 2015–2016 Zika Virus Outbreak." *Cyberpsychology, Behavior, and Social Networking* 21, no. 8 (August): 485–90. doi:10.1089/cyber.2017.0669.

World Health Organization. 2020. "Infodemics." Accessed January 13, 2022. https://www.who.int/health-topics/infodemic#tab=tab_1.

Wu, Liang, Fred Morstatter, Kathleen M. Carley, and Huan Liu. 2019. "Misinformation in Social Media: Definition, Manipulation, and Detection." *ACM SIGKDD Explorations Newsletter* 21, no. 2 (December): 80–90. doi:10.1145/3373464.3373475.

Xiao, Xizhu, Porismita Borah, and Yan Su. 2021. "The Dangers of Blind Trust: Examining the Interplay among Social Media News Use, Misinformation Identification, and News Trust on Conspiracy Beliefs." *Public Understanding of Science* 30, no. 8 (March): 977–92. doi:10.1177/0963662521998025.

Xu, Qian, Shi Chen, and Lida Safarnejad. 2020. "Effects of Information Veracity and Message Frames on Information Dissemination: A Case Study of 2016 Zika Epidemic Discussion on Twitter." *Health Communication* 36, no. 12 (June): 1560–70. doi:10.1080/10410236.2020.1773705.

Yang, Qinghua, Angeline Sangalang, Molly Rooney, Erin Maloney, Sherry Emery, and Joseph N. Cappella. 2018. "How Is Marijuana Vaping Portrayed on YouTube? Content, Features, Popularity and Retransmission of Vaping Marijuana YouTube Videos." *Journal of Health Communication* 23, no. 4 (March): 360–69. doi:10.1080/10810730.2018.1448488.

Yetley, Elizabeth A., Amanda J. MacFarlane, Linda S. Greene-Finestone, Cutberto Garza, Jamy D. Ard, Stephanie A. Atkinson, Dennis M. Bier et al. 2017. "Options for Basing Dietary Reference Intakes

(DRIs) on Chronic Disease Endpoints: Report from a Joint US-/Canadian-sponsored Working Group." *The American Journal of Clinical Nutrition* 105, no. 1 (December): 249S–285S. doi:10.3945/ajcn.116.139097.

Yoon, Sunmoo, Michelle Odlum, Peter Broadwell, Nicole Davis, Hwayoug Cho, Nanyi Deng, Maria Patrao, Deborah Schauer, Michael E. Bales, and Carmela Alcantara. 2020. "Application of Social Network Analysis of COVID-19 Related Tweets Mentioning Cannabis and Opioids to Gain Insights for Drug Abuse Research." *Studies in Health Technology and Informatics* 272 (June): 5–8. doi:10.3233/SHTI200479.

Zhang, Shuai, Wenjing Pian, Feicheng Ma, Zhenni Ni, and Yunmei Liu. 2021. "Characterizing the COVID-19 Infodemic on Chinese Social Media: Exploratory Study." *JMIR Public Health and Surveillance* 7, no. 2 (February): e26090. doi:10.2196/26090.

Zhang, Yafei, Lin Wang, Jonathan J. H. Zhu, and Xiaofan Wang. 2021. "Conspiracy vs Science: A Large-Scale Analysis of Online Discussion Cascades." *World Wide Web* 24, no. 2 (January), 585–606. doi:10.1007/s11280-021-00862-x.

2

The Ecology of Online Health Information and COVID-19 Misinformation

David R. Kaufman, Adiebonye E. Jumbo, and Tonya N. Taylor

We are not just fighting an epidemic; we're fighting an infodemic.

–General Director, World Health Organization
(Ghebreyesus 2020)

PARALLEL TO THE COVID-19 pandemic, the greatest public health crisis of our generation, is an equally lethal *infodemic* of politicized disinformation. Conspiracy theories about its origins and exaggerated severity raged unabated on the internet, in discussion groups, and on social media platforms. Fueled by populist opposition to science, the government, social elites, or the establishment (Naeem, Bhatti, and Khan 2021), the COVID-19 *infodemic* is the largest threat to vaccine uptake and efforts to end the pandemic (Depoux et al. 2020; Larson 2018). The federal COVID-19 response was not prompt, accurate, or consistent, resulting in confusion and misunderstandings. It undermined the credibility of institutions and trust in public health response and opened a window for misinformation. The search for credible and reliable COVID-19 information is further complicated by deficits in critical thinking, media, and information literacy skills, as well as selective access to channels of information (Bekalu 2014; Lin, Jung, et al. 2014; Lin, Savoia, et al. 2014; Ramanadhan and Viswanath 2008).

Political discourses promoting "fake news" and "alternative facts" fostered enormous mistrust in mainstream media and the dismissal of information that contradicts existing beliefs (Howard et al. 2019). A Pew survey found that half of US adults get their news from social media (Shearer and Mitchell 2021). Misinformation is inaccurate, false, or misleading information believed to be true. Individuals often share misinformation with the intent to help educate others or to provoke "fear and suspicion" (Chen et al. 2015). Disinformation is the intentional dissemination of false or misleading information to deceive or for financial gain. Alex Jones's malicious lie that the Sandy Hook massacre was a hoax is classic disinformation (Lazer et al. 2018; Swire-Thompson and Lazer 2019; Caramancion 2020). The intentional use of disinformation to cause harm or political, personal, or financial gain is a significant threat to democracy and public health.

In this exposition of the ecology of COVID-19 misinformation, disinformation, and conspiracy theories, we first describe the online health information (OHI) environment and the shift to social media. Through the omnipresent smartphone, billions of users engage in OHI seeking, using a variety of digital media platforms that include online news media, social media (e.g., Facebook, Twitter, and Instagram), mobile social networking apps (MSNs) (e.g., WhatsApp and WeChat), and new social live steaming services (SLS), such as YouTube Now and Facebook Live, Tok-tok Live, and Instagram. We describe the evolution of COVID-19 misinformation, disinformation, and conspiracy theories and a review of psychological theories that might explain why individuals are predisposed to these beliefs. To guide our discussion, we use Williamson's (1998) ecological model of information seeking developed to explain how individuals use a variety of information sources to meet their everyday information needs and adapt it to the consumption and dissemination of COVID-19 misinformation (see figure 2.1). We explore the complex interactions between (1) the psychological predispositions toward conspiracy theories and disinformation, (2) the pursuit of OHI that are often influenced by (3) preexisting social networks and manipulative algorithms. The negative effects (i.e., antiscience and antiestablishment views) were reinforced by (4) trusted institutions (e.g., Fox News) and sources of information that had (5) a negative impact on the adoption of mitigation or prevention behaviors, such as masks and vaccination (Baral et al. 2013).

We propose that across psychological, interpersonal, community/organizational, and policy levels and information structures, politically charged ecologies of disinformation have hurt COVID-19 prevention and vaccine uptake efforts. Consumers and producers of COVID-19

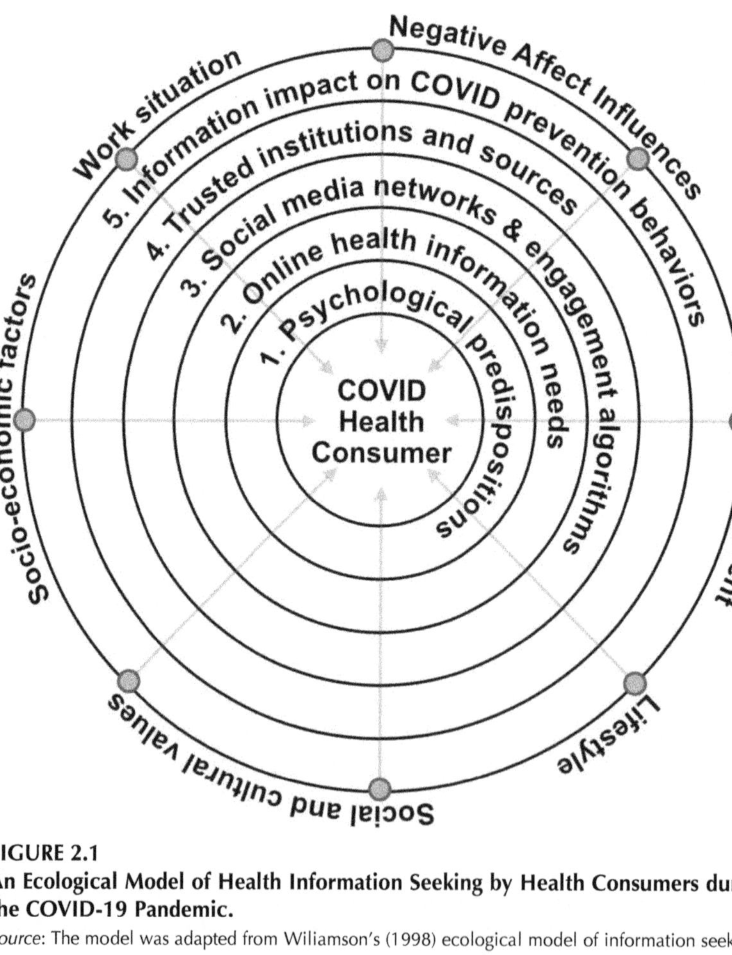

FIGURE 2.1
An Ecological Model of Health Information Seeking by Health Consumers during the COVID-19 Pandemic.
Source: The model was adapted from Wiliamson's (1998) ecological model of information seeking.

mis- and disinformation have thus become subject to rambling and incoherent public discourse, political situations, economic circumstances, and increasing globalization with deadly consequences (Ginsburg 2002). Conspiratorial thinking and the use of disinformation to obfuscate information are not unique to COVID-19; these alternative explanatory models and scapegoating techniques have existed for centuries. Using lessons learned from the AIDS pandemic in the 1980s (Jaiswal, LoSchiavo, and Perlman 2020), we show how disinformation, conspiratorial thinking, and blaming immigrants are common, albeit dangerous, societal responses to the existential threats of unknown contagions.

Scapegoating, Misinformation, and Conspiracy Theories: Parallels between the COVID-19 and AIDS Pandemics

The global spread of AIDS and its parallel pandemic of mis- or disinformation, much like COVID-19, was triggered by a dangerous epidemic of blame and racial prejudice. Attributing the source of a pandemic (or social ailment) outside the boundaries of national identity (e.g., foreigners, immigrants, or marginalized populations in society) is a common explanatory model used throughout history for events such as the plague of Athens, the Bubonic plague in the fourteenth century that blamed Jews, the 1918 influenza pandemic, or the 1832 cholera epidemic in the United States (Dionne and Turkmen 2020; Markel and Stern 2002). Dr. Jonathan Mann, the former head of the WHO Global Program on AIDS, called this process of shifting blame to others the third level of the AIDS pandemic. The first level of the AIDS pandemic was the "silent" and undetectable transmission of HIV, followed by the clinical presentation of the disease itself (Mann 1988). According to Dr. Mann (1988), the third level of blame and accusation made the "social, cultural, economic and political reactions to AIDS . . . central to the global AIDS challenge as the disease itself (131)."

Countries affected by the AIDS pandemic, just like COVID-19, first blamed those deemed as societal "others," such as African or Black immigrants or marginalized groups (e.g., homosexuals and drug users). Racist beliefs of primitiveness around the trade and consumption of bushmeat fueled AIDS and COVID-19 discrimination directed toward Africans and Asians, respectively (Hirsch et al. 1989; King et al. 2021). Nationals from heavily affected countries, such as Uganda, were detained in airports or refused visas. African students studying in Russia and China were forced to leave because of growing hostilities due to fears of infection (Farmer 1990; Sabatier and Tinker 1988). Similarly, with COVID-19, racist rhetoric about the "China Virus" or "Kung-Flu" shifted the blame of the pandemic to China (Walker and Daniel Anders 2021). This racist scapegoating resulted in the rise of anti-Asian hate crimes (Gover, Harper, and Langton 2020).

AIDS misinformation, or *denialism*, promotes alternative beliefs about the origins and relationship between HIV and AIDS despite thirty years of international scientific consensus. The Duesberg hypothesis, developed by Peter Duesberg, a cell biologist at the University of California, Berkeley, proposed that the combined use of recreational and pharmaceutical drug use was the underlying cause of AIDS, not HIV, which he considered to be an innocuous passenger virus (Cohen 1994). Duesberg was a respected scientist who espoused an alternative hypothesis. Proponents of AIDS denialism employed the persuasive strategy of citing sources perceived as credible with advanced degrees. Regrettably, South African President Tabo Mbeki was an AIDS denialist and believed AIDS was caused by poverty, malnutrition, and environmental factors, such as polluted water, and not HIV (Nattrass 2008). This delayed the allocation of resources for testing and surveillance. Similarly, COVID-19 denialists contended that COVID-19 was "just the flu" and a hoax created by Democratic elites trying to undermine Donald Trump's presidency. These claims were further fueled on social media by a small group of fringe medical doctors who were savvy conmen peddling pseudoscience (Hotez 2021) and twelve anti-vaxxers (the "disinformation dozen") who were found to be responsible for perpetuating the vast majority of lies about the COVID-19 vaccines (Martin 2021).

Conspiracy theories are explanatory models driven by beliefs that powerful agents in the world are covertly acting for their benefit or profit and against the common good (Uscinski, Klofstad, and Atkinson 2016). Conspiratorial thinking is often associated with periods of crisis, fear, and uncertainty. AIDS conspiracy theories, all of which have been discredited, primarily revolve around beliefs that powerful entities manufactured AIDS using vaccines to exterminate certain populations (e.g., homosexuals, immigrants, and Blacks/Africans). In *Blaming Others: Prejudice, Race and Worldwide AIDS*, Sabatier and Tinker (1988) explore the racialized conspiracy beliefs that AIDS is an "imperialist plot to destroy the Third World." The United States' most popular AIDS conspiracy theory was that HIV was manufactured at Fort Detrick, Maryland, by the US Defense Department as a biological weapon (Operation INFEKTION) to exterminate racial and ethnic minorities (Farmer 1990). Many Black Americans continue to believe that AIDS was created in government laboratories or spread by the CIA because of the US's long history of medical abuse (e.g., Tuskegee Experiment) (Elders et al. 2011). These beliefs continue to undermine HIV prevention efforts. Similarly, the Chinese Communist Party pushed conspiracy theories of US laboratory leaks and COVID-19 as a US bioweapon (Knight 2021). In the United States, theories tried to frame Dr. Fauci as the COVID pandemic mastermind because he approved NIH research funding for the Wuhan lab (Knight 2021; Kuperjanov 2021). Although disinformation, conspiratorial thinking, and the assignment of blame on immigrants are not unique to COVID-19, the rapid dissemination of these beliefs via social media has created an enormous threat to public health and safety.

The Ecology of OHI and Shift to Social Media

The internet provides unprecedented consumer access to OHI and serves as a mediator of health education, decision-making, and management (Cronin, Jimison, and Johnson 2021). The rapid growth in access to internet-mediated information has created new possibilities for individuals, especially vulnerable uninsured and rural populations, to become proactive in their health and health care (Bundorf et al. 2006). The increasing use and reliance on ehealth applications are due to the exponential growth of internet users worldwide, access to the internet through mobile devices, the development of participative health care models (Gerber and Eiser 2001), the difficulty for physicians to keep pace with rapidly changing clinical guidelines, reduction of physician time with patients due to managed care cost constraints (Forrest et al. 2002), and the promotion of self-care management and prevention, especially for chronic diseases (Cronin, Jimison, and Johnson 2021). The Pew Internet Project, which surveys consumers about their OHI seeking habits, has found that most respondents not only search for health information online but use the information to inform treatment decisions (Fox 2008). Popular online health care websites, such as WebMD and the Mayo Clinic, can be highly effective for providing health-related information to large audiences on a wide scale (Gesualdo et al. 2010; Xavier et al. 2013). Despite the benefits of promoting consumer health, the highly variable quality of OHI impacts individuals' understanding of health-related issues (Keselman, Kaufman, and Patel 2002; Keselman et al. 2019; Kaufman, Mirkovic, and Chan 2017).

Prior to the COVID-19 pandemic, health care professionals advocated for the use of social media to bolster the dissemination of public health information (Chou et al. 2009; Moorhead et al. 2013; Vance, Howe, and Dellavalle 2009), leading many to argue that social media has become a ubiquitous part of health care (Hawn 2009). There has also been extensive debate regarding the disadvantages of using social media to communicate and disseminate health care information (Hudson and Mackenzie 2019; O'Brien, Moore, and McNicholas 2020; Schwenk et al. 2020; Wong, Capel, and Malbrain 2019). During the emergency crisis of the pandemic, medical and public health use of social media accelerated the rapid dissemination of critical care and prevention information (Wong et al. 2021). COVID-19 web-based resources developed during the pandemic include the *Internet Book of Critical Care: COVID-19, Intensive Care Society COVID-19 Hub, European Society of Intensive Medicine (ESICM) COVID-19* blog, and *New England Journal of Medicine (NEJM) COVID-19.* The COVID-19 Marathon Webinar had 64,115 YouTube views, 78,100 Facebook views, and 7,277 website views (Wong et al. 2021).

Social Media Infrastructure and the Proliferation of Bots

Social media infrastructure includes physical structures such as telecommunications, internet connectivity, and broadband access to commodities and services essential to enable, sustain, or improve living conditions and quality of life (Fulmer 2009). Open technology standards are available for many applications and support many innovations. They also create a window of opportunity for those peddling mis- and disinformation related to health. All social media platforms employ content-recommendation algorithms that selectively push content to users, based in part on user preference and attitudes. However, platforms also increase the visibility of popular posts more to increase engagement without considering the quality or accuracy metrics. Troll farms are groups that work in a deliberate and coordinated fashion to post provocative content to social networks. Facebook enabled Eastern Europe disinformation campaigns to reach about 50 percent of all Americans (focusing on Christian and Black American pages) in the run-up to the 2020 presidential election using Facebook's engagement-driven algorithm for newsfeeds (Hao 2021). Collectively, these troll-farm pages reached 140 million US users monthly and 360 million global users weekly. These Eastern European troll farms were state actors or *cyber troops* defined as "government, military or political party teams committed to manipulating public opinion over social media" (Howard and Bradshaw 2017). Since 2010, different countries have employed large numbers of cyber troops to influence public opinion, targeting both domestic and foreign audiences.

Software bots are automated tools (scripts) that can free developers by automating tedious tasks (Eslahi, Salleh, and Anuar 2012). These bots are also cyber weapons for sowing disinformation or assaulting networked computers through denial-of-service attacks. Approximately, 94 percent of websites have encountered a bot attack (Imperva 2021). Overall, bad bots, which account for 26 percent of all internet traffic, mimic human interactions making them harder to detect and block; they also facilitate attacks on websites, mobile apps, and APIs and enable bot operators, disreputable competitors, and swindlers to perform a vast range of malicious activities (Imperva 2021). Imperva Cyber Security reports globally a 372 percent increase in bad bot traffic on health care websites since September 2020; one bot was observed making as many as 12,000 vaccine appointment requests per hour (Imperva 2021). Overall, bad bots amounted to 25.6 percent of all internet traffic (Imperva 2021). Bots have transformed the social media landscape, creating the illusion of popularity and mass endorsement or unrealistically exaggerating the importance of topics (Dow et al. 2021b). Social media bots are tools for spreading conspiracy theories and the false impression that others widely endorse information.

COVID-19 Disinformation in the OHI Ecosystem

The pandemic led to a dramatic increase in social media usage in part because of the disruption in life. Individuals were greatly restricted in their movements and efforts to socialize face-to-face (Dow et al. 2021a). The year 2020 witnessed tremendous global social media growth with 330 million new users, which raised the total number of users to 4.7 billion (Kemp 2021). Social media became the primary source of COVID-19 disinformation in the United States and worldwide. For social and computer scientists, the pandemic provided an opportunity to explore novel methods to understand the problem of disinformation on social media.

Fondazione Bruno Kessler analyzed over 100 million social media posts related to COVID-19 and determined that more than 40 percent contained information from unreliable sources and 42 percent were circulated by bots (Lupi 2020). Lee et al. (2020) found that 68 percent of adults have been exposed to COVID-19-related disinformation through social networking services or instant messaging. Naeem, Bhatti, and Khan (2021) analyzed 1,225 pieces of fake news stories about COVID-19 and found that social media accounted for spreading over 50 percent of the stories. Sources of disinformation about vaccines gained 4.5 billion views on social media in just one month, undermining the impact of vaccination campaigns (Naeem, Bhatti, and Khan 2021). In a study with over 126,000 online news stories, researchers found that falsehoods, rumors, and hoaxes far eclipsed more trustworthy information (Vosoughi, Roy, and Aral 2018). Naeem and colleagues identified three types of COVID-19 fake news: (a) *false claims*, such as "coronavirus can be transmitted through houseflies or mosquito bites," (b) *conspiracy theories*, such as the ones about 5G cellular phone networks and coronavirus, and (c) *pseudoscientific health therapies*, such as "colloidal silver solution can help with coronavirus" (Naeem, Bhatti, and Khan 2021). False claims that diminished the threat posed by COVID-19 ("it's just like the flu" or "the number of COVID-19 deaths is grossly exaggerated") and the promotion of pseudoscientific therapies, such as Ivermectin, an antiparasitic drug commonly used in animals, as a cure for COVID-19 proliferated across social media. Loomba and colleagues (2021) demonstrated that exposure to false information reduced intent to vaccinate by more than 6 percent in United Kingdom and United States sample populations. Scientific-sounding statements, such as "the vaccine will literally alter your DNA," had the greatest negative impact.

In a comparative study of COVID-19 posts on Facebook and Twitter at the beginning of the pandemic, Yang et al. (2021) found that low-credibility posts were associated with removed or banned YouTube links; that Twitter exhibited a higher percentage of low-credibility information than Facebook (32 percent vs. 21 percent) on average; and that small groups of "superspreaders," or influential, high-profile, official, and verified accounts, were responsible for disseminating most of the COVID-19 disinformation. Yang et al. (2021) also found that low-credibility information on both platforms surpassed all high-credibility accounts. Interestingly, the primary drivers of low-credibility content tend to be high-profile and verified accounts, rather than low-credibility domains. Facebook and Twitter platforms have different models of diffusion that allow certain users to exploit the model and amplify the spread of disinformation. Cross-platform coordination, including those controlled by influential organizations, increases harmful disinformation potency and can reinforce malevolent messaging.

Psychological Predispositions to Disinformation and Conspiracy Theories

The pandemic has caused enormous disruptions in people's lives. For more than two years, we have been operating under dark clouds of uncertainty, which has led to high levels of anxiety, paranoia, and delusional thinking (Grimes 2021). It also provided the ideal conditions for disinformation, conspiratorial thinking, and the assignment of blame to immigrants to thrive (Dow et al. 2021b; Grimes 2021). Humans respond to existential threats by engaging in compensatory mechanisms that restore psychological equilibrium (Simchon et al. 2021). Social and cognitive biases that lead to thinking that is not rational have been the subject of research for years. This is best exemplified by the heuristic and biases program pioneered by Tversky and Kahneman (Kahneman et al. 1982). There has also been a long history of research investigating misconceptions in science (Vosniadou 2020) and susceptibility to believe in pseudoscience (Keselman, Kaufman, and Patel 2004). However, the study of fake online news has greatly accelerated in the wake of the COVID-19 pandemic. This section briefly examines psychological theories that endeavor to explain external conditions that lead to receptivity to disinformation and conspiracy theories and the psychological states that predispose individuals to process information selectively.

Dow and colleagues sketch a rather broad explanatory framework of how social and cognitive disruptions during the pandemic made some receptive to respond to conspiracy theories in harmful ways (Dow et al. 2021b). Cognitive disruptions due to lockdowns, business closures, and mask mandates led to a perceived loss of control or diminished agency. Increased consumption of social media is evidenced by the 25 percent rise in internet traffic after the lockdown (Rizzo and Click 2020). Social media created an oasis for users to share experiences and opinions, to seek information, and for some to restore a measure of control over their lives (Dow et al. 2021b). Although the pandemic diminished face-to-face interactions, fractured social bonds, and increased feelings of isolation and loneliness, engagement with social media helped many achieve "basic needs for affiliation and belonging" (Dow et al. 2021a).

Conspiracy theories are appealing because they provide simplicity, clarity, and a consistent way to understand the world (Dow et al. 2021a). The prevalence of disinformation, bad bots, and algorithms that spread disinformation created a perfect storm. Fake news spreads rapidly on social media. For example, research suggests that false rumors on Twitter moved six times faster than the truth (Vosoughi, Roy, and Aral 2018). Anti-vaccine advocates have a well-documented and significant presence in social media, with anti-vaccine tweets accounting for 50 percent of vaccine-related tweets (Broniatowski et al. 2018). High-status social influencers have an inordinate impact on the spread of disinformation. A study by the Center for Countering Digital Hate (Ahmed 2021) found that 65 percent of anti-vaccine social media posts could be traced back to just twelve influencers. Dow et al. (2021a) argue that people become trapped in homogenous information echo chambers with others having similar interests and beliefs. Members of such a community receive social reinforcement with shared posts, likes, and followers, creating a continuous feedback loop for greater engagement with like-minded individuals and social cohesion among the conspiracy-minded subgroup or subculture. Evidence also supports that conspiracy beliefs reduce healthy behaviors and promote harmful practices, resulting in diminished health outcomes (Dow et al. 2021a). Dow and colleagues make a compelling argument that fractured social and cognitive structures create an opening for conspiratorial thinking and increase the likelihood of becoming a member of a social media community that propagates this disinformation.

The seminal heuristics and biases program of Kahneman et al. (1982) laid the foundation for studying how people make decisions based on flawed reasoning. This, in part, gave rise to interesting new lines of research investigating how social beliefs inform science-related decisions. It is widely accepted that belief in fake political news is driven by partisanship (Kahan 2017). Purveyors of false information persuade or dissuade people from weighing evidence in science-related decisions. Zhao, Da, and Yan (2021) found a correlation between people's preferences for particular media outlets when seeking health-related information and their behaviors during the pandemic in the United States. For example, people who considered Fox News a more trustworthy information source than mainstream media exhibited a higher number of risky behaviors and less preventive behaviors related to COVID-19 (e.g., not wearing face masks). Kahan proposes the "identity protective cognition" (IPC) mechanism as an explanatory device. IPC refers to the tendency of a group of individuals to selectively accept and reject evidence in patterns that reflect the beliefs associated with their group. This is consistent with evidence that people join conspiracy-minded others in forums that amplify scientifically specious claims about vaccines, global warming, genetically modified food, and a host of other issues (Hmielowski et al. 2014). Kahan reviewed a range of research on decisions related to matters of science (Kahan 2017) and found that people process information in a manner oriented to generating or preserving identity-consistent rather than factually accurate beliefs. Receptiveness to fracking or global warming information generates predictable responses along the liberal-conservative continuum. However, beliefs related to less politically charged issues like genetically modified food were not influenced by political disposition.

Pennycook and colleagues contest the assumptions that IPC is the primary cognitive mechanism underlying receptivity to fake news (Pennycook, Cannon, and Rand 2018; Pennycook and Rand 2019). They draw on the dual-process theory associated with the work of Kahneman (2011). The theory distinguishes between System-1 thinking, which is fast, intuitive, and nearly effortless, and System-2 thinking, which is meticulous, analytic, and effortful, imposing significant demands on attention and memory. In their studies, Pennycook and Rand employed the Cognitive Reflection Test (CRT), a measure of an individual's predisposition to engage in analytic thinking (Pennycook and Rand 2019). The study presented participants with fifteen factually accurate news and fifteen fake news (headlines news). The stories were selected to be Democrat-consistent, Republican-consistent, and politically neutral. They found that a predisposition toward analytical thinking was positively correlated with the ability to differentiate fake news from real news. The alignment of the headlines with individuals' political points of view had no discernible impact. The authors conclude that the vulnerability of individuals to fake news is driven more by lazy System-1-type thinking rather than politically motivated reasoning. However, it is important to keep in mind that these are experimental studies and are subject to real-world validation. It is reasonable to speculate that both IPC mechanisms and lazy System-1 thinking make individuals more or less susceptible to misinformation. A higher degree of personal engagement in a controversy may be more likely to engage IPC-like thinking in evaluating the veracity of a claim.

Conclusions

This chapter explored problems and consequences associated with COVID-19 disinformation and conspiracy theories, including growing mistrust of medical, scientific, and public health institutions and lower uptake of COVID-19 prevention and mitigation efforts. The COVID-19 pandemic revealed that the social determinants of health (SDoH), such as racism, poverty, crowded housing, employment in essential services, inability to quarantine or socially distance, and differential access to the internet, created higher burdens of disease and death among vulnerable populations (Hooper, Nápoles, and Pérez-Stable 2020; Laurencin and McClinton 2020; Van Dorn, Cooney, and Sabin 2020). In New York City, the first COVID-19 epicenter in the United States, Black and Hispanic people accounted for 77 percent of nonfatal hospitalization and 90 percent of mortalities in the first few months of the pandemic (Holtgrave et al. 2020). A *syndemic* is characterized by biological and social interactions between conditions and states that increase a person's susceptibility to suboptimal health outcomes (Horton 2020). The syndemic of racial and ethnic inequalities in the United States is inextricably linked to differential exposure, vulnerability, and susceptibility to COVID-19 among Black and Hispanic people. Disparities in COVID-19 outcomes (infection rates, symptom severity, and death) are driven by high infection risks, higher burdens of chronic health conditions (diabetes, hypertension, cardiovascular diseases, and obesity), and the SDoH mentioned earlier (Upshaw et al. 2021; Baidal et al. 2020). COVID-19 disparities were also driven by communication inequalities that include differential access or exposure to COVID-19 prevention information, comprehension, and capacity to act on information (Viswanath, Lee, and Pinnamaneni 2020); limited access to the internet, broadband, and computers (Bodie and Dutta 2008; Beaunoyer, Dupéré, and Guitton 2020; Khilnani, Schulz, and Robinson 2020; Robinson et al. 2020); and low levels of education and health literacy (Abel and McQueen 2020; Nguyen et al. 2020; Sentell, Vamos, and Okan 2020).

In this chapter, we used the ecological model of information seeking as a rubric to describe different dimensions of health disinformation at various system levels. COVID-19 *communication ecologies* across the individual, interpersonal, organizational, community, and policy levels include a complex web of interconnected social networks and communicative resources to report, access, and disseminate perceived accurate and credible information. Myriad circumstances laid the groundwork for an *infodemic* with grave consequences for health behavior. The once-in-a-lifetime crisis of a lethal global pandemic created fertile soil and ample opportunity for voices of scapegoating and disinformation to be heard by a fearful and receptive audience. Members of the audience further amplified the message and created a chorus of similarly minded conspiracy espousing contrarians rejecting mainstream views such as the need for vaccines and mask mandates.

Vaccines have long been the target of conspiracy theorists (Broniatowski et al. 2018). In 2018, Heidi Larson (WHO vaccine initiative) predicted that "the deluge of conflicting information, disinformation and manipulated information on social media" would adversely impede global vaccine efforts (Larson 2018). Social media has been a primary source for disseminating many anti-vax conspiracies where anti-vaccine advocates have a significant presence (Broniatowski et al. 2018). These conspiracies can have real-world consequences. Vaccine-hesitant parents are more likely to have faith in the internet for information and less likely to trust health care providers and public health experts on the subject (Jones et al. 2012). Exposure to the vaccine debate often suggests that there is no scientific consensus, thus reducing confidence in vaccination (Witteman and Zikmund-Fisher 2012). In other words, the science remains equivocal, and the health decision remains a matter of personal choice. Evidence suggests that a false vaccine narrative across platforms tends to drive hesitancy, making it more difficult for the public health strategies needed to drive collective behavioral changes (Loomba et al. 2021). Such information can stoke preexisting fears, seeding doubt and cynicism over new vaccines, and limit public uptake of COVID-19 vaccines. There has been ample social science research endeavoring to understand how disinformation is perceived and appropriated. Collectively, it constitutes an interesting body of research spanning different disciplines that examine various facets of the problem. But there is much research yet to be done to understand how and why people engage views contrary to those of science. The understanding could inform us on how to mitigate these challenges and the risks to public health.

References

Abel, Thomas, and David McQueen. 2020. "Critical Health Literacy and the COVID-19 Crisis." *Health Promotion International* 35 (6): 1612–1613.

Ahmed, Imran. 2021. "Dismantling the Anti-Vaxx Industry." *Nature Medicine* 27 (3): 366–366.

Baidal, Jennifer Woo, Amanda Y. Wang, Katarina Zumwalt, Dahsan Gary, Yael Greenberg, Ben Cormack, Stephanie Lovinsky-Desir, Kelsey Nichols, Neil Pasco, Andres Nieto et al. 2020. "Social Determinants of Health and COVID-19 Among Patients in New York City." Research Square [preprint]. doi: 10.21203/rs.3.rs-70959/v1.

Baral, Stefan, Carmen H. Logie, Ashley Grosso, Andrea L. Wirtz, and Chris Beyrer. 2013. "Modified social ecological model: a tool to guide the assessment of the risks and risk contexts of HIV epidemics." BMC Public Health 13, (1): 1–8.

Beaunoyer, Elisabeth, Sophie Dupéré, and Matthieu J Guitton. 2020. "COVID-19 and Digital Inequalities: Reciprocal Impacts and Mitigation Strategies." *Computers in Human Behavior* 111: 106424.

Bekalu, Mesfin Awoke. 2014. "Communication Inequalities and Health Disparities." *Information Development* 30 (2): 189–191.

Bodie, Graham D., and Mohan Jyoti Dutta. 2008. "Understanding Health Literacy for Strategic Health Marketing: Ehealth Literacy, Health Disparities, and the Digital Divide." *Health Marketing Quarterly* 25 (1–2): 175–203.

Broniatowski, David A., Amelia M. Jamison, SiHua Qi, Lulwah AlKulaib, Tao Chen, Adrian Benton, Sandra C. Quinn, and Mark Dredze. 2018. "Weaponized Health Communication: Twitter Bots and Russian Trolls Amplify the Vaccine Debate." *American Journal of Public Health* 108 (10): 1378–1384. doi: 10.2105/ajph.2018.304567.

Bundorf, M. Kate, Todd H. Wagner, Sara J. Singer, and Laurence C. Baker. 2006. "Who Searches the Internet for Health Information?" *Health Services Research* 41 (3p1): 819–836.

Caramancion, Kevin Matthe. 2020. "An Exploration of Disinformation as a Cybersecurity Threat." 3rd International Conference on Information and Computer Technologies (ICICT): 440–444, doi: 10.1109/ICICT50521.2020.00076.

Chen, Xinran, Sei-Ching Joanna Sin, Yin-Leng Theng, and Chei Sian Lee. 2015. "Why Students Share Misinformation on Social Media: Motivation, Gender, and Study-Level Differences." *The Journal of Academic Librarianship* 41 (5): 583–592.

Chou, Wen-Ying Sylvia, Yvonne M. Hunt, Ellen B. Beckjord, Richard P. Moser, and Bradford W. Hesse. 2009. "Social Media Use in the United States: Implications for Health Communication." *Journal of Medical Internet Research* 11 (4): e48.

Cohen, Jon. 1994. "The Duesberg Phenomenon." *Science* 266 (5191): 1642.

Cronin, Robert M., Holly Jimison, and Kevin B. Johnson. 2021. "Personal Health Informatics." In *Biomedical Informatics: Computer Applications in Health Care and Biomedicine*, edited by James J. Cimino Edward H. Shortliffe, Michael F. Chiang, 363–389. Springer.

Depoux, Anneliese, Sam Martin, Emilie Karafillakis, Raman Preet, Annelies Wilder-Smith, and Heidi Larson. 2020. *The Pandemic of Social Media Panic Travels Faster than the COVID-19 Outbreak.* Oxford University Press.

Dionne, Kim Yi, and Fulya Felicity Turkmen. 2020. "The Politics of Pandemic Othering: Putting COVID-19 in Global and Historical Context." *International Organization* 74 (S1): E213-E230.

Dow, Benjamin J., Amber L. Johnson, Cynthia S. Wang, Jennifer Whitson, and Tanya Menon. 2021a. "The COVID-19 Pandemic and the Search for Structure: Social Media and Conspiracy Theories." *Social and Personality Psychology Compass* 15 (9): e12636.

Dow, Benjamin J., Amber L. Johnson, Cynthia S. Wang, Jennifer Whitson, and Tanya Menon. 2021b. "The COVID⊠19 Pandemic and the Search for Structure: Social Media and Conspiracy Theories." *Social and Personality Psychology Compass* 15 (9). doi: 10.1111/spc3.12636.

Elders, M. Joycelyn, Rueben C. Warren, Vivian W. Pinn, James H. Jones, Susan M. Reverby, David Satcher, Mary E. Northridge, Ronald Braithwaite, Mario DeLaRosa, and Luther S. Williams. 2011. *The Search for the Legacy of the USPHS Syphilis Study at Tuskegee: Reflective Essays Based upon Findings from the Tuskegee Legacy Project.* Lexington Books.

Eslahi, Meisam, Rosli Salleh, and Nor Badrul Anuar. "Bots and Botnets: An Overview of Characteristics, Detection and Challenges." Presented at the International Conference on Control System, Computing and Engineering, 2012.

Farmer, Paul Edward. 1990. *AIDS and Accusation: Haiti and the Geography of Blame.* Harvard University.

Forrest, Christopher B., Leiyu Shi, Sarah Von Schrader, and Judy Ng. 2002. "Managed Care, Primary Care, and the Patient⊠Practitioner Relationship." *Journal of General Internal Medicine* 17 (4): 270–277.

Fox, Susannah. 2008. *The Engaged e-Patient Population.* Washington, DC: Pew Internet & American Life Project.

Fulmer, Jeffrey. 2009. "What in the World Is Infrastructure." *PEI Infrastructure Investor* 1 (4): 30–32.

Gerber, Ben S., and Arnold R. Eiser. 2001. "The Patient-Physician Relationship in the Internet Age: Future Prospects and the Research Agenda." *Journal of Medical Internet Research* 3 (2): e15.

Gesualdo, Francesco, Mariateresa Romano, Elisabetta Pandolfi, Caterina Rizzo, Lucilla Ravà, Daniela Lucente, and Alberto E. Tozzi. 2010. "Surfing the Web During Pandemic Flu: Availability of World Health Organization Recommendations on Prevention." *BMC Public Health* 10 (1): 1–8.

Ghebreysus, Tedros A. (2020). "Munich Security Conference." https://www.who.int/director-general/speeches/detail/munich-security-conference.

Ginsburg, Faye. 2002. "Introduction: The Social Practice of Media." In *Media Worlds: Anthropology on New Terrain.* Berkeley: University of California Press. pp. 16–49.

Gover, Angela R., Shannon B. Harper, and Lynn Langton. 2020. "Anti-Asian Hate Crime During the COVID-19 Pandemic: Exploring the Reproduction of Inequality." *American Journal of Criminal Justice* 45 (4): 647–667.

Grimes, David Robert. 2021. "Medical Disinformation and the Unviable Nature of COVID-19 Conspiracy Theories." *PLOS ONE* 16 (3): e0245900. doi: 10.1371/journal.pone.0245900.

Hao, Karen. 2021. "Troll Farms Reached 140 Million Americans a Month on Facebook before 2020 Election, Internal Report Shows." *MIT Technology Review.*

Hawn, Carleen. 2009. "Take Two Aspirin and Tweet Me in the Morning: How Twitter, Facebook, and Other Social Media are Reshaping Health Care." *Health Affairs* Volume 28 (2): 361–368.

Hirsch, Vanessa M., Robert A. Olmsted, Michael Murphey-Corb, Robert H. Purcell, and Philip R. Johnson. 1989. "An African Primate Lentivirus (SIV sm Closely Related to HIV-2)." *Nature* 339 (6223): 389–392.

Hmielowski, Jay D., Lauren Feldman, Teresa A. Myers, Anthony Leiserowitz, and Edward Maibach. 2014. "An Attack on Science? Media Use, Trust in Scientists, and Perceptions of Global Warming." *Public Understanding of Science* 23 (7): 866–883. doi: 10.1177/0963662513480091.

Holtgrave, David R., Meredith A. Barranco, James M. Tesoriero, Debra S. Blog, and Eli S. Rosenberg. 2020. "Assessing Racial and Ethnic Disparities Using a COVID-19 Outcomes Continuum for New York State." *Annals of Epidemiology* 48: 9–14.

Hooper, Monica Webb, Anna María Nápoles, and Eliseo J Pérez-Stable. 2020. "COVID-19 and Racial/Ethnic Disparities." *JAMA* 323 (24): 2466–2467.

Horton, Richard. 2020. "Offline: COVID-19 Is Not a Pandemic." *The Lancet* 396 (10255): 874.

Hotez, Peter J. 2021. "Anti-Science Kills: From Soviet Embrace of Pseudoscience to Accelerated Attacks on US Biomedicine." *PLOS Biology* 19 (1): e3001068.

Howard, Philip N., Bharath Ganesh, Dimitra Liotsiou, John Kelly, and Camille François. 2019. The IRA, Social Media and Political Polarization in the United States, 2012–2018. In *Project on Computational Propaganda*. Oxford, UK.

Howard, Phillip, and S. Bradshaw. 2017. "Troops, Trolls and Troublemakers: A Global Inventory of Organized Social Media Manipulation." *Oxford: Computational Propaganda Project*. Accessed February 6, 2022. http://governance40.com/wp-content/uploads/2018/11/Troops-Trolls-and-Troublemakers.pdf.

Hudson, Sarah, and Graham Mackenzie. 2019. "'Not Your Daughter's Facebook': Twitter Use at the European Society of Cardiology Conference 2018." *Heart* 105 (2):169-170.

Imperva. 2021. "Bad Bot Report 2021: The Pandemic of the Internet." Accessed February 6, 2022. https://www.imperva.com/blog/bad-bot-report-2021-the-pandemic-of-the-internet/.

Jaiswal, J., C. LoSchiavo, and D. C. Perlman. 2020. "Disinformation, Misinformation and Inequality-Driven Mistrust in the Time of COVID-19: Lessons Unlearned from AIDS Denialism." *AIDS and Behavior* 24: 2776–2780.

Jones, Abbey M., Saad B. Omer, Robert A. Bednarczyk, Neal A. Halsey, Lawrence H. Moulton, and Daniel A. Salmon. 2012. "Parents' Source of Vaccine Information and Impact on Vaccine Attitudes, Beliefs, and Nonmedical Exemptions." *Advances in Preventive Medicine* 2012: 1–8. doi: 10.1155/2012/932741.

Kahan, Dan M. 2017. Misconceptions, Misinformation, and the Logic of Identity-Protective Cognition. In *Cultural Cognition Project Working Paper*. Yale Law School.

Kahneman, Daniel. 2011. *Thinking, Fast and Slow*. McMillan/Farrar, Straus and Giroux.

Kahneman, Daniel, Stewart Paul Slovic, Paul Slovic, and Amos Tversky. 1982. *Judgment Under Uncertainty: Heuristics and Biases*. Cambridge University Press.

Kaufman, David R., Jelena Mirkovic, and Connie Chan. 2017. "eHealth Literacy as a Mediator of Health Behaviors." In *Cognitive Informatics in Health and Biomedicine*, 271–297. Springer.

Kemp, Simon. 2021. "Digital 2021: April Global Statshot." *Erişim Adresi*. https://datareportal.com/reports/digital-2021-april-global-statshot.

Keselman, A., C. Arnott Smith, A. C. Murcko, and D. R. Kaufman. 2019. "Evaluating the Quality of Health Information in a Changing Digital Ecosystem." *Journal of Medical Internet Research* 21 (2): e11129. doi: 10.2196/11129.

Keselman, Alla, David R. Kaufman, and Vimla L. Patel. 2002. "Barriers to Adolescent Ability to Evaluate the Accuracy of Information about HIV." In *Proceedings of the AMIA Symposium*.

Keselman, Alla, David R. Kaufman, and Vimla L. Patel. 2004. "'You Can Exercise Your Way Out of HIV' and Other Stories: The Role of Biological Knowledge in Adolescents' Evaluation of Myths." *Science Education* 88 (4): 548–573.

Khilnani, Aneka, Jeremy Schulz, and Laura Robinson. 2020. "The COVID-19 Pandemic: New Concerns and Connections Between eHealth and Digital Inequalities." *Journal of Information, Communication and Ethics in Society* 18(3) 393–403.

King, Michelle T., Jia-Chen Fu, Miranda Brown, and Donny Santacaterina. 2021. "Rumor, Chinese Diets, and COVID-19: Questions and Answers about Chinese Food and Eating Habits." *Gastronomica: The Journal for Food Studies* 21 (1): 77–82.

Knight, Dacre. 2021. "COVID-19 Pandemic Origins: Bioweapons and the History of Laboratory Leaks." *Southern Medical Journal* 114 (8): 465.

Kuperjanov, Maris. 2021. "Early Days of the Novel Coronavirus: Public Response in Social Media During the First Month of the Outbreak." *Folklore: Electronic Journal of Folklore* (82): 159–182.

Larson, Heidi J. 2018. "The Biggest Pandemic Risk? Viral Misinformation." *Nature* 562 (7726): 309–310.

Laurencin, Cato T., and Aneesah McClinton. 2020. "The COVID-19 Pandemic: A Call to Action to Identify and Address Racial and Ethnic Disparities." *Journal of Racial and Ethnic Health Disparities* 7 (3): 398–402.

Lazer, D. M. J., M. A. Baum, Y. Benkler, A. J. Berinsky, K. M. Greenhill, F. Menczer, and J. L. Zittrain. 2018. "The Science of Fake News." *Science* 359 (6380): 1094–1096.

Lee, Jung Jae, Kyung-Ah Kang, Man Ping Wang, Sheng Zhi Zhao, Janet Yuen Ha Wong, Siobhan O'Connor, Sook Ching Yang, and Sunhwa Shin. 2020. "Associations between COVID-19 Misinformation Exposure and Belief with COVID-19 Knowledge and Preventive Behaviors: Cross-Sectional Online Study." *Journal of Medical Internet Research* 22 (11): e22205.

Lin, Leesa, Minsoo Jung, Rachel F. McCloud, and Kasisomayajula Viswanath. 2014. "Media Use and Communication Inequalities in a Public Health Emergency: A Case Study of 2009–2010 Pandemic Influenza A Virus Subtype H1N1." *Public Health Reports* 129 (6_suppl4): 49–60.

Lin, Leesa, Elena Savoia, Foluso Agboola, and Kasisomayajula Viswanath. 2014. "What Have We Learned About Communication Inequalities during the H1N1 Pandemic: A Systematic Review of the Literature." *BMC Public Health* 14 (1): 1–13.

Loomba, Sahil, Alexandre De Figueiredo, Simon J. Piatek, Kristen De Graaf, and Heidi J. Larson. 2021. "Measuring the Impact of COVID-19 Vaccine Misinformation on Vaccination Intent in the UK and USA." *Nature Human Behaviour* 5 (3): 337–348. doi: 10.1038/s41562-021-01056-1.

Lupi, Viviana. 2020. COVID-19 and Fake News in the Social Media. Bruno Kessler Foundation. https://www.fbk.eu/en/press-releases/covid-19-and-fake-news-in-the-social-media/.

Mann, Jonathan M. 1988. "Statement at an Informal Briefing on AIDS to the 42nd Session of the United Nations General Assembly." *Journal of the Royal Statistical Society. Series A (Statistics in Society)* 151 (1): 131–136.

Markel, Howard, and Alexandra Minna Stern. 2002. "The Foreignness of Germs: The Persistent Association of Immigrants and Disease in American Society." *The Milbank Quarterly* 80 (4): 757–788.

Martin, Brian. 2021. "COVID Information Struggles." *Social Epistemology Review and Reply Collective* 10 (6): 16–26.

Moorhead, S. Anne, Diane E. Hazlett, Laura Harrison, Jennifer K. Carroll, Anthea Irwin, and Ciska Hoving. 2013. "A New Dimension of Health Care: Systematic Review of the Uses, Benefits, and Limitations of Social Media for Health Communication." *Journal of Medical Internet Research* 15 (4):e1933.

Naeem, Salman Bin, Rubina Bhatti, and Aqsa Khan. 2021. "An Exploration of How Fake News Is Taking Over Social Media and Putting Public Health at Risk." *Health Information and Libraries Journal* 38 (2): 143–149. doi: 10.1111/hir.12320.

Nattrass, Nicoli. 2008. "AIDS and the Scientific Governance of Medicine in Post-Apartheid South Africa." *African Affairs* 107 (427): 157–176.

New York City Department of Health. 2020. "Age-Adjusted Rates of Lab Confirmed COVID-19 Non-hospitalized Cases, Estimated Non-Fatal Hospitalized Cases, and Persons Known to Have Died per 100,000 by Race/Ethnicity Group." https://www1.nyc.gov/assets/doh/downloads/pdf/imm/covid-19-deaths-race-ethnicity-04242020-1.pdf.

Nguyen, Hoang C., Minh H. Nguyen, Binh N. Do, Cuong Q. Tran, Thao T.P. Nguyen, Khue M. Pham, Linh V. Pham, Khanh V. Tran, Trang T Duong, and Tien V. Tran. 2020. "People with Suspected COVID-19 Symptoms Were More Likely Depressed and Had Lower Health-Related Quality of Life: The Potential Benefit of Health Literacy." *Journal of Clinical Medicine* 9 (4): 965.

O'Brien, Michael, Kathleen Moore, and Fiona McNicholas. 2020. "Social Media Spread During COVID-19: The Pros and Cons of Likes and Shares." *Irish Medical Journal* 113 (4): 52.

Pennycook, Gordon, and David G. Rand. 2019. "Lazy, Not Biased: Susceptibility to Partisan Fake News Is Better Explained by Lack of Reasoning than by Motivated Reasoning." *Cognition* 188: 39-50.

Pennycook, Gordon, Tyrone D. Cannon, and David G. Rand. 2018. "Prior Exposure Increases Perceived Accuracy of Fake News." *Journal of Experimental Psychology: General* 147 (12): 1865.

Ramanadhan, Shoba, and K. Viswanath. 2008. "Communication Inequality." *The International Encyclopedia of Communication* https://doi.org/10.1002/9781405186407.wbiecc076.

Rizzo, L., and S. Click. 2020. "How COVID-19 Changed Americans' Internet Habits." *Wall Street Journal,* August 15, 2020. https://www.wsj.com/articles/coronavirus-lockdown-tested-internets-backbone-11597503600.

Robinson, Laura, Jeremy Schulz, Aneka Khilnani, Hiroshi Ono, Shelia R. Cotten, Noah Mcclain, Lloyd Levine. et al. 2020. "Digital Inequalities in Time of Pandemic: COVID-19 Exposure Risk Profiles and New Forms of Vulnerability." *First Monday* 25, no. 10. https://firstmonday.org/article/view/10845/9563.

Sabatier, Renée, and Jon Tinker. 1988. "Blaming Others: Prejudice, Race and Worldwide AIDS." In *Blaming Others: Prejudice, Race and Worldwide AIDS*, vii, 168-vii, 168.

Schwenk, Eric S., Kellie M. Jaremko, Brian H. Park, Marjorie A. Stiegler, Jamison G. Gamble, Larry F. Chu, Audun Utengen, and Edward R. Mariano. 2020. "I Tweet, Therefore I Learn: An Analysis of Twitter Use Across Anesthesiology Conferences." *Anesthesia & Analgesia* 130 (2): 333–340.

Sentell, Tetine, Sandra Vamos, and Orkan Okan. 2020. *Interdisciplinary Perspectives on Health Literacy Research Around the World: More Important Than Ever in a Time of COVID-19*. Multidisciplinary Digital Publishing Institute.

Shearer, Elisa, and Amy Mitchell. 2021. *News Use Across Social Media Platforms in 2020*. Pew Research Center. Survey.

Simchon, Almog, Chaya Leibman, Tal Svoray, Itai Kloog, and Michael Dorman. 2021. "Beyond Doubt in a Dangerous World: The Effect of Existential Threats on Certainty Expressions in Societal Discourse." [Preprint] PsyArXiv. https://europepmc.org/article/ppr/ppr378846.

Swire-Thompson, Briony, and David Lazer. 2019. "Public Health and Online Misinformation: Challenges and Recommendations." *Annual Review of Public Health* 41: 433–451.

Upshaw, Tara L., Chloe Brown, Robert Smith, Melissa Perri, Carolyn Ziegler, and Andrew D. Pinto. 2021. "Social Determinants of COVID-19 Incidence and Outcomes: A Rapid Review." *PLOS ONE* 16 (3): e0248336.

Uscinski, Joseph E., Casey Klofstad, and Matthew D. Atkinson. 2016. "What Drives Conspiratorial Beliefs? The Role of Informational Cues and Predispositions." *Political Research Quarterly* 69 (1): 57–71.

Van Dorn, Aaron, Rebecca E. Cooney, and Miriam L. Sabin. 2020. "COVID-19 Exacerbating Inequalities in the US." *Lancet (London, England)* 395 (10232): 1243.

Vance, Karl, William Howe, and Robert P. Dellavalle. 2009. "Social Internet Sites as a Source of Public Health Information." *Dermatologic Clinics* 27 (2): 133–136.

Viswanath, K., Edmund WJ Lee, and Ramya Pinnamaneni. (2020). "We need the lens of equity in COVID-19 communication." Health Communication 35 (14): 1743–1746.

Vosniadou, Stella. 2020. "Students' Misconceptions and Science Education." In *Oxford Research Encyclopedia of Education*. New York: Oxford University Press.

Vosoughi, Soroush, Deb Roy, and Sinan Aral. 2018. "The Spread of True and False News Online." *Science* 359 (6380): 1146–1151. doi:10.1126/science.aap9559.

Walker, Denetra, and Allison Daniel Anders. 2021. "'China Virus' and 'Kung-Flu': A Critical Race Case Study of Asian American Journalists' Experiences During COVID-19." *Cultural Studies↔ Critical Methodologies* 22(1): 76–88. https://doi.org/10.1177/15327086211055157.

Williamson, Kirsty. 1998. "Discovered by chance: The role of incidental information acquisition in an ecological model of information use." Library & Information Science Research 20 (1): 23–40.

Witteman, Holly O., and Brian J. Zikmund-Fisher. 2012. "The Defining Characteristics of Web 2.0 and Their Potential Influence in the Online Vaccination Debate." *Vaccine* 30 (25): 3734–3740. doi:10.1016/j.vaccine.2011.12.039.

Wong, Adrian, Ifor Capel, and Manu Malbrain. 2019. "Social Media in Critical Care: Fad or a New Standard in Medical Education? An Analysis of International Critical Care Conferences Between 2014 and 2017." *Journal of the Intensive Care Society* 20 (4):341–346.

Wong, Adrian, Serene Ho, Olusegun Olusanya, Marta Velia Antonini, and David Lyness. 2021. "The Use of Social Media and Online Communications in Times of Pandemic COVID-19." *Journal of the Intensive Care Society* 22 (3): 255–260.

Xavier, Andre Junqueira, Eleonora d'Orsi, Jane Wardle, Panayotes Demakakos, Samuel G. Smith, and Christian von Wagner. 2013. "Internet Use and Cancer-Preventive Behaviors in Older Adults: Findings from a Longitudinal Cohort Study." *Cancer Epidemiology and Prevention Biomarkers* 22 (11): 2066–2074.

Yang, Kai-Cheng, Francesco Pierri, Pik-Mai Hui, David Axelrod, Christopher Torres-Lugo, John Bryden, and Filippo Menczer. (2021). "The covid-19 infodemic: Twitter versus facebook." Big Data & Society 8 (1): 20539517211013861.

Zhao, Yuehua, Jingwei Da, and Jiaqi Yan. 2021. "Detecting Health Misinformation in Online Health Communities: Incorporating Behavioral Features into Machine Learning Based Approaches." *Information Processing & Management* 58 (1): doi: 10.1016/j.ipm.2020.102390.

3

The Health Misinformation Ecosystem on Social Media

Emerging Evidence and Research Gaps

Wen-Ying Sylvia Chou, Anna Gaysynsky, and Yuki Lama

According to the Pew Research Center, over 72 percent of American adults reported using social media in 2021—a dramatic increase from just fifteen years ago when only about 5 percent of Americans were using these platforms (Pew Research Center 2021). As social media use increases, the real-world impact of these platforms cannot be underestimated. Online interactions reflect, perpetuate, and shape personal relationships and social networks, as well as attitudes, decisions, and behaviors regarding everything from health to politics.

The current social media landscape is characterized by several key features. First, social media users have become more diverse over time. Social media use is highly prevalent across gender, racial/ethnic groups, and education and income levels; and although significant differences by age remain (with older adults being less likely to use social media than younger individuals), social media use is relatively high even among older adults (Pew Research Center 2021). Second, an increasing percentage of the population relies on social media for news and information; in 2020, approximately half of adults in the United States reported getting news from social media at least "sometimes" (Shearer and Mitchell 2021), which represents a significant shift in the information landscape. This may not necessarily be a positive development, as a 2020 Pew Research Center report finds that individuals who rely on social media for news are less likely to have accurate knowledge about important topics like the COVID-19 pandemic (Mitchell et al. 2020).

Third, the unprecedented ability of social media platforms to collect user data and deploy sophisticated algorithms based on that data has further shifted the information ecosystem. The algorithms through which platforms suggest content and accounts to users are often based on user data (e.g., search history and geolocation) and past engagement behaviors. Consequently, algorithms may be less likely to surface or recommend content that contains an opposing viewpoint, contradictory information, or topics the user has not yet shown interest in. Although the goal of these algorithms is to increase user engagement and time spent on the platform, in practice, they may help reinforce "echo-chambers" where users encounter mostly information that they are familiar with or that confirms their existing views, and in some cases these algorithms may even push users toward more extreme content. Lastly, visuals (e.g., photos, videos, and emoticons) are an essential aspect of the social media landscape today. In fact, some of the leading platforms (e.g., Pinterest and Instagram) are primarily focused on visual content rather than text (Russmann and Svensson 2017).

Given the high penetration of social media, and the above-mentioned characteristics of the social media environment, it is vital to better understand how social media use affects health—in ways both good and bad. For example, social media platforms make it easy to find and share health information on topics ranging from chronic disease management (Paige et al. 2015) to mental health (Devendorf, Bender, and Rottenberg 2020) and provide a means for connecting with others to exchange social support (Gavrila et al. 2019). Social media can also benefit public health efforts by enabling public health surveillance (Allem et al. 2017; Masri et al. 2019) and serving as a channel for delivering health promotion interventions (Chou et al. 2013). However, these benefits may not accrue equitably across the population, as studies have shown that certain groups (e.g., younger individuals and women) are more likely to engage in social media for both general and health-specific purposes (Chou et al. 2021).

In addition, social media use also has the potential to cause harm, which is alarming given the expansive reach of these platforms. For instance, studies have found that many social media posts encourage and normalize harmful behaviors, including eating disorders (Bert et al. 2016), self-harm (Arendt, Scherr, and Romer 2019), and tobacco product use (Albarracin et al. 2018). Furthermore, although concerns about the quality of health information online have been long-standing (Moorhead et al. 2013), social media as an important source of health misinformation (which we define as "any health-related claim of fact that is false based on current scientific consensus" [Chou, Gaysynsky, and Cappella 2020]) has only recently come to the attention of government leaders, scholars, and health care practitioners. Studies have documented the spread of misinformation on these platforms across many important public health topics, including vaccines, medical treatments, and infectious disease pandemics (Suarez-Lledo and Alvarez-Galvez 2021).

Alarmingly, misinformation has been found to spread more widely and more quickly than accurate information. In a large study, Vosoughi, Roy, and Aral (2018) examined the diffusion of both verified and false news stories on Twitter between 2006 and 2017, finding that false information spread significantly further, faster, and more broadly than true news stories across all information domains studied (including politics, science, and finance), possibly due to the "novel" nature of falsehoods and their ability to elicit emotions such as fear, disgust, and surprise. Some research on health misinformation has found similar patterns. For example, a study of Zika information on Facebook found that misleading posts garnered far more views and were shared more often than posts containing accurate public health information (Sharma et al. 2017).

Unfortunately, despite the potential for significant harm, mitigating the spread of misinformation on social media has been difficult for several reasons. To begin with, much of the misinformation found on these platforms may not be provably false but simply misleading based on framing, insinuation, word choice, omission, or exaggeration (Nan, Wang, and Thier 2020), which makes it far more difficult to identify and address. Misinformation content on social media also often relies on anecdotal evidence or personal narratives (Guidry et al. 2015; Kearney et al. 2019) that cannot be as easily refuted, which further underscores the difficulty of both identifying and addressing social media misinformation. The use of automated "bots" to disseminate false information may also pose a challenge, as bots can increase the volume and the speed of misinformation spread at a low cost, and humans are often unable to distinguish bots from genuine accounts (Memon and Carley 2020; Shao et al. 2018).

Another important challenge concerns the tension between content moderation practices aimed at addressing the spread of misinformation (particularly content or account removal) and considerations around individuals' freedom of expression. Some have argued that widespread removal of content and de-platforming of accounts would amount to censorship and "threaten the democratic cornerstone of freedom of speech" (Armitage 2021). Those who place a premium on free speech believe that all ideas should be debated "in the marketplace of ideas" (Armitage 2021) and often posit that *more* speech (i.e., more accurate information in these spaces) is the best way to deal with misinformation (Wardle and Singerman 2021). However, those advocating for a more robust response from social media platforms point out that "freedom of speech" is not the same as "freedom of reach" (Wardle and Singerman 2021), and note that the substantial individual and societal harm that could be caused by misinformation must be balanced against freedom of expression considerations (Yang, Broniatowski, and Reiss 2019).

Social media platforms are private companies and are therefore able to restrict speech that violates their terms of service without running afoul of the First Amendment (Yang, Broniatowski, and Reiss 2019). However, not everyone is comfortable with allowing social media platforms to decide what should be classified as misinformation (Bode 2019). This is especially true in light of reports that platforms often apply their content moderation policies inconsistently or incorrectly (Broniatowski, Dredze, and Ayers 2021). There are substantial technical and conceptual challenges to ensuring that content moderation works well. For example, identifying health misinformation can be difficult because, as mentioned previously, misinformation can be quite nuanced; furthermore, what is considered "misinformation" can shift as new research emerges, and conflicting information can reflect genuine disagreement and lack of consensus among experts (Wardle and Singerman 2021). Given these conceptual challenges, it is difficult for humans, let alone classification models, to accurately identify, flag, or remove misinformation. While this lack of accuracy will likely allow a significant amount of misinformation to continue circulating, it also means that some unproblematic content may be incorrectly labeled as misinformation and removed (Bode 2019).

Even if these conceptual and technical limitations could be resolved—allowing misinformation to be identified and removed with absolute precision—there is some concern that these efforts might still generate unintended consequences. Some experts have argued that de-platforming anti-vaccine groups would feed into the conspiracies and narratives these groups promote and further deepen mistrust among individuals who are receptive to their messages (Broniatowski, Dredze, and Ayers 2021; Armitage 2021). Removing misinformation agents from mainstream platforms could also drive them to alternative platforms where it will be much more difficult to monitor their activity (Armitage 2021). There is also concern that the removal of malicious content and bad actors will stifle relevant discussion and discourage the sharing of legitimate questions (Armitage 2021; Mills and Sivelä 2021). Lastly, simply removing problematic content and malicious accounts without archiving them would hamper researchers' ability to study misinformation (Yang, Broniatowski, and Reiss 2019).

Although a sizeable body of research has emerged over the past few years focusing on health misinformation on social media, important gaps remain in our understanding of the nature and consequences of this phenomenon. Many studies have examined misinformation in the context of specific health topics and have assessed the spread of misinformation on individual social media platforms. While these studies generate important insights, more research is needed to comprehensively evaluate the landscape of health misinformation on social media (including how falsehoods spread within and across platforms and whether patterns of misinformation diffusion differ based on topic) to better understand the real-world impact of misinformation exposure and to evaluate the effectiveness of interventions and policies to mitigate the impact of misinformation.

In this chapter, we provide an overview of the state of research on health misinformation—presenting examples across a wide variety of health topics and platforms—and discuss what current research tells us about the health misinformation ecosystem. We then delve into remaining scientific gaps and identify research priorities that will need to be tackled if we are to keep pace with an evolving social media landscape and stem the tide of health misinformation.

What We Know about Health Misinformation on Social Media: Current Evidence

Although there are no comprehensive data on the overall prevalence of health misinformation on social media, studies focused on specific health topics suggest that there is a *substantial amount of misinformation* present on these platforms. A review conducted by Suarez-Lledo and Alvarez-Galvez (2021) found a very high prevalence of misinformation about drugs/tobacco and vaccines on social media (as well as lower, but still moderate, levels of misinformation on eating disorders, noncommunicable diseases, and pandemics). Research has also shown that information about urologic conditions is often inaccurate, biased, and/or false across a wide range of social media platforms (Loeb et al. 2020). Cancer misinformation on social media is also a concern: an analysis of 200 popular social media articles on common cancers found that a high proportion (32.5 percent) contained misinformation and that the median number of engagements with articles containing misinformation was greater than that of articles containing accurate information (Johnson et al. 2021). Additionally, an analysis of breast cancer information on Pinterest found that 11.4 percent of the sample contained misinformation related to breast cancer prevention or treatment (Wilner and Holton 2020). Substantial levels of COVID-19-related misinformation have also been documented on social media: early in the pandemic, Kouzy et al. (2020) found that approximately 25 percent of non-humorous COVID-19 tweets contained misinformation, while Southwick et al. (2021) found that 27 percent of TikTok videos contained incorrect, misleading, or incomplete health information about COVID-19.

In addition to tracking misinformation on social media, research has also attempted to understand characteristics that may make users more or less susceptible to misinformation. Scherer et al. (2021) examined social media posts across three different health topics and found that susceptibility to misinformation was consistently predicted by lower educational attainment and limited health literacy, distrust in the health care system, and positive attitudes toward alternative medicine. Similarly, a study using a global sample found that higher trust in scientists and higher numeracy were consistently associated with lower susceptibility to COVID-19-related misinformation—and further showed that susceptibility to misinformation could reduce willingness to comply with public health measures (Roozenbeek et al. 2020). Other characteristics that have been found to be associated with receptivity to misinformation include certain cognitive styles and political ideology (Scherer and Pennycook 2020; Sindermann, Cooper, and Montag 2020; Garrett and Bond 2021)—although it is possible that certain psychological variables (e.g., lower tolerance for ambiguity) may be associated with both conservative ideology and susceptibility to misinformation (Salvi et al. 2021). There are also factors such as analytical thinking (Sindermann, Cooper, and Montag 2020) and the need for cognition (i.e., an individual's tendency to engage in and enjoy effortful cognitive activity)

(Leding and Antonio 2019) that seem to improve accuracy perceptions and protect against susceptibility to misinformation.

Several studies have also been conducted to evaluate the impact of policies enacted by social media platforms to address misinformation. For example, Guidry et al. (2020) assessed changes in human papillomavirus (HPV) vaccine-related search results on Pinterest after the platform adopted a policy in 2019 to moderate vaccine-related search results. They found that although the policy was largely successful in reducing anti-vaccine results and increasing the number of pins from reputable health sources, it also seemed to have an unintended consequence: the way the search restrictions were implemented limited the overall amount of HPV vaccination content available in search results, potentially creating an "information vacuum" on the topic (Guidry et al. 2020). In a different attempt to assess the impact of platform misinformation mitigation efforts, Geeng et al. (2020) surveyed users about the perceived helpfulness of measures adopted by social media platforms to address COVID-19 misinformation (e.g., banners linking to authoritative resources and warning labels on specific posts). The results indicate that while users generally perceived these interventions positively, a majority of participants reported that they discovered information was false through alternative means (e.g., web searches, seeking out trusted sources, and seeing a correction in a comment). Only a small number of participants learned something was false (whether or not they initially believed it) because the social media platform had labeled it as misinformation, raising questions about how much impact these initiatives are really having.

Although these results suggest that current social media policies are falling short, research also provides cause for optimism concerning the possibility of successfully addressing misinformation. For example, emerging evidence suggests that a relatively small number of actors are responsible for a large proportion of the misinformation on social media—at least for certain health topics, like vaccines. A study examining vaccine conversations on Twitter found that a total of 129 "top authors" (those with the highest levels of engagement) were responsible for driving over half of all vaccine opposition conversations and that these actors tended to employ a relatively small set of anti-vaccine themes, which may make monitoring, identifying, and responding to anti-vaccine content more feasible than might be expected given the sheer volume of tweets (Bonnevie et al. 2020). Similarly, the Center for Countering Digital Hate (2021) performed an analysis of URLs included in anti-vaccine posts retrieved from thirty anti-vaccine Facebook groups and found that 73 percent of the anti-vaccine content shared can be traced back to only twelve influential individuals, suggesting that removing their accounts could be an efficient way to reduce the dissemination of misinformation about vaccines on the platform. More generally, research has shown that diffusion of information online is largely driven by "broadcast" (where a single influential source shares information with many individuals), rather than person-to-person cascades, further suggesting that monitoring and targeting influential accounts may be an effective—and efficient—strategy to reduce the spread of misinformation (Swire-Thompson and Lazer 2019).

In addition to removing content and banning influential accounts, a growing body of research provides evidence for *a range of interventions* that can be adopted in addressing misinformation on social media. In fact, several studies to date have shown that *corrections can be effective* in reducing belief in misinformation. Strategies that have proven effective include providing related stories that correct false information in a post (Bode and Vraga 2015), citing expert sources in the correction itself, providing corrections from an expert source (Vraga and Bode 2017), and providing logic-based corrections (Vraga et al. 2020). However, corrections may not be as effective for polarizing issues or when views on a topic have become entrenched

(Vraga and Bode 2020; Bode and Vraga 2015), and although several methods can be used to increase the effectiveness of corrections (e.g., repetition and presentation of an alternative explanation), research generally suggests that corrections have limitations—they can *reduce* reliance in misinformation, but they may not be able to eliminate it entirely (Lewandowsky et al. 2012; Walter and Tukachinsky 2020). Due to these limitations, researchers are also investigating alternative approaches, including "inoculating" *users against misinformation*. These kinds of proactive strategies aim to prevent misinformation from gaining traction in the first place rather than trying to correct misinformation once it has already been accepted (Lewandowsky and Van Der Linden 2021). Studies suggest that inoculating individuals by warning them that they might be misinformed and then providing them with a refutational preemption (i.e., "prebunking") can increase resilience and reduce vulnerability to misinformation (Lewandowsky and Van Der Linden 2021). For example, an inoculation intervention aimed at preventing smoking initiation might first warn adolescents that they may be exposed to peer pressure in middle school (Pfau, Bockern, and Kang 1992) and then present a few of the arguments they might be pressured with (e.g., "just trying a cigarette isn't a big deal"), before refuting, or "prebunking," those statements with evidence (e.g., "actually, nicotine is a highly addictive drug and some adolescents experience tobacco dependence within a day of first inhaling"). Although prebunking efforts can target individual pieces of misinformation, broader strategies that target the general techniques of manipulation (e.g., teaching individuals to identify flawed argumentation) are especially promising as they could be more scalable (Lewandowsky and Van Der Linden 2021). For example, an online game designed by Roozenbeek and van der Linden (2019) that teaches players about six common manipulation techniques used in misinformation campaigns was found to improve the ability to identify and resist misinformation across education level, age, political ideology, and cognitive style.

Research Gaps and Future Priorities

Although the knowledge base regarding social media health misinformation is expanding rapidly, there are notable limitations to the research conducted to date, which need to be addressed in order to improve our understanding of health misinformation and how to best mitigate its harms. First, there is a need to expand research into a more diverse range of social media platforms. A systematic review by Suarez-Lledo and Alvarez-Galvez (2021) found that the most common platforms used in health misinformation studies were Twitter, YouTube, and Facebook, while other platforms like Instagram and Pinterest were far less frequently used. Although researchers are beginning to study health misinformation on Instagram and Pinterest, many other social media platforms have received limited scholarly attention, including TikTok, Tumblr, and Reddit. This may be problematic because the usage of platforms varies by sociodemographic factors including age, race, and gender (e.g., a much larger percentage of women report using Pinterest compared to men) (Pew Research Center 2021). This lack of attention to smaller and emerging platforms risks missing important information about specific populations and their exposure to misinformation.

Additionally, much of the research conducted to date has focused on platforms popular in Western countries (and on English language posts on those platforms), which may be limiting our knowledge of *misinformation spread in immigrant communities* who may be using platforms popular in their home countries (e.g., WeChat, Weibo, and Vkontakte) or engaging with non-English language content on mainstream platforms (to illustrate, in an analysis of nationally representative data, Hispanic individuals were found to be more likely to watch health-related videos on YouTube compared to non-Hispanic whites (Chou et al. 2021)). A study by Madraki et al. (2021) found that the nature of COVID-19 misinformation varied across countries and languages, likely due to factors such as differences in culture, beliefs, and government restrictions, suggesting that research on English language and US-based platforms will not necessarily generalize to other contexts. Furthermore, the fact that social media misinformation research lacks linguistic diversity (e.g., only 10 percent of studies in the Suarez-Lledo and Alvarez-Galvez [2021] review included posts written in more than one language) is concerning because non-English-speaking individuals may face more barriers to obtaining accurate information from expert sources, and the quality of misinformation *monitoring and moderation of non-English content* may be more limited on social media platforms (Wilson and Land 2020; Bond 2021), potentially putting non-English speakers at greater risk of misinformation exposure.

Comparing patterns of misinformation sharing across different platforms is also an important avenue for additional research. An analysis of COVID-19 information on Twitter, Instagram, YouTube, Reddit, and Gab found substantial differences in the volume of information from questionable sources on different platforms (Cinelli et al. 2020), suggesting that unique platform features and userbases need to be taken into account. However, while analyses that compare individual platforms can be useful, conceptualizing the social media ecosystem as decentralized but interconnected might help improve understanding of the *movement of misinformation—and actors—across platforms*. For example, a study found that hate groups form interconnected networks across independent platforms, which makes them very resilient and allows them to quickly adapt in response to attempts to limit their activity—particularly in the absence of coordinated cross-platform policing (Johnson et al. 2019). An analysis by Velasquez et al. (2021) showed that the existence of such networks enabled COVID-19 misinformation to spread quickly between platforms and circumvent moderation efforts.

There is also a more general need to expand the methods and approaches used in misinformation research. Literature reviews have shown that the dominant methodological approaches used in misinformation studies are quality evaluation, social network analysis, and content/text analysis (Suarez-Lledo and Alvarez-Galvez 2021; Wang et al. 2019)—a greater diversity of approaches (e.g., longitudinal cohort studies, real-time rumor detection, and ethnographic case studies) could lead to additional insights about the nature of health misinformation. Development of automated methods that can be applied at a large scale to identify and analyze misinformation is also needed, given the sheer volume of content posted to social media sites (Singh, Ghosh, and Sonagara 2021). Several automated methods have been developed for misinformation detection, including creator/user analysis (focused on factors like posting frequency and behavior), social context analysis (focused on user networks or dissemination patterns), and content analysis (focused on specific linguistic, semantic, or stylistic features of text) (Zhang and Ghorbani 2020). However, automated methods for visual content have been limited, and this is a major gap as the social media environment is increasingly multimodal (comprising both visuals and text). An analysis of COVID-19-related misinformation posts suggests that visuals may serve specific functions in communicating misinformation, including illustrating and selectively emphasizing arguments, providing "evidence" for claims, and impersonating supposedly authoritative sources (Brennen, Simon, and Nielsen 2021). *Multimodal approaches* combining text and visual features are an especially promising direction for automated detection techniques. Work conducted by Singh, Ghosh, and Sonagara (2021) demonstrates the potential of this type of approach; the researchers identified the text and visual features most strongly associated with fake news articles and built classification algorithms that combined these features, finding that multimodal models were better able to detect false news articles compared to single-modality approaches (especially text-only models).

However, perhaps the most critical gap in the social media misinformation literature is the lack of research on the consequences of exposure to health misinformation. Research that systematically elucidates the extent to which misinformation exposure affects attitudes, decisions, behaviors, and health outcomes both at the individual and population level is needed to understand how online misinformation impacts health in the real world. This area of inquiry has been hampered by the technical challenges of linking online exposure and offline behavior, as well as the limitations of standard self-report measures (e.g., surveys) in assessing both harm and exposure (Swire-Thompson and Lazer 2019). Therefore, the development of innovative approaches to advance this area of research is crucial.

Relatedly, research is needed to better understand disparities in susceptibility to, and therefore potential harm from, misinformation. To date, findings are mixed on certain factors that influence vulnerability. For example, although some research suggests older age might increase vulnerability to online misinformation (possibly due to cognitive decline or lower levels of digital literacy) (Brashier and Schacter 2020), other studies have shown that older adults might in fact be less vulnerable to misinformation (Roozenbeek et al. 2020). Such inconsistent findings may be due to the different contexts studied (politics vs. health), suggesting that the association between demographic characteristics and misinformation vulnerability might be context-dependent (Bode and Vraga 2021). Additional research is also needed on a number of *understudied factors*, including emotions (Martel, Pennycook, and Rand 2020), personality traits (e.g., conscientiousness) (Calvillo et al. 2021; Sindermann, Cooper, and Montag 2020), and conspiracy mind-set (Landrum and Olshansky 2019; Uscinski et al. 2020).

A better understanding of who is vulnerable to believing and sharing misinformation could also allow counter messages and mitigation efforts to be more effectively targeted. For example, Ghenai and Mejova (2018) built a classifier based on factors like user attributes and linguistic features that was capable of identifying users likely to tweet about unproven cancer treatments. This information could enable interventionists to deploy strategically targeted measures to prevent misinformation from being posted and allow them to focus on monitoring high-risk accounts so they can more quickly act to limit the spread of misinformation once it is posted (Ghenai and Mejova 2018).

More work also needs to be done to evaluate existing efforts and develop additional mitigation measures. Specifically, the impact of different social media policies regarding misinformation needs to be carefully and iteratively evaluated by independent social science researchers. The consequences of the measures adopted by platforms, such as removal, downranking, and flagging of certain health misinformation, are largely unknown outside the companies themselves. *More data access and transparency* would enable researchers to evaluate the overall impact of changing policies and interventions, as well as their differential effects (e.g., whether they generate backfire effects, confusion, or greater mistrust and cynicism among certain groups). This knowledge could then facilitate the development of more effective and targeted strategies to counter misinformation. However, as noted in a 2021 Surgeon General Advisory, responding to misinformation will require a whole-of-society effort that goes beyond social media platforms (Office of the Surgeon General 2021). *Multilevel and multisector efforts* that involve government, health organizations, health care providers, journalists, communities, and individuals also need to be developed and evaluated. For example, digital and health literacy programs implemented in both school and community settings (e.g., libraries) could make individuals less vulnerable to misinformation. Government efforts could also help reduce the amount of health misinformation circulating on social media and remove some of the financial incentives driving misinformation. For instance, during the COVID-19 pandemic, the Food and Drug Administration and the Federal Trade Commission targeted companies making deceptive or scientifically unsupported health claims about products they promoted and sold online (Federal Trade Commission 2020). In combination, such efforts by different societal actors could help reduce the volume and impact of misinformation and produce a healthier information environment.

Conclusion

As we have outlined in this chapter, due to its enormous reach, health misinformation on social media poses a potentially significant threat to public health, and further efforts to increase our understanding of the online misinformation environment and develop effective strategies to mitigate the impact of health misinformation are urgently needed. The evidence base is growing with respect to the nature and prevalence of health misinformation on social media, traits that increase susceptibility to misinformation, and effective intervention strategies, but there is still more to be learned. Several key actions will be critical to mitigating the spread and impact of misinformation, including (1) enhancing surveillance (by advancing automated detection methods, conducting research across a greater array of platforms and languages, and paying more attention to visual content), (2) assessing the consequences of health misinformation exposure (concerning both the impact of specific misinformation on health-related attitudes and behaviors, as well as the more global impact of the misinformation environment on outcomes such as disengagement, apathy, and skepticism), (3) identifying individuals and groups who are most vulnerable to misinformation or most likely to spread it, and (4) developing and evaluating effective multilevel response measures (Chou, Gaysynsky, and Cappella 2020).

References

Albarracin, Dolores, Daniel Romer, Christopher Jones, Kathleen Hall Jamieson, and Patrick Jamieson. 2018. "Misleading Claims About Tobacco Products in Youtube Videos: Experimental Effects of Misinformation on Unhealthy Attitudes." *Journal of Medical Internet Research* 20 (6): e229.

Allem, Jon-Patrick, Emilio Ferrara, Sree Priyanka Uppu, Tess Boley Cruz, and Jennifer B. Unger. 2017. "E-cigarette Surveillance with Social Media Data: Social Bots, Emerging Topics, and Trends." *JMIR Public Health and Surveillance* 3 (4): e98.

Arendt, Florian, Sebastian Scherr, and Daniel Romer. 2019. "Effects of Exposure to Self-Harm on Social Media: Evidence From a Two-Wave Panel Study Among Young Adults." *New Media & Society* 21 (11–12): 2422–2442.

Armitage, R. 2021. "Online 'Anti-Vax' Campaigns and COVID-19: Censorship is Not the Solution." *Public Health* 190: e29.

Bert, Fabrizio, Maria Rosaria Gualano, Elisa Camussi, and Roberta Siliquini. 2016. "Risks and Threats of Social Media Websites: Twitter and The Proana Movement." *Cyberpsychology, Behavior, and Social Networking* 19 (4): 233–238.

Bode, Leticia. 2019. "User Correction as a Tool in the Battle against Social Media Misinformation." *Georgetown Law Tech Review* 4: 367.

Bode, Leticia, and Emily Vraga. 2021. "Value for Correction: Documenting Perceptions about Peer Correction of Misinformation on Social Media in the Context of COVID-19." *Journal of Quantitative Description: Digital Media* 1.

Bode, Leticia, and Emily K Vraga. 2015. "In Related News, That Was Wrong: The Correction of Misinformation Through Related Stories Functionality in Social Media." *Journal of Communication* 65 (4): 619–638.

Bond, Shannon. 2021. "'Ya Basta Facebook' Says Company Must Curb Misinformation in Spanish." *NPR*, March 16, 2021. https://www.npr.org/2021/03/16/977613561/ya-basta-facebook-says-company-must-curb-misinformation-in-spanish?sc=18&f=1001.

Bonnevie, Erika, Jaclyn Goldbarg, Allison K. Gallegos-Jeffrey, Sarah D. Rosenberg, Ellen Wartella, and Joe Smyser. 2020. "Content Themes and Influential Voices within Vaccine Opposition on Twitter, 2019." *American Journal of Public Health* 110 (S3): S326–S330.

Brashier, Nadia M., and Daniel L. Schacter. 2020. "Aging in an Era of Fake News." *Current Directions in Psychological Science* 29 (3): 316–323.

Brennen, J Scott, Felix M Simon, and Rasmus Kleis Nielsen. 2021. "Beyond (Mis) Representation: Visuals in COVID-19 Misinformation." *The International Journal of Press/Politics* 26 (1): 277–299.

Broniatowski, David A., Mark Dredze, and John W. Ayers. 2021. "'First Do No Harm': Effective Communication About COVID-19 Vaccines." *American Journal of Public Health* 111(6): 1055–1057.

Calvillo, Dustin P., Ryan J. B. Garcia, Kiana Bertrand, and Tommi A Mayers. 2021. "Personality Factors and Self-Reported Political News Consumption Predict Susceptibility to Political Fake News." *Personality and Individual Differences* 174: 110666.

Center for Countering Digital Hate. 2021. *The Disinformation Dozen.* Accessed February 7, 2022. https://www.counterhate.com/_files/ugd/f4d9b9_b7cedc0553604720b7137f8663366ee5.pdf.

Chou, Wen-Ying Sylvia, Anna Gaysynsky, and Joseph N. Cappella. 2020. "Where We Go from Here: Health Misinformation on Social Media." *American Journal of Public Health* 110 (S3): S273–S275.

Chou, Wen-Ying Sylvia, Anna Gaysynsky, Neha Trivedi, and Robin C. Vanderpool. 2021. "Using Social Media for Health: National Data from HINTS 2019." *Journal of Health Communication* 26 (3): 184–193.

Chou, Wen-ying Sylvia, Abby Prestin, Claire Lyons, and Kuang-yi Wen. 2013. "Web 2.0 for Health Promotion: Reviewing the Current Evidence." *American Journal of Public Health* 103 (1): e9–e18.

Cinelli, Matteo, Walter Quattrociocchi, Alessandro Galeazzi, Carlo Michele Valensise, Emanuele Brugnoli, Ana Lucia Schmidt, Paola Zola, Fabiana Zollo, and Antonio Scala. 2020. "The COVID-19 Social Media Infodemic." *Scientific Reports* 10 (1): 1–10.

Devendorf, Andrew, Ansley Bender, and Jonathan Rottenberg. 2020. "Depression Presentations, Stigma, and Mental Health Literacy: A Critical Review and YouTube Content Analysis." *Clinical Psychology Review* 78: 101843.

Federal Trade Commission. 2020."FTC, FDA Send Warning Letters to Seven Companies about Unsupported Claims that Products Can Treat or Prevent Coronavirus." Accessed February 7, 2022. https://www.ftc.gov/news-events/press-releases/2020/03/ftc-fda-send-warning-letters-seven-companies-about-unsupported.

Garrett, R. Kelly, and Robert M. Bond. 2021. "Conservatives' Susceptibility to Political Misperceptions." *Science Advances* 7 (23): eabf1234.

Gavrila, Valerie, Ashley Garrity, Emily Hirschfeld, Breann Edwards, and Joyce M. Lee. 2019. "Peer Support through a Diabetes Social Media Community." *Journal of Diabetes Science and Technology* 13 (3): 493–497.

Geeng, Christine, Tiona Francisco, Jevin West, and Franziska Roesner. 2020. "Social Media COVID-19 Misinformation Interventions Viewed Positively, But Have Limited Impact." Preprint, *arXiv*. https://arxiv.org/abs/2012.11055.

Ghenai, Amira, and Yelena Mejova. 2018. "Fake Cures: User-Centric Modeling of Health Misinformation in Social Media." *Proceedings of the ACM on Human-Computer Interaction* 2 (CSCW): 1–20.

Guidry, Jeanine P. D., Kellie Carlyle, Marcus Messner, and Yan Jin. 2015. "On Pins and Needles: How Vaccines are Portrayed on Pinterest." *Vaccine* 33 (39): 5051–5056.

Guidry, Jeanine P. D., Emily K. Vraga, Linnea I. Laestadius, Carrie A. Miller, Aurora Occa, Xiaoli Nan, Hannah M. Ming, Yan Qin, Bernard F. Fuemmeler, and Kellie E. Carlyle. 2020. "HPV Vaccine Searches on Pinterest: Before and After Pinterest's Actions to Moderate Content." *American Journal of Public Health* 110 (S3): S305–S311.

Johnson, Nicola F., R. Leahy, N. Johnson Restrepo, Nicolas Velasquez, Ming Zheng, P. Manrique, P. Devkota, and Stefan Wuchty. 2019. "Hidden Resilience and Adaptive Dynamics of the Global Online Hate Ecology." *Nature* 573 (7773): 261–265.

Johnson, Skyler B., Matthew Parsons, Tanya Dorff, Meena S. Moran, John H. Ward, Stacey A. Cohen, Wallace Akerley, Jessica Bauman, Joleen Hubbard, and Daniel E. Spratt. 2021. "Cancer Misinformation and Harmful Information on Facebook and Other Social Media: A Brief Report." *JNCI: Journal of the National Cancer Institute*. https://pubmed.ncbi.nlm.nih.gov/34291289/.

Kearney, Matthew D., Preethi Selvan, Michael K. Hauer, Amy E. Leader, and Philip M. Massey. 2019. "Characterizing HPV Vaccine Sentiments and Content on Instagram." *Health Education & Behavior* 46 (2_suppl): 37S–48S.

Kouzy, Ramez, Joseph Abi Jaoude, Afif Kraitem, Molly B. El Alam, Basil Karam, Elio Adib, Jabra Zarka, Cindy Traboulsi, Elie W. Akl, and Khalil Baddour. 2020. "Coronavirus Goes Viral: Quantifying the COVID-19 Misinformation Epidemic on Twitter." *Cureus* 12 (3).

Landrum, Asheley R., and Alex Olshansky. 2019. "The Role of Conspiracy Mentality in Denial of Science and Susceptibility to Viral Deception about Science." *Politics and the Life Sciences* 38 (2): 193–209.

Leding, Juliana K., and Lilyeth Antonio. 2019. "Need for Cognition and Discrepancy Detection in the Misinformation Effect." *Journal of Cognitive Psychology* 31 (4): 409–415.

Lewandowsky, Stephan, and Sander Van Der Linden. 2021. "Countering Misinformation and Fake News through Inoculation and Prebunking." *European Review of Social Psychology* 32(2): 348–384. doi: 10.1080/10463283.2021.1876983.

Lewandowsky, Stephan, Ullrich K. H. Ecker, Colleen M. Seifert, Norbert Schwarz, and John Cook. 2012. "Misinformation and Its Correction: Continued Influence and Successful Debiasing." *Psychological Science in the Public Interest* 13 (3): 106–131.

Loeb, Stacy, Jacob Taylor, James F. Borin, Rada Mihalcea, Veronica Perez-Rosas, Nataliya Byrne, Austin L. Chiang, and Aisha Langford. 2020. "Fake News: Spread of Misinformation about Urological Conditions on Social Media." *European Urology Focus* 6 (3): 437–439.

Madraki, Golshan, Isabella Grasso, Jacqueline M. Otala, Yu Liu, and Jeanna Matthews. 2021. "Characterizing and Comparing COVID-19 Misinformation across Languages, Countries and Platforms." Companion Proceedings of the Web Conference 2021. Ljubljana, Slovenia.

Martel, Cameron, Gordon Pennycook, and David G. Rand. 2020. "Reliance on Emotion Promotes Belief in Fake news." *Cognitive Research: Principles and Implications* 5 (1): 1–20.

Masri, Shahir, Jianfeng Jia, Chen Li, Guofa Zhou, Ming-Chieh Lee, Guiyun Yan, and Jun Wu. 2019. "Use of Twitter Data to Improve Zika Virus Surveillance in the United States During the 2016 Epidemic." *BMC Public Health* 19 (1): 1–14.

Memon, Shahan Ali, and Kathleen M. Carley. 2020. "Characterizing COVID-19 Misinformation Communities Using a Novel Twitter Dataset." Preprint, *arXiv*. https://arxiv.org/abs/2008.00791

Mills, Melinda C., and Jonas Sivelä. 2021. "Should Spreading Anti-Vaccine Misinformation Be Criminalised?" *BMJ* 372.

Mitchell, A., M. Jurkowitz, J. B. Oliphant, and E. Shearer. 2020. "Americans Who Mainly Get Their News on Social Media Are Less Engaged, Less Knowledgeable." *Pew Research Center: Journalism & Media.* https://www.pewresearch.org/journalism/2020/07/30/americans-who-mainly-get-their-news-on-social-media-are-less-engaged-less-knowledgeable/.

Moorhead, S. Anne, Diane E. Hazlett, Laura Harrison, Jennifer K. Carroll, Anthea Irwin, and Ciska Hoving. 2013. "A New Dimension of Health Care: Systematic Review of the Uses, Benefits, and Limitations of Social Media For Health Communication." *Journal of Medical Internet Research* 15 (4): e85.

Nan, Xiaoli, Yuan Wang, and Kathryn Thier. 2020. "Health Misinformation." In *The Routledge Handbook of Health Communication*, edited by Teresa Thompson and Nancy Harrington. New York: Routledge, pp. 318–332.

Office of the Surgeon General. 2021. *Confronting Health Misinformation: The U.S. Surgeon General's Advisory on Building a Healthy Information Environment.* Washington DC: US Department of Health and Human Services. https://www.hhs.gov/sites/default/files/surgeon-general-misinformation-advisory.pdf.

Paige, Samantha R., Michael Stellefson, Beth H. Chaney, and Julia M. Alber. 2015. "Pinterest as a Resource for Health Information on Chronic Obstructive Pulmonary Disease (COPD): A Social Media Content Analysis." *American Journal of Health Education* 46 (4): 241–251.

Pew Research Center. 2021. "Social Media Fact Sheet." Accessed February 7, 2022. https://www.pewresearch.org/internet/fact-sheet/social-media/.

Pfau, Michael, Steve Van Bockern, and Jong Geun Kang. 1992. "Use of Inoculation to Promote Resistance to Smoking Initiation Among Adolescents." *Communications Monographs* 59 (3): 213–230.

Roozenbeek, Jon, Claudia R. Schneider, Sarah Dryhurst, John Kerr, Alexandra L.J. Freeman, Gabriel Recchia, Anne Marthe Van Der Bles, and Sander Van Der Linden. 2020. "Susceptibility to Misinformation about COVID-19 around the World." *Royal Society Open Science* 7 (10): 201199.

Roozenbeek, Jon, and Sander van der Linden. 2019. "Fake News Game Confers Psychological Resistance Against Online Misinformation." *Palgrave Communications* 5 (1): 1–10.

Russmann, Uta, and Jakob Svensson. 2017. "Introduction to Visual Communication in the Age of Social Media: Conceptual, Theoretical and Methodological Challenges." *Media and Communication* 5 (4): 1–5.

Salvi, Carola, Paola Iannello, Mason McClay, Sabrina Rago, Joseph E. Dunsmoor, and Alessandro Antonietti. 2021. "Going Viral: How Fear, Socio-Cognitive Polarization and Problem-Solving Influence Fake News Detection and Proliferation during COVID-19 Pandemic." *Frontiers in Communication* 5: 127.

Scherer, Laura D., and Gordon Pennycook. 2020. "Who Is Susceptible to Online Health Misinformation?" *American Journal of Public Health* 110(Suppl 3): S276–S277.

Scherer, Laura D., Jon McPhetres, Gordon Pennycook, Allison Kempe, Larry A. Allen, Christopher E. Knoepke, Channing E. Tate, and Daniel D. Matlock. 2021. "Who Is Susceptible to Online Health Misinformation? A Test of Four Psychosocial Hypotheses." *Health Psychology* 40 (4): 274–284.

Shao, Chengcheng, Giovanni Luca Ciampaglia, Onur Varol, Kai-Cheng Yang, Alessandro Flammini, and Filippo Menczer. 2018. "The Spread of Low-Credibility Content by Social Bots." *Nature Communications* 9 (1): 1–9.

Sharma, Megha, Kapil Yadav, Nitika Yadav, and Keith C. Ferdinand. 2017. "Zika Virus Pandemic—Analysis of Facebook as a Social Media Health Information Platform." *American Journal of Infection Control* 45 (3): 301–302.

Shearer, Elisa, and Amy Mitchell. 2021. News Use Across Social Media Platforms in 2020. Pew Research Center. Accessed February 7, 2022. https://www.journalism.org/wp-content/uploads/sites/8/2021/01/PJ_2021.01.12_News-and-Social-Media_FINAL.pdf.

Sindermann, Cornelia, Andrew Cooper, and Christian Montag. 2020. "A Short Review on Susceptibility to Falling for Fake Political News." *Current Opinion in Psychology* 36: 44–48.

Singh, Vivek K., Isha Ghosh, and Darshan Sonagara. 2021. "Detecting Fake News Stories via Multimodal Analysis." *Journal of the Association for Information Science and Technology* 72 (1): 3–17.

Southwick, Lauren, Sharath C. Guntuku, Elissa V. Klinger, Emily Seltzer, Haley J. McCalpin, and Raina M. Merchant. 2021. "Characterizing COVID-19 Content Posted to TikTok: Public Sentiment and Response During the First Phase of the COVID-19 Pandemic." *Journal of Adolescent Health* 69 (2): 234–241.

Suarez-Lledo, Victor, and Javier Alvarez-Galvez. 2021. "Prevalence of Health Misinformation on Social Media: Systematic Review." *Journal of Medical Internet Research* 23 (1): e17187.

Swire-Thompson, Briony, and David Lazer. 2019. "Public Health and Online Misinformation: Challenges and Recommendations." *Annual Review of Public Health* 41: 433–451.

Uscinski, Joseph E., Adam M. Enders, Casey Klofstad, Michelle Seelig, John Funchion, Caleb Everett, Stefan Wuchty, Kamal Premaratne, and Manohar Murthi. 2020. "Why Do People Believe COVID-19 Conspiracy Theories?" *Harvard Kennedy School Misinformation Review* 1 (3).

Velasquez, Nicolas, Rhys Leahy, N. Johnson Restrepo, Yonatan Lupu, Richard Sear, Nicholas Gabriel, O. K. Jha, Beth Goldberg, and N. F. Johnson. 2021. "Online Hate Network Spreads Malicious COVID-19 Content Outside the Control of Individual Social Media Platforms." *Scientific Reports* 11 (1): 1–8.

Vosoughi, Soroush, Deb Roy, and Sinan Aral. 2018. "The Spread of True and False News Online." *Science* 359 (6380): 1146–1151.

Vraga, Emily K., and Leticia Bode. 2017. "Using Expert Sources to Correct Health Misinformation in Social Media." *Science Communication* 39 (5): 621–645.

Vraga, Emily K., and Leticia Bode. 2020. "Correction as a Solution for Health Misinformation on Social Media." *American Journal of Public Health* 110 (S3): S278–S280.

Vraga, Emily K., Sojung Claire Kim, John Cook, and Leticia Bode. 2020. "Testing the Effectiveness of Correction Placement and type on Instagram." *The International Journal of Press/Politics* 25 (4): 632–652.

Walter, Nathan, and Riva Tukachinsky. 2020. "A Meta-Analytic Examination of the Continued Influence of Misinformation in the Face of Correction: How Powerful Is It, Why Does It Happen, and How to Stop It?" *Communication Research* 47 (2): 155–177.

Wang, Yuxi, Martin McKee, Aleksandra Torbica, and David Stuckler. 2019. "Systematic Literature Review on The Spread of Health-Related Misinformation on Social Media." *Social Science & Medicine* 240: 112552.

Wardle, Claire, and Eric Singerman. 2021. "Too Little, Too Late: Social Media Companies' Failure to Tackle Vaccine Misinformation Poses a Real Threat." *BMJ* 372.

Wilner, Tamar, and Avery Holton. 2020. "Breast Cancer Prevention and Treatment: Misinformation on Pinterest, 2018." *American Journal of Public Health* 110 (S3): S300–S304.

Wilson, Richard Ashby, and Molly K. Land. 2020. "Hate Speech on Social Media: Towards a Context-Specific Content Moderation Policy." *Connecticut Law Review* 52 (3): 1029–1076.

Yang, Y. Tony, David A. Broniatowski, and Dorit Rubinstein Reiss. 2019. "Government Role in Regulating Vaccine Misinformation on Social Media Platforms." *JAMA Pediatrics* 173 (11): 1011–1012.

Zhang, Xichen, and Ali A. Ghorbani. 2020. "An Overview of Online Fake News: Characterization, Detection, and Discussion." *Information Processing & Management* 57 (2): 102025.

4

Flies in the Ointment

Vaccine Hesitancy and Bad Medical Advice during the Russian COVID-19 Pandemic

Alexandra Arkhipova and Ian Brodie

—Don't get vaccinated!

—Why?

—They put Lucifer's gene inside it. Everybody who got the vaccine starts to hate God. Better stay home and drink more hot tea; this is a good prevention against COVID.

THIS IS A PARAPHRASE of a conversation accidentally overheard by one of the authors in a Moscow grocery store in September of 2021. The brief exchange intertwines two fragments of inaccurate information—an anti-vaccination belief with a religious content (*the vaccine contains Lucifer's gene*) and a piece of folk medicine common to many countries (*hot water or tea is a good protection*) extended toward COVID-19—alongside a sanctioned and official medical protocol (*stay at home*). Such fragments are easily transmitted from person to person, in informal situations, typically between people in some kind of relationship of goodwill. We see these fragments in different combinations in different performance contexts, from China to Canada, from the United States to Australia: they are conspicuous, stylized, and recurrent, comprising what folklorists refer to as motifs (Georges and Jones 1995, 24), similar to the motif in music or the decorative arts. Motifs thus constitute building blocks that can be used in new constructions. Because these particular motifs are in stark contradiction to the advice of both emerging medical and scientific consensus and public health policy that is (hopefully) rooted therein, they contribute to the ongoing "infodemic," the term coined by the World Health Organization (WHO) in February of 2020 referring to the "global epidemic of misinformation . . . [posing] a serious problem for public health" (Zaracostas 2020); we thus refer to these as "infodemic motifs." They appear alone or in combination, sometimes also amid motifs of sanctioned medical advice and frequently illustrated with purported real-world examples.

Almost two years into the COVID-19 pandemic, most of us are familiar with a host of spurious ideas about the disease, including its very existence, its origins, its severity, the risks of official treatments, the benefits of vernacular treatments, and many more. They can take many forms, in word and image, from a retelling of what a neighbor said about heavy metals in vaccines to a pseudo-scientific text, where incorrect medical information about COVID-19 is attributed to some kind of authoritative voice, often adjacent to prescribed advice derived from traditional folk medical practices. Individually each infodemic motif poses a potential risk by suggesting a counterproductive course of action; collectively they create powerful "networks of doubt" and compose a body of knowledge set in opposition to official information as if both were on equal footing. As such, they have been blamed for high levels of vaccine hesitancy and medical mistrust (Islam et al. 2021).

The standard narrative of progress would suggest that, as greater understanding is made available through the findings of the scientific community, previously held assumptions that cannot be reconciled with the new information are dropped, perhaps charitably allowed to continue if firmly and constantly reaffirmed as mere metaphor. By extension, to hold fast to those assumptions is to remove oneself from the table of serious matters, and the binaries of reason/superstition, science/magic, and progress/tradition serve to further dichotomize. In this thinking, as better medical information is discovered and made known to the public, more people should trust it and use it for their good. This positivistic idea can clearly no longer be assumed in the twenty-first century, as we encounter how people react ambiguously to new scientific data and do not believe or heed medical recommendations.

The question of why this is happening is often asked by medical professionals and politicians during the COVID-19 epidemic, but perhaps it is not doctors who are best equipped to answer. Social anthropologists and folklorists studying vernacular perceptions of risk have studied how and why people might accept, act upon, and share infodemic motifs. To explain these reasons, we need to find out exactly what people are saying about COVID-19—and especially those concerning treatment and vaccines—and then how people negotiate them. Only then can we ask why these infodemic motifs are spread.

Context, Methodology, and Data

This study was carried out on Russian material from 2020 through 2021, but one will find these observations applicable to other countries. There is remarkable consistency among infodemic motifs found internationally; yet, region by region, they are very much manifested in particular ways, along with local outliers that don't appear to have many further parallels on the level of motif yet, in their circulation, speak to comparable social concerns, fears, prejudices, and allegiances.

As elsewhere, the COVID-19 epidemic hit Russia in March 2020, and the concurrent infodemic was exacerbated by the peculiar context of information in the Putin era: the active measures of propaganda and fake news within an institutional media landscape where a proclaimed support of freedom of speech allows for any viewpoint to be given a platform, obscuring by cacophony the effort to discern what is valid (Fedchenko 2016) and heavy participation in unregulated social media. Russian officials tried to fight false information by actively censoring it and introducing criminal penalties by amending its "fake news laws" (Arkhipova and Peigin 2021).[1] More than 500 people were punished with severe fines for spreading infodemic motifs in the first year; even under such harsh circumstances, rumors continued unabated. Russia is thus a good test case to help understand the social function of infodemic motifs.

To address this problem, we compiled a corpus of infodemic motifs, drawn from their circulation in social networks and in oral communication. At first, we carried out a qualitative analysis of social media (the Social Media Listening method, developed by our colleague Daria Radchenko),[2] complemented by texts sent to us by volunteers, namely users of social networks and mailing lists (Telegram channels, Facebook pages, and so forth). From this initial collection exercise of over a thousand examples, we identified not only a number of different texts—ranging from short narratives to mere fragments of asserted fact—but most of them also in multiple versions, suggesting either transmission or polygenesis (multiple independent origins), both of which intimate some level of resonant value for the teller. We also noted many motifs that are common places of contagion narratives: Patient Zeros, ethnicities with purported natural immunity, deliberate infectors, and so forth (Goldstein 2004).

From these, we abstracted keywords in an effort to identify the elemental motif, from which we could construct search terms to feed into *Medialogia* (https://www.mlg.ru/), the Russian social media aggregator. The search terms were constructed in a manner broad enough to capture analogues while precise enough to focus on one particular motif: for example, "The vaccine contains heavy metals" became "[vaccine OR Sputnik-V OR Pfizer] +/3+ [contains OR includes OR has] +/3+ [heavy metals OR mercury OR aluminum]." The initial findings of computational folklorist Timothy Tangherlini and his colleagues at UCLA began to appear in preprint publications in the summer of 2020, doing similar work on COVID-19 rumors and conspiracy theories in the United States (Shahsavari et al. 2020; Tangherlini 2021). Our team was even more confident that we were on the right track, needing to refine our methodology only a little before running the numbers. The search was tuned in such a way as to get the maximum number of relevant—and the minimum number of irrelevant—texts.

This is also, most likely, the tip of the iceberg. For both ethical and technical reasons, data extraction occurred only from the open segments of platforms (public channels, groups, and accounts), but not private messages or protected groups and accounts. One can surmise the amount and types of infodemic motifs shared in these more interpersonal media, but for now we leave them uncounted. For motifs to have moved from the private to the public sphere, within the context of the fake news laws and the possibility of persecution, it means that their public discussion is important enough to warrant that risk. At the same time, their public discussion invited refutation and ridicule. Thus, belief narratives (*Bill Gates will kill us all!*) can be reformulated with disbelief narratives (*These stupid people really believe that Bill Gates would kill us all!*). Our method does not automatically distinguish belief/disbelief narratives, so we take the numbers to show the degree of public discussion rather than real attitudes.

The database anonymizes what is collected: it contains messages in text form and metadata about the posting time, the specific platform, key post metrics (the number of likes, comments, and reposts), as well as basic information about the account that posted it (gender, age, city), if its owner made this information public. As new motifs emerge, we continue to search, and the process will be ongoing.

Since collection began in January 2020, as of this writing we have identified more than 300 motifs based on over 10 million discrete reposts from Russian social media.[3] We have clustered them into seven main categories: infodemic motifs about vaccination (comprising 41 percent of the reposts); medicine and treatment (24 percent), including pseudo-medical advice; COVID-19's origin and spread (15 percent); governmental dysfunction (infrastructural shortages, medical malpractice, army, and police violence) (10 percent); governmental misinformation (*COVID-19 is not even real* or has been exaggerated as a disease; false statistics) (4 percent); disinfection and PPE (*masks are dangerous*) (4 percent); and quarantine and social distancing (2 percent). Clearly, the largest cluster of infodemic motifs concerns vaccination and treatment (65 percent of the total), and these are the fastest spreading (see figure 4.1). In terms of absolute numbers, the vaccination group comprises 126 distinct motifs, and together they were reposted 1.4 million times in 2021 alone; medicine and treatment include 52 motifs reposted over 472,000 times in the same period.

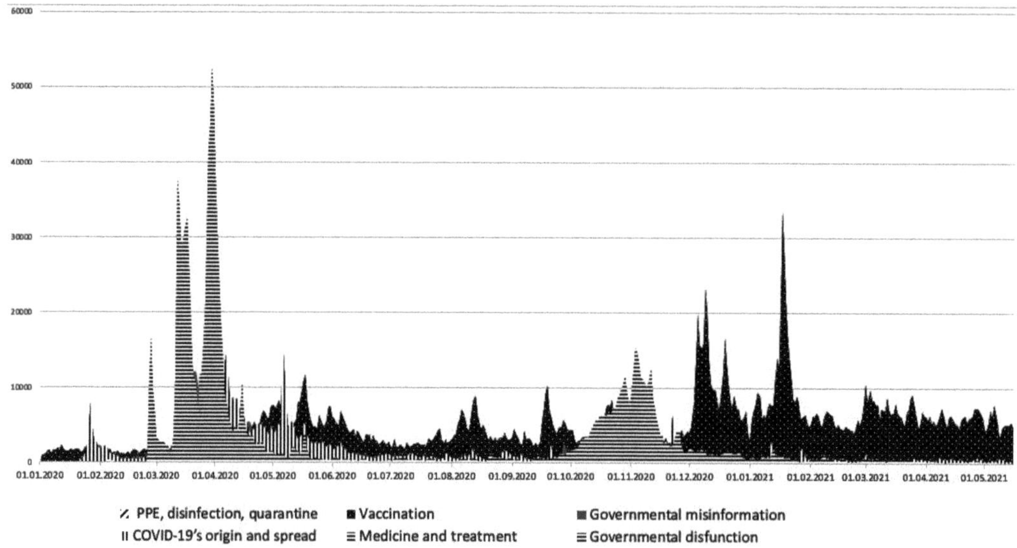

FIGURE 4.1
Dynamics of Thematic Groups of Infodemics in Social Networks from January 1, 2020, to May 16, 2021 (Absolute Figures).

A Question of When

Intuitively, one might have assumed that the "explosion" of rumors and other infodemic narratives would come at a time when first the epidemiological and then the socioeconomic situation in Russia had become truly dangerous: a large number of COVID-19 cases, the introduction of quarantines and their repercussions, hospitals working to the limit, an acute shortage of personal protective equipment for doctors and ordinary citizens, the deprivation of many Russians of work, not to mention the significant changes to the average citizen's daily routine. In other words, we expected a surge in the spread of rumors in April 2020 and the first ten days of May 2020, leading up to the peak of the new infections for the Russian pandemic, when, on May 10, 2020, 11,656 people fell ill in one day.

But infodemic motifs about the coronavirus did not begin their rapid spread at this moment. Instead, the growth of their popularity began back in February and March, when almost no cases of infection in Russia had yet been reported (see figure 4.2). However, at this time, disturbing news had begun to flow first from China and then from Europe. In Italy, the epidemic situation was growing more serious. This was all happening against the backdrop of official statements that Russia did not and most likely would not have a COVID-19 outbreak.

It is vital to remember the context in which these are shared and that infodemic motifs are the content of communicative acts. The study of contemporary (or "urban") legend provides insight. Legend scholars suggest that in the wake of change when unprecedented circumstances prove previously held expectations wanting and a new consensus has yet to emerge, particularly when official pronouncements are either absent or mistrusted, the void is filled with rumors and legends. They purport to be informed statements with implied or explicit suggestions for action, often rooted in a narrative of actual events. Demographic changes (like immigration), seismic historical events, and new diseases often reveal deeply held but buried convictions for how the world ought to be, challenged by the unprecedented.[4] Even in the semi-broadcast register of social media posts, legends are told mostly out of concern for the

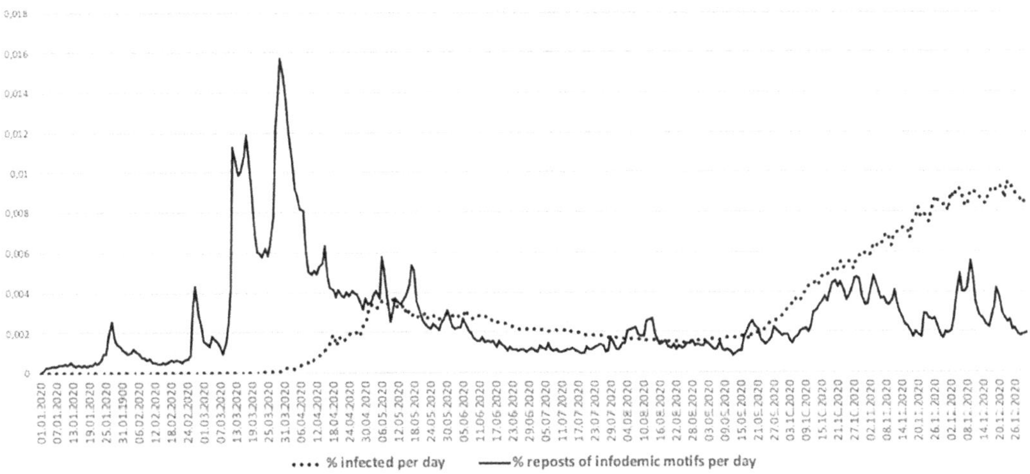

FIGURE 4.2
The Ratio of the Proportion of Infected (of the Total Amount in the Period from January 1, 2020, to May 16, 2021) and the Share of Reposts of Infodemic Narratives (of the Total Amount in the Same Period).

recipient and, indeed, invite the recipient not simply to accept but to negotiate and test their credibility. Over time they become either accepted or not, especially when the moment of the most pressing uncertainty has passed; more experiences and encounters are had; and, for those disposed to trust authorities, official pronouncements come forward.

Contemporary legends of contagion are prospective and proactive: they suggest what will (or might) come for the listener, based in part on what the teller had heard about what is (or was) happening elsewhere. February and March of 2020 were periods of maximum uncertainty: China and Europe—both having fraught histories with Russia—were affected, but, so far, Russia was spared. Should things shut down or stay open? Is the disease even really dangerous? All Russian cases were linked to travel from abroad, not locally transmitted. When community spread was first reported in late March 2020, and particularly when the self-isolation regime was introduced on March 30, the situation became much more definite and real, and the number of infodemic narratives sharply declined.

Psychology also provides insights into why it is times of uncertainty, and not necessarily danger, when rumors and legends are most actively spread. In an experiment, Jennifer Whitson and Adam Galinsky (2008) made participants feel a loss of control over events (e.g., by making them reflect on a childhood trauma). The participants would then demonstrate an increased propensity to find nonexistent patterns in a random set of data, as well as a willingness to retell theories about a powerful enemy who affects everyday life. Outside of the lab, Kelly Greenhill and Ben Oppenheim (2017) studied rumors in civil conflict zones in the Philippines and Thailand and discovered that rumors spread best in areas where strong political instability was recorded, and respondents' susceptibility to rumors is determined by the greater degree of the insolubility of the conflict. Thus, in the life cycle of an infodemic motif, it is as important to determine *when* it is as *what* it is (Ellis 1989).

A Question of What

Which infodemic motifs appeared at the beginning of the epidemic, at the moment of greatest uncertainty? Perhaps, one would have expected concern about the coronavirus' origins (*it was designed as a bioweapon*) or how it is spread (*you can get the virus from Chinese bananas*). These infodemic motifs are popular, but they are not *the most* popular. As happened elsewhere,[5] for Russia, pseudo-medical advice—incorrect medical information framed to suggest authoritativeness somehow withheld—came first (see figure 4.1). In autumn 2020, the second COVID-19 wave hit Russia, and the situation repeated: pseudo-medical motifs were again the first to appear. They provided remarkable certainty amid the ambiguity, explaining what coronavirus is (*just a flu* and *pneumonia*), describing what the symptoms are and are not and thus how to determine if you have it, and prescribing simple preventive measures and treatments (*garlic*, *fresh air*, and *hot water*). By offering "proven," "time-tested" treatments that can be done at home, they put people at ease.

The most popular pseudo-medical advice shared on Russian social media was first noted on February 23, 2020, concerning a young Russian doctor, Yura Klimov, and his advice for both self-diagnosis and treatment. Here is one of the shorter examples:

> Klimov Yura—a young doctor from the Russian Federation, working in a hospital in Shenzhen—was transferred to the study of the Wuhan pneumonia virus. He called my relatives and gave an explanation. If you have a runny nose and phlegm from a cold, you cannot be a carrier of coronavirus infection. Coronavirus pneumonia is a dry cough without a runny nose. This is the easiest way to determine what kind of infection you have. The Wuhan virus is not heat-resistant and dies at a temperature of 26-27 degrees. Therefore, drink more hot water. Be in the sun more often and longer. Hot water is not a cure, but it is healthy and effective against all viruses. (Collected from Facebook March 11, 2020; see Yablokov 2021)

The text contains internal claims to Klimov's authority: not only a doctor, but a Russian doctor with a direct connection to China and Chinese research, and thus the firsthand knowledge. A further chain of authority is established between Klimov and the ostensible narrator: "he called my relatives," which is akin to the "friend of a friend" chain commonplace in contemporary (or "urban") legends (Dale 1984, 12). Plausible sounding terminology (*coronavirus pneumonia*) and specific data that resonates with what is generally understood about some other viruses (*dies at a temperature of 26–27 degrees*) provide additional touchstones of credibility, as does the inversion of the last and first names at the very beginning, echoing the same practice in official communications. Between February and November of 2020, the post was shared over 700,000 times across social media; this is the most popular pseudo-medical motif in the database.

Where did it come from? Asking it in this manner almost suggests a solitary author composing a complete text de novo with, as might be implied, full knowledge that what it contains is false. Contemporary legend scholarship reminds us that a precedent for a narrative does not necessarily suggest a strict genetic relationship between versions. Motifs are part of a group's collective repertoire while also rarely being wholly unique to that group. They can cover topics such as who comprises authority, the nature of particular communities, conventionalized wisdom, and so on, and they can be the basis for jokelore, for invocation in both popular and elite cultural forms, and as the basis for practices of implicit or explicit bias. Apart, they comprise "in ectoplasmic form elements that go to make up the legend: what is lacking is the catalyst that will bind and shape them into narrative" (Buchan 1992, 96).

"Yura Klimov" supplanted an earlier Chinese text with advice from somebody's nephew from a Shenzhen hospital, which was also circulating on Russian social media. Indeed for one week both versions existed on the Russian internet simultaneously:

> My own nephew completed his master's degree and worked at a Shenzhen hospital. He was transferred to research the Wuhan virus. . . . He just asked me to tell everyone that if you catch a cold and have a runny nose, as well as a wet cough, it cannot be a new coronavirus, because coronavirus pneumonia is a dry cough without a runny nose. (Collected from Weibo, January 29, 2020)

> Hospital chief Zhenxing [a name shared by a doctor at the Emergency Department of Hong Kong's Queen Mary Hospital] reports that the current Wuhan virus is not heat-resistant, and dies in an environment with a temperature of 26-27 degrees. (Collected from Taiwanese communities on Facebook, February 1–10, 2020)

It is clear why the regime change took place: why should the Russians trust some Chinese nephew? The advice from a Shenzhen hospital was a direct Google translation of one circulating through social media channels in east Asia starting at the end of January, catalyzed by the stress of the emerging pandemic.[6] In this context, the advice to drink hot water is completely understandable, as it is common advice in Chinese traditional medicine. (It is also persistent; independent of the Dr. Klimov narrative, the advice to drink hot water was reposted over 169,000 times in the calendar year 2021.)

But Dr. Klimov was not the only circulating narrative that appears to have emerged from that same confluence. In the United States a similar legend cycle, citing east Asian expertise, also emerged. One such example:

> SERIOUS EXCELLENT ADVICE by Japanese doctors treating COVID-19 cases. Everyone should ensure your mouth & throat is moist, never DRY. Take a few sips of water every 15 mins at least. WHY? Even if the virus gets into your mouth . . . drinking water or other liquids will WASH them down through your oesophagus and into the stomach. Once there in tummy . . . your stomach ACID will kill all the virus. If you don't drink enough water more regularly . . . the virus can enter your windpipes and into the LUNGS. That's very dangerous. (Collected from Facebook, March 10, 2020; see AAP FactCheck 2020)

Arguably, the Japanese and, in other versions, Taiwanese experts—conspicuously, not Chinese, especially given the tenor of American sinophobia at this stage of the pandemic (Fordham 2020; Shafer 2020)—provide not only close-to-the-frontlines experience but also the perceived authority of "Eastern" medical practices that integrate traditional and institutional medicine, tapping into what Kimbery Lau refers to as the "popular orientalism" of alternative health and the critique of modernity (2000, 7–10). Eventually, however, the advice became attributed not to a frontline doctor close to the outbreak's point of origin and passed along through a chain of personal transmission, but instead with the apparent imprimatur of trusted American institutions, notably the motifically authoritative Stanford University, working within an international community of experts:

> Info from Stanford University:
> The new Coronavirus may not show sign of infection for many days. How can you know if you are infected? By the time you have fever and/or cough and go to the hospital, the lung is usually 50% fibrosis.

> Taiwan experts provide a simple self-check that we can do every morning: Take a deep breath and hold it for more than 10 seconds. If you do this successfully without coughing, without discomfort, stiffness or tightness, there is no fibrosis in the lungs; it basically indicates no infection. In critical times, please self-check every morning in an environment with clean air.

> Serious excellent advice by Japanese doctors treating COVID-19 cases: Everyone should ensure your mouth & throat are moist, never dry. Take a few sips of water every 15 minutes at least. Why? Even if the virus gets into your mouth, drinking water or other liquids will wash them down through your throat and into the stomach. Once there, your stomach acid will kill all the virus. If you don't drink enough water regularly, the virus can enter your windpipe and then the lungs. That's very dangerous. (Collected from Facebook March 10, 2020; see Weinberg 2020)

It is important to consider why what is essentially the same set of motifs became, on Russian social media, attributed to a young Russian doctor who revealed the real situation to his relatives, while in the United States it became advice from a well-known authoritative institution. Who is more trusted: personal contacts or official culture? Contemporaneous sociological data confirms this position: the majority of respondents to a survey conducted from March 27 to 29, 2020 (when our data shows pseudo-medical advice at its zenith) said that in the situation of epidemic one can rely only on oneself and collective responsibility, and not on the state (Stepantsov and Vileikis 2020). Most Russians would heed the private advice of an insider who either knows the situation better than state representatives or has no agenda.

The stressor of a new disease that was spreading unabated, despite the apparent efforts of official medical interventions, catalyzed the emergence of narratives born of the clustering of elements already present within the culture, slowly cohering into something of a consistent (yet still subject to variation) text that was communicated through informal channels and adapted when new contexts required new cultural referents.

A Question of Whence

Where did the mistrust of officialdom come from? Russia was the first country to develop a vaccine (Sputnik-V) and start the vaccination rollout. Despite this, polls conducted from May to August of 2021 indicated that 55–65 percent of respondents were choosing not to vaccinate (Levada 2021). Indeed, by the start of October 2021, only 35 percent of Russians were vaccinated (in contrast to the United States at 65 percent), despite how in Russia the daily death and infection rates were at the time at their highest since the beginning of the epidemic.

And it was predictable. In June of 2020, two comparative surveys on the readiness to vaccinate were conducted. The first (Lazarus et al. 2021) revealed that, of the twenty countries surveyed, Russians gave the highest proportion (41 percent) of negative responses to the question of their future readiness to vaccinate; in the second (Solís Arce et al. 2021), only 30.4 percent of Russians were ready to be vaccinated (among twelve countries).

Hesitancy is not only for new COVID-19 vaccines; in Russia, only 48 percent of the population believe that vaccines are safe, despite how almost 100 percent of the population is vaccinated against tuberculosis, diphtheria, and measles (Solís Arce et al. 2021). This skepticism is characteristic of the entire post-communist world in general. Several Central and Eastern European countries have experienced decreasing vaccine uptake and delayed vaccinations following the fall of the Soviet Union, and some of these countries experienced outbreaks of vaccine-preventable diseases, such as diphtheria and measles (Akmatov et al. 2008).

This is in part attributable to the official Soviet medical attitude and the legacy of resistance against it. In the years following the Second World War, there were several infectious disease outbreaks that caused a significant infant mortality (Filtzer 2010). Systematic vaccination was a way to defeat diseases and child mortality, and, starting in the 1960s, it was almost impossible to avoid. Children began receiving their vaccines as infants in the maternity ward, followed up later with shots administered in the state schools. It was difficult for parents to refuse vaccination; a doctor needed to be convinced that vaccination for this particular child was dangerous. Those with access and influence, such as families of the Soviet intelligentsia (including families of doctors), could quietly get exemptions. Refusal to vaccinate became a disguised privilege, and parents regained agency and the right to decide for their children within an otherwise harsh, uncompromising Soviet medical system.

This form of medical dissent was close to, and sometimes combined with, political dissent; stories about the dangers of vaccines were a way to rationalize not getting vaccinated. In our interviews with contributors to the first phase of our data collection, almost one in three former Soviet citizens told us about the fear of a possible allergic reaction to the vaccine, and the conviction "my child had allergies" was immediately coupled with "and Soviet vaccination policy did not take this into account." Pleading the child's special circumstances is a redress to the lack of individuation, let alone individual agency, in Soviet medicine. This was greatly facilitated, of course, by the success of the vaccination program: infectious childhood diseases became a rarity and parents ceased to see the benefits of vaccination. Why expose a child to the hazards of the polio vaccine when the probability of contracting the disease is so low?

In a different context, folklorist Andrea Kitta (2012) studied the attitudes of educated middle-class Canadians about vaccinations and vaccine skepticism, years before the concerns about vaccination for COVID-19. In anxious efforts of due diligence, parents (who are not already committed anti-vaccinators) try to assess the arguments both for and against vaccination, accumulating a large number of questions. When they turn to health care providers for further clarification, the very act of seeking verification is met with hostility. As a consequence, parents often begin to resist vaccines, half out of spite and half out of concern that there is an agenda.

Vaccine resistance as regime resistance continued after the fall of the Soviet Union and the relative increase in personal liberties that brought, prepared for the new freedoms in part through the established habit of carving out agency within the seemingly Soviet monolith. Ongoing justification came via the circulation of infodemic motifs about the dangers of the vaccine, comprising at first a "hidden transcript" of resistance, a means of pushing against the authoritative system without exposing oneself to the genuine risks of overt protest, until its subsequent public declaration (Scott 1990, 202ff).

In their study of people during disease outbreak situations, Julii Brainard and Paul Hunter (2019) noted how, regardless of the level of education, gender, and age, people react poorly to "disease avoidance actions recommended by public health authorities" (366), but at the same time willingly follow the pseudo-medical advice of their networks. In this same study, however, they described a mathematical model that mimics "infection" with "bad advice" in the same way that epidemics of infectious diseases spread. According to this model, if one carrier of information "infected" another with pseudo-medical advice, then the probability of following the correct medical advice fell. In general, the risk of contracting an infectious disease in such a situation increased by 40 percent for the population (Brainard and Hunter 368).

Given the historical precedent, Russia's low rates of vaccination and high rates of vaccine skepticism in the COVID-era are less surprising; a generation of people has grown up for whom vaccination is a dubious matter. The ill-conceived 2020–2021 vaccination campaign only made the situation worse. Unlike every other industrial country, the Russian government provided conspicuously little transparency about either the Sputnik-V clinical trials or the progress of the vaccination campaign. No official statistics indicating the numbers or percentages of infected and vaccinated people were made available until October of 2021. In their absence, ordinary citizens took the initiative to make vaccine information more transparent. As early as January 2020, an anonymous group created a website, Gogov.ru, with statistics aggregated from local authorities and sources; it still remains the main scientific source for these statistics (including for the *New York Times*; see Holder 2022). A combination of the Russian government's insistence on vaccine compliance, ineffectual explanation of the science behind the vaccine, and WHO's refusal to recognize Sputnik-V only served to worsen the situation and give infodemic motifs about vaccines even more resonance.

Our data bears this out. Infodemic motifs about COVID-19 vaccines appeared before a pandemic was even declared and had an initial surge in May of 2020, when the discussion was turning toward the need for and possibility of a vaccine as an alternative to a persistent self-isolation regime. In December, when the Sputnik-V vaccination program began, the biggest wave of anti-vaccination rumors appeared and have been the most persistent since (see figure 4.1). We have clustered the 126 distinct vaccine infodemic motifs into five subcategories: (a) the rationale for vaccination (conspiracies on who created vaccines and why, comprising twenty-one distinct motifs), (b) dangerous features and side effects of vaccines (thirty-three, including rumors of suspicious deaths), (c) the problems of vaccination in Russia (twenty, such as *Expired vaccines are sent to the non-metropolitan regions*), (d) the consequences for vaccinated/unvaccinated people (thirty-four, including advice on how to neutralize the vaccine), and (e) Western vaccines and geopolitics (seven, such as *Women who have sex with men who have received the Pfizer vaccines start to have malfunctioning reproductive systems*) (see figure 4.3). They were mostly analogous to ones found internationally (see Bodner et al. 2021; Uibu 2021); only C contains specifically Russian rumors. In 2021, vaccine infodemic motifs were reposted 1.4 million times.

In January and February of 2021, in what was effectively the first two months of vaccine rollout, there was a surge in subcategory B—dangerous features and side effects of vaccines: a certain person had died, or contracted a serious disease, or was rendered infertile. But the

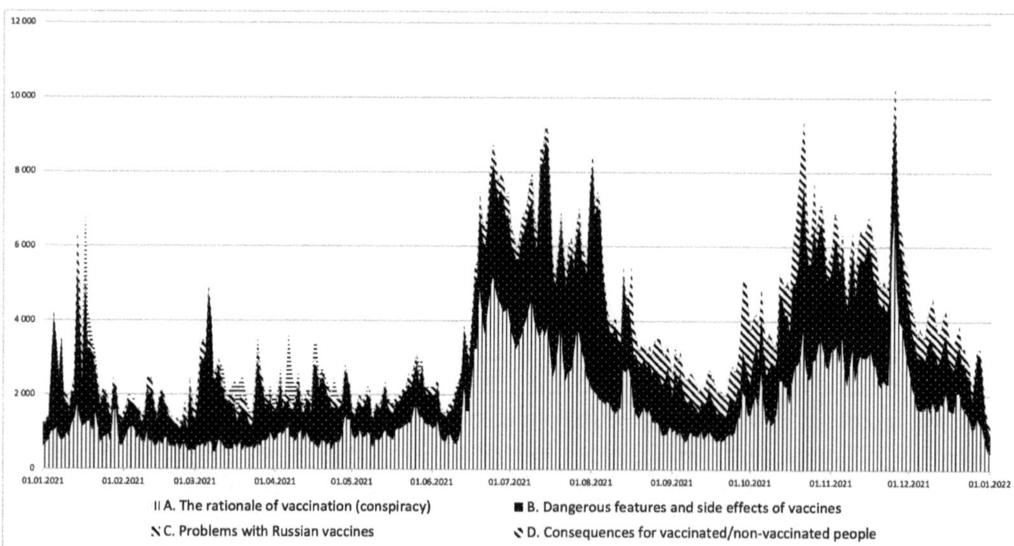

FIGURE 4.3
Dynamics of Vaccine Infodemic Motifs in Social Media from January 1, 2021, to January, 1 2022 (Absolute Figures).

number of those vaccinated at this point was surprisingly small; barely 3 percent of the adult population of Russia had been vaccinated by the end of February. This subcategory subsided for a while, beginning to surge again in late March when gift cards were announced as inducements for those who had yet to vaccinate. In late June, when authorities insisted that service workers were required to have at least one dose of the vaccine, the backlash was accompanied by the largest and most prolonged surge in side-effect motifs, sustained into early autumn with the dramatic rise of the delta variant. In October 2021, the Russian government proposed two new laws that would introduce a national system of QR codes to limit access to public transport and most public spaces (bars, restaurants, and theaters) to those who were vaccinated; after great public outcry, including street protests, the proposed laws were withdrawn.

Not surprisingly, this moment saw yet another surge in side-effect motifs, but they were also accompanied by ones about the consequences of a segregated society of the vaccinated and unvaccinated (category D). Furthermore, conspiratorial motifs about the real motivation behind the vaccine and its rollout (category A) brought the entire enterprise into question, with the most popular one being "vaccination is an experiment on people."

With some caution we can say the following: medical fears about vaccines were very common among Russians long before the pandemic and re-emerged when the COVID-19 vaccine was only an abstraction. When it became a reality, motifs of its deadly side effects were quick to circulate when only a fraction of the population had even received it. But the more the option to remain unvaccinated is made untenable by the state and the more polarized the population, the more conspiracies about the vaccine's actual rationale are in circulation.

A Question of Why

A prevailing opinion is that people who share, entertain, and heed infodemic information that is so easily disproven are somehow merely stupid; certainly, commentary and jokes by pro-vaccination people frame them as such. But while sociologist and evolutionary psychologist Pascal Boyer stresses the self-evident benefit of "epistemic vigilance"—regularly testing information and developing specialties, like the institution of science itself, to do so—he also notes the (perhaps ironic) evolutionary advantage of *not* always doing that (2018, 89). Coalitions, and by extension communities, are built on trust, and information taken as true and not held up to scrutiny (i.e., "taken on faith") is part of the coalition-building processes between teller and listener. Such is the case for information passed along that happens to be independently and verifiably true as much as it is for the false, and we base much of its validity on how we perceive the judgment of the person we heard it from (McNeill 2018). We *can* trace "practice social distancing," "wash your hands thoroughly," and "wear your mask in public" back to official sources, but that doesn't mean that we *do*. "By contrast," Boyer adds, "those who ask for evidence, or debate the plausibility of your claims, signal that any solidarity with you would be conditional, which is of course not what we want of coalitional allies" (2018, 87). Recalling Andrea Kitta and the Canadian parents seeking advice, their questioning of the science was effectively taken by doctors as conditional solidarity and were treated as such; in turn, any sense of allyship from the parent to the doctor and, by proxy, to medical expertise was similarly damaged (Kitta 2012).

Moreover, in times of uncertainty and within the perception of threat, we will often "turn down our epistemic vigilance mechanisms" (Boyer 2018, 81), not simply in the "better safe than sorry" approach to practices but, when uncertainty and threat undermine the sense of a community, coalitions are (re-)affirmed through taking the information on faith.[7] If we frame the willingness to accept infodemic motifs as occurring within the context of coalition building, consider the consequences to the community since the pandemic started. The quotidian opportunities for social interaction and phatic communication—passing moments of "How are you?" that are less about exchanging statuses and more about affirming mutual respect—have, for epidemiologically defensible reasons, been largely taken away: schools, offices, places of worship, third spaces, and the public square. A destruction of ties both strong (like with work colleagues) and weak (like with the coffee barista) causes social tension; we need people to whom we express support with a phatic conversation and who will do the same for us.

This does not provide an immediate answer to how to combat infodemic information, but it does suggest that the issue is not mere ignorance, so "more" information might not be the most productive redress. The sharing of infodemic motifs is inherently detrimental, and bad actors do exist. Nevertheless, it is useful to begin with a more holistic approach, that for the most part, those who share are doing so not in an effort to deceive but in an earnest effort at communicating what they take to be important information in times of urgency and that they do so when authoritative answers are absent or considered unsatisfactory or suspect. Giving serious consideration to the various motivations behind the infodemic is neither equivocating nor playing devil's advocate; rather, if we are trying to change minds, it is best to understand what those reasons are, not what we project them to be.

Acknowledgments

Thanks go to Sergey Shpilkin for his help with statistics; to Daria Radchenko for her Social Media Listening method; to Aglaya Starostina for assistance with Chinese language materials; to Ira Kozlova, Boris Peygin, and Maria Govrilovsa for help with the index; to Andrea Kitta, Willow Mullins, and Shelley Ingram for suggestions for vernacular health belief; and to Artem Yukhin and Asya Levadnaya for their hospitality during an earlier stage of this writing.

Notes

1. In March of 2019, Article 13.15 of the Code of Administrative Offenses, covering "abuse of freedom of the media," was amended with three additional parts—which in the vernacular became known as "the fake news laws"—to prosecute those responsible for the dissemination of fake news. On April 1, 2020, the Criminal Code of the Russian Federation was supplemented with a new Article (207.1) on the "public dissemination of knowingly false information about circumstances posing a threat to the life and safety of citizens."
2. Research methods are described in more detail in Arkhipova et al. 2020.
3. We limited our database to infodemic motifs, but the same method could be applied to discover how, which, and when constructive and sanctioned information was communicated through these same channels.
4. For a sampling of examples of legend and demographic changes, see Buchan 1992; for seismic historical events, see Goldstein 2009 and Turner 2022; and for new diseases, see Goldstein 2004.
5. Matteo Cinelli and colleagues (2020), studying the distribution of English-language infodemic texts in February and March 2020, noticed that "protection advice" turned out to be the most popular on almost all platforms.
6. Thanks go to sinologist Dr. Aglaya Starostina for advice on this issue and for collecting and translating the original texts for our team.

7. Our research also notes how often questions were asked on search engines either about the veracity of an infodemic motif or, more intriguingly, what one should do since it is true, which suggests some ongoing efforts at vigilance.

References

AAP FactCheck. 2020. "COVID-19 Drinking Water Advice Dry on Evidence." Accessed January 23, 2022. https://www.aap.com.au/factcheck/covid-19-drinking-water-advice-dry-on-evidence.

Akmatov, Manas K., Mirjam Kretzschmar, Alexander Krämer, and Rafael T. Mikolajczyk. 2008. "Timeliness of Vaccination and Its Effects on Fraction of Vaccinated Population." *Vaccine* 26(31): 3805–3811. doi: 10.1016/j.vaccine.2008.05.031.

Arkhipova, Alexandra, and Boris S. Peigin. 2021. In Russian. "Ministry of Truth: How the Russian State Fights Fake News during the COVID-19 Pandemic." *Shagi/Steps* 7(4): 124–150. doi: 10.22394/2412-9410-2021-7-4-124-150.

Arkhipova, Alexandra S., Daria A. Radchenko, Irina V. Kozlova, Boris S. Peigin, Maria V. Gavrilova, and Nikit V. Petrov. 2020. In Russian. "Specifics of Infodemic in Russia: From WhatsApp to the Investigative Committee." *Monitoring of Public Opinion: Economic and Social Changes*, 6: 4–38. doi: 10.14515/monitoring.2020.6.1778.

Bodner, John, Wendy Welch, Ian Brodie, Anna Muldoon, Donald Leech, and Ashley Marshall. 2021. *COVID-19 Conspiracy Theories. QAnon, 5G, the New World Order and Other Viral Ideas.* Jefferson: McFarland & Company.

Boyer, Pascal. 2018. *Minds Make Societies: How Cognition Explains the World Humans Create.* New Haven, CT: Yale University Press.

Brainard, Julii, and Paul R. Hunter. 2019. "Misinformation Making a Disease Outbreak Worse: Outcomes Compared for Influenza, Monkeypox, and Norovirus." *Simulation: Transactions of the Society for Modeling and Simulation International* 96(4): 365–374. doi: 10.1177/0037549719885021.

Buchan, David. 1992. Folkloristic Methodology and a Modern Legend. In *Folklore Processed: in Honour of Lauri Honko on his 60th Birthday*, edited by Reimund Kvideland, 89–103. Helsinki: Suomalaisen Kirjallisuuden Seura.

Cinelli, Matteo, Walter Quattrociocchi, Alessandro Galeazzi, Carlo Michele Valensise, Emanuele Brugnoli, Ana Lucia Schmidt et al. 2020. "The COVID-19 Social Media Infodemic." *Scientific Reports* 10: 16598. doi: 10.1038/s41598-020-73510-5.

Dale, Rodney. 1984. *It's True . . . It Happened to a Friend.* London: Duckworth.

Ellis, Bill. 1989. "When Is a Legend? An Essay in Legend Morphology." In *The Questing Beast: Perspectives on Contemporary Legend IV*, edited by Gillian Bennett and Paul Smith, 31–53. Sheffield: Sheffield Academic Press.

Fedchenko, Yevhen. 2016. "Kremlin Propaganda: Soviet Active Measures by Other Means." *Sojateadlane (Estonian Journal of Military Studies)* 2: 141–170. http://ekmair.ukma.edu.ua/handle/123456789/11622.

Filtzer, Donald. 2010. *The Hazards of Urban Life in Late Stalinist Russia: Health, Hygiene, and Living Standards, 1943-1953.* New York: Cambridge University Press.

Fordham, Evie. 2020. "China 'Still Lying' About Coronavirus Outbreak: Sen. Tom Cotton." *Fox Business*, February 24, 2020. https://www.foxbusiness.com/politics/coronavirus-covid-outbreaktom-cotton.

Georges, Robert A., and Michael Owen Jones. 1995. *Folkloristics: An Introduction.* Bloomington and Indianapolis: Indiana University Press.

Goldstein, Diane E. 2004. *Once Upon a Virus: AIDS Legends and Vernacular Risk Perception.* Logan: Utah State University Press.

Goldstein, Diane E. 2009. "9/11 . . . And After: Folklore in Times of Terror." *Western Folklore* 68(2/3). https://www.jstor.org/stable/i40026241.

Greenhill, Kelly M., and Ben Oppenheim. 2017. "Rumor Has It: The Adoption of Unverified Information in Conflict Zones." *International Studies Quarterly* 61(3): 660–676. doi: 10.1093/isq/sqx015.

Holder, Josh. 2021. "Tracking Coronavirus Vaccinations Around the World." *New York Times* January 29, 2021. Last modified February 1, 2022. https://www.nytimes.com/interactive/2021/world/covid-vaccinations-tracker.html.

Islam, Md Saiful, Abu-Hena Mostofa Kamal, Alamgir Kabir, Dorothy L. Southern, Sazzad Hossain Khan, S. M. Murshid Hasan, Tonmoy Sarkar et al. 2021. "COVID-19 Vaccine Rumors and Conspiracy Theories: The Need for Cognitive Inoculation Against Misinformation to Improve Vaccine Adherence." *PLOS ONE* 16(5): e0251605. doi: 10.1371/journal.pone.0251605.

Kitta, Andrea. 2012. *Vaccination and Public Concern in History: Rumor, Legend and Risk Perception.* New York: Routledge.

Lau, Kimberly J. 2000. *New Age Capitalism: Making Money East of Eden.* Philadelphia: University of Pennsylvania Press.

Lazarus Jeffrey V., Scott C. Ratzan, Adam Palayew, Lawrence O. Gostin, Heidi J. Larson, Kenneth Rabin, Spencer Kimball et al. 2021. "A Global Survey of Potential Acceptance of a COVID-19 Vaccine." *Nature Medicine* 27: 225–228. doi: 10.1038/s41591-020-1124-9.

Levada. 2021. Коронавирус, вакцина и меры [Coronavirus, vaccine and measures]. Accessed January 25, 2022. https://www.levada.ru/2021/11/01/koronavirus-vaktsina-i-mery.

McNeill, Lynne S. 2018. "'My Friend Posted It and That's Good Enough for Me!': Source Perception in Online Information Sharing." *Journal of American Folklore* 131(522): 493–499. doi: 10.5406/jamerfolk.131.522.0493.

Scott, James C. 1990. *Domination and the Arts of Resistance: Hidden Transcripts.* New Haven: Yale University Press.

Shafer, Ronald G. 2020. "Spain Hated Being Linked to the Deadly 1918 Flu Pandemic. Trump's 'Chinese Virus' Label Echoes That." *Washington Post,* March 23, 2020. https://www.washingtonpost.com/history/2020/03/23/spanish-flu-chinese-virus-trump/.

Shahsavari, Shadi, Pavan Holur, Tianyi Wang, Timothy R. Tangherlini, and Vwani Roychowdhury. 2020. "Conspiracy in the Time of Corona: Automatic Detection of Emerging COVID-19 Conspiracy Theories in Social Media and the News." *Journal of Computational Social Science* 3(2): 279–317. doi: 10.1007/s42001-020-00086-5.

Solís Arce, Julio S., Shana S. Warren, Niccolò F. Meriggi, Alexandra Scacco, Nina McMurry, Maarten Voors, Georgiy Syunyaev et al. 2021. "COVID-19 Vaccine Acceptance and Hesitancy in Low- and Middle-Income Countries." *Nature Medicine* 27: 1385–1394. doi: 10.1038/s41591-021-01454-y.

Stepantsov, Vileikis, and Vileikis Alekdsandr. 2020. "Coronavirus and Society. How Russians React to the Epidemic." *Knife*, April 1, 2020. https://knife.media/corona-sociology-1/.

Tangherlini, Timothy. 2021. "Using Big Data in Folklore Scholarship." In *What Folklorists Do: Professional Possibilities in Folklore Studies*, edited by Timothy Lloyd, 16–20. Bloomington and Indianapolis: Indiana University Press.

Turner, Patricia A. 2022. *Trash Talk: Anti-Obama Lore and Race in the 21 Century.* Berkeley, CA: University of California Press.

Uibu, Marko. 2021. "'Doctors Just Don't Care about People!' How Medical Specialists Are Depicted in a Vaccine-Critical Estonian Facebook Group." *Folklore* (Estonia) 82: 215–238. doi:10.7592/FEJF2021.82.uibu.

Weinberg, Abigail. 2020. "There's a Facebook Coronavirus Post Going Viral Claiming to Be from Stanford. Don't Believe It." *Mother Jones*, March 12, 2020. https://www.motherjones.com/politics/2020/03/theres-a-facebook-coronavirus-post-going-viral-claiming-to-be-from-stanford-dont-believe-it/.

Whitson, Jennifer A., and Adam D. Galinsky. 2008. "Lacking Control Increases Illusory Pattern Perception." *Science* 322(5898): 115–117. doi: 10.1126/science.1159845.

Yablokov, Ilya. 2021. "How the Kremlin's Years of Conspiracy Spreading Are Biting Back." *The Moscow Times,* March 1, 2021. https://www.themoscowtimes.com/2021/03/01/how-the-kremlins-years-of-conspiracy-spreading-are-biting-back-a73111.

Zarocostas, John. 2020. "How to Fight an Infodemic." *The Lancet* 395(10225): 676. doi: 10.1016/S0140-6736(20)30461-X.

II

SUSCEPTIBILITY TO MISINFORMATION; LITERACIES AS SAFEGUARDS

5

Let the Reader and Viewer Beware

Quality Markers for Health Information

Catherine Arnott Smith

The Case of Wisconsin Health Literacy

THE NONPROFIT Wisconsin Health Literacy, one of the seventy community-based literacy programs in the state, offers a range of services, from customized communication workshops to full-day training sessions and three-day retreat, as well as holding "the Midwest's largest health literacy summit" conference every year (Wisconsin Health Literacy 2021). Since 2018, supported by funding from the Network of the National Library of Medicine, Wisconsin Health Literacy has facilitated sixty-two workshops and nine train-the-trainer sessions for librarians (Wisconsin Health Literacy, n.d.). All programs focused on digital health literacy: "Health Online: Finding Information You Can Trust." Wisconsin Health Literacy will soon implement a new train-the-trainer program targeting "COVID-19 information, misinformation and vaccination hesitancy in thirty-five communities statewide" (Wisconsin Literacy 2021).

Participants in these workshops are consumers deemed at highest risk for low health literacy, particularly "refugees, immigrants, indigenous peoples, LGBT communities and those with low literacy"—that is, low general literacy in the domains required for everyday life. These consumers are educated in the core elements of effective health information seeking online, while library staff attend train-the-trainer sessions on similar topics, such as "how to spot unreliable sources; determine the purpose of a webpage; and evaluating a site based on accuracy, authority, bias, currency, and coverage" (Wisconsin Health Literacy 2021).

Wisconsin Health Literacy instructors emphasize that searchers need to look for unbiased, evidence-based research, authored by providers writing from their own expertise. Critical questions are recommended for web-based information seekers:

- Who is providing the information?
- Why did they create the website?
- Do they want personal information? If so, what will they do with it?
- Who is paying for the website?
- Is the information up-to-date?

Session handouts point participants to these specific markers of credibility that can help answer the questions mentioned:

- "About Us" page
- Specific domains (.com, .gov, etc.)
- Dates
- Sponsors
- Credits (Wisconsin Health Literacy, n.d.)

Why are programs like Wisconsin Health Literacy necessary? How bad is the problem of online health misinformation? Medical informatics researchers have attempted to quantify the extent of the problem for as long as there has been public access to the internet. The first systematic review of health information quality online appeared in 2000; it revealed forty-one published studies, twenty-nine of them specific to websites (Eysenbach 2000). By 2013, the evaluation itself had become a booming research field. Investigators found 1,611 evaluation studies of online health information indexed in just one health sciences database; 69 percent of these focused on content quality "such as accuracy and currency of the information" (Tieman and Bradley 2013). Replicating this search on PubMed yielded 9,714 such studies in September 2021. These ongoing statistics attest to widespread and long-standing concern about the problem.

One systematic review of research focused specifically on health *mis*information, defined expansively as "all forms of false information related to health" (Wang et al. 2019, 2). These authors found 131 research studies published between 2012 and 2018, mostly about communicable diseases, particularly influenza and viruses. Unfortunately, research into online health information quality remains a growing industry.

The challenges posed by COVID-19 for health literacy are new ones, but the importance of evaluation skills in a health information environment has been recognized for at least a century. In fact, the evaluative benchmarks, standards, quality metrics, and skills currently taught by organizations like Wisconsin Health Literacy originated in a world of print. All the aforementioned evaluation criteria are derived from a National Library of Medicine web-based tutorial titled "Evaluating Internet Health Information" (National Library of Medicine 2020). Although Wisconsin Health Literacy has no librarians on staff, this tutorial both expresses and encodes librarian values articulated since at least the 1930s.

This chapter examines the evolution of health information criteria in an evolving context of misinformation. It begins with the early twentieth-century origins of health information evaluation and human mediators called "librarians." Librarians selected materials for the general public based on professional principles that transmitted long-standing quality markers. The web then accelerated the urgency of the problem as information began to be deployed in new media. The vast new volumes of health information and a growing audience required new strategies—from quality filters to human taggers to computer automation—but with the same goal as the old strategies: enabling health information seekers to find answers, then to assess and understand what they found.

Origins: Quality Health Information and Access by the Public

Researchers can have short memories. A common misconception expressed in the literature on health care is that public interest in health topics began with the World Wide Web—where it became "a source of anxiety almost since its first appearance" (Purcell, Wilson, and Delamothe 2002, 557). For example, Hanif et al. (2009) write that, prior to the internet, the physician was the conduit to health information as well as health: "outside of layman press articles, individual contact with a physician was the only way a patient was educated regarding medical information. This was followed by books like 'Family Doctor' and health programmes on various television channels" (234).

This perspective positions the physician as vitally necessary, not only for patient education in the clinic but also for consumer health information seeking outside the clinic. In fact, one important location of medical information has always been the public library (Smith 2015). In 1899, there were forty-five "medical departments" in public libraries (Wannarka 1968). Physicians were the primary assumed user demographic for these departments. But even in 1898, the general public, in the sense of "laypeople," was already being referred to as a secondary audience for these medical collections; they were clearly using the physicians' materials (Getchell 1898). The public library was by definition more open to consumers and patients, and open in a way that didn't require either physician intervention or physician interpretation. Instead, the reader's most important—yet invisible—relationship was with the librarian who had selected the material.

Depending on local institutional culture and policy, librarians might serve as guides but also as guardians at the medical department gates. The development of selection criteria for print materials allowed for both roles. What titles were deemed acceptable for the public to see in print collections, and what quality criteria were used to determine acceptability?

Books of Information

Evaluation criteria for medical information in public libraries first appeared in a very early textbook published by the American Library Association. *Book Selection* referred to medical books only very briefly but commented on them as a special kind of "books of information" (Drury 1930, 77). Helen Haines's classic text (1950) later explained why these books had to be assessed in different ways than books of fiction:

> [Evaluation of] books of information give weight to factual values of knowledge and accuracy, and to method of treatment. Tests for author's qualifications and physical features are of less importance in consideration of books that are inspirational and recreational—essays, plays, poetry, novels are judged by their own qualities, not by the author's scholarly attainments or specialized experience. (55)

Library "selection criteria" were originally developed not for library users but for the professionals who decide how best to meet the needs of these users now and in the future. However, selection decisions have a considerable impact beyond the user. In the world of print, the librarian selects not only for individuals but also for the communities and contexts in which these users live. As "books of information" increased in popularity, new policies became necessary to establish what books, on what topics, and by what authors would be collected. A panel on "questionable medical literature in the library" was convened in 1963 at the National Library of Medicine. A panelist from the Skokie, Illinois Public Library called out "faddist and quackery categories" as particularly problematic because they "may not only leave the reader with half-truths, but frequently give him misinformation" (Radmacher 1963, 464). Her examples included not only *Calories Don't Count* but books by popular nutritionist Adele Davis. Another panelist pointed to "pseudotechnical" books as "truly dangerous" (Connor 1963, 468).

A physician and lawyer similarly wrote of ethical dilemmas for public librarians if the author's motivation might be to "sell books . . . vitamin pills . . . or . . . diet preparations" (Charney 1982, 100). Librarians began partnering with health professionals to investigate the depth of the problem. In 1975, an expert panel composed of a lawyer, a pharmacology professor, a public librarian, and a hospital librarian assessed the Worcester, Massachusetts, public library's print-based health information with depressing results:

> [M]any of the titles were challenged and criticized by panelists as being deceptive, out-of-date, totally worthless or even harmful . . . this list is typical of library holdings and this in turn reflects a need for librarians to examine and evaluate their own collections. (Crocker 1978, 24–25)

In 1981, Syracuse, New York, librarians asked local physicians to perform a similar analysis. The doctors examined the print reference sources used to answer real patron questions collected at the Onondaga County Public Library. This team had happier results than the one at Worcester: 82 percent of the sources used to answer reference questions were found sufficiently accurate to answer the question. However, the physician judges deemed 14 percent of the sources to be "somewhat sketchy, slightly misleading" and 3 percent to be "very oversimplified, misleading, inaccurate" (Yellott and Barrier 1986, 117).

Selection Criteria for Print

The selection criteria initially articulated in 1930 and 1950 would remain not only stable but consistent for decades. An exemplar is the *Book Selection Policies for Baltimore's Enoch Pratt Free Library*, compiled in 1963 (Enoch Pratt Free Library 1963). Library staff listed these elements for selectors in medicine to consider:

- Author
- Physical characteristics/format
- Scope and subject
- Style/tone/purpose
- Publisher
- Sources
- Target audience

By the 1960s, an additional professional criterion had emerged for assessing medical books: readability, defined as the ease with which they could be read and understood by the general public (Radmacher 1963; Severns 1962). Compare the Enoch Pratt selection criteria with those from another classic text published in 1995:

- Format (printed/microform/electronic, physical makeup, illustrations)
- Scope (purpose, coverage, timeliness)
- Relation to similar works ("uniqueness")
- Authority ("authorship, publisher/sponsor, sources of information")
- Treatment ("accuracy, objectivity, style/audience") (Bopp and Smith 1995, 297)

Librarians recognized, even before the web happened, that these elements of evaluation were useful beyond the medium of print: "much of it is applicable to other reference forms, including machine-readable records" (Katz 1982, 21–22). McKiernan explicitly translated these quality criteria to the internet for his pioneering Cyberstacks, an internet-based virtual reference library developed just before the web, writing:

> In considering the general principles which would guide the selection of World Wide Web (WWW) and other internet resources for Cyberstacks, we decided to adopt the same philosophy and general criteria used by libraries in the selection of non-Internet Reference resources. (References Adult Services Division 1992, 3)

Cyberstacks' criteria were:

1. Authority of the source
2. Accuracy of information
3. Clarity of presentation
4. Uniqueness within the total collection
5. Recency or timeliness
6. Favorable reviews
7. Community needs

Note that the context in which an individual item of information is located was considered important and that *community* needs for the information, not just individual needs, had to be taken into account. As every librarian knows, understanding the user group, the community in which the individual information seeker sits, is almost as important as understanding the seeker's need for the information. Thus, the librarian as a selector has to think about more than one user at a time. These elements have proved long-lasting. The concept of an "intended audience" and health information's goodness of fit to that audience has been an important facet of quality since the 1960s, when it began to appear as a requisite for print collections. By 1996, one researcher of web content could say that "it would be as inappropriate to criticize an openly 'gossipy' and partisan pop star fan site for a lack of attribution or referencing, as it would be to complain that Surgerydoor does not include cartoons" (Trochim 1996, 100). By 2002, the fit to a "target user group" had become an established part of website assessment (Craan and Oleske 2002; Williams et al. 2002).

Health Misinformation Moves Online

Quality criteria for health information accessed via the new "reference form" called the World Wide Web were first articulated in 1997, in an article subtitled "*Caveant Lector et Viewor*: Let the Reader and Viewer Beware." This impactful piece from the AMA appeared in the *Journal of the American Medical Association:*

> [T]he basic issues involved in presenting information on the Internet have changed little since Gutenberg first pulled the lever on his printing press . . . there are standards by which to judge the quality of editorial content, to differentiate author from shill, editorial from advertising, education from promotion, evidence from opinion, science from hype. Those who follow these conventions develop a respected brand identity, establish a level of trust with their readers, and serve as a forum for the kind of informed, intelligent discourse that advances the scientific process and benefits the public health. (Silberg, Lundberg, and Musacchio 1997, 1244)

The authors outlined specific "core standards" by which the quality of health information on the internet could be maintained. These were authorship, attribution, disclosure (of financing and overall sponsorship), and currency.

The authors had perceived an important difference between web- and print-based medical information: the absence of an intermediary who could guarantee certain quality standards on the shelf, guide the information seeker in the use of the information, and interpret information for the user as necessary. This relates to another significant difference: Silberg et al. (1997) seem to have been thinking of *health care professionals* as intermediaries, guides, and interpreters; the librarians who wrote earlier about the problem and articulated guidelines for other librarians had clearly been thinking of librarians in this role. No matter who the intermediator, online, it was entirely possible for a user to either encounter the wrong information or believe they had discovered all the right information—in both cases, never knowing what they were missing—hence the potential for misinformation and the "Viewer Beware" of Silberg's subtitle.

A very early report in *Searcher* magazine (Piper 2000) defined misinformation simply as "wrong information" and presented a general taxonomy of misinformation found on contemporary websites. This taxonomy illustrates the range of content considered problematic:

- Malicious (sponsored by hate groups)
- Fictitious ("not true parodies")
- Questionable (blend of "paranoia and fantasy")
- Spoof ("light parody")
- Counterfeit (political, humorous, or instructional; purports to be a real website)
- Product (commercial)
- Subject-specific (medical, business)

The health domain was an "area in which misinformation can cause critical damage" (Piper 2000, 2). Piper's examples, all unfortunately relevant today, included sites promoting a "cure for cancer" (9), aspartame as a cause of multiple sclerosis and lupus, and AIDS denialism.

Fear of physical or psychological harm caused by misinformation became a common theme in the medical literature. "Snake oil" online was "medical misinformation, and by extension . . . medical products with unproven efficacy or unproven safety" (Culver et al. 1997, 469). Inaccuracy itself was described as actively harmful to patients. Biermann et al. (1999) reviewed 371 websites about Ewing's sarcoma and found "major errors" in 6 percent, for example, survival rates cited as 5 percent when the accurate answer was over 75 percent. "The devastating effect these postings would have on vulnerable patients is incalculable," commented Biermann (385). Patients might be victimized by "widespread practice of fraud" online (Risk and Dzwenowagis 2001, 2). The sheer *volume* of misinformation was cause for alarm because the problem affected the community, not just the individual: "a substantial proportion of clinical information on the Internet might be inaccurate, erroneous, misleading, or fraudulent, and thereby pose a threat to public health" (McLeod 1998, 1663)· Complementary and alternative medicine was frequently mentioned in all these contexts. One very typical warning piece of the 1990s focused on Quackwatch, the controversial website maintained by a psychiatrist and longtime consumer advocate and educator Stephen Barrett. On the list of Quackwatch's things to avoid are the sites that featured "secret cures, pseudomedical jargon" and "any product claimed to be effective against a wide range of unrelated diseases" (Kennedy 1997, 40).

Professional angst was inevitable as physicians recognized more and more that the web was the world's largest vanity press, with no accountability for content (Silberg et al. 1997).

By the early 2000s, concern over the effect of poor information on patients was widespread enough that physicians in the European MEDCERTAIN initiative developed the DAERI database to record adverse events caused by health misinformation (Eysenbach et al. 2000; Köhler and Eysenbach 2002). The database team defined internet "harm" expansively and paid physicians a small honorarium to report adverse events via an online form. The options available for reporting provide a taxonomy of potential harms to patients and/or physician fears of the same:

- Patient has been harmed (psychologically or physically) by misinformation on the internet
- Patient has misinterpreted information on the internet, leading to considerable harm
- Patient was seeing a physician too late because of internet research or internet diagnosis
- Patient misdiagnosed him/herself or received a wrong diagnosis on the internet
- Patient consulted his/her physician recurrently or needlessly due to internet searches ("cyberhypochondria")
- Patient ordered drugs or products, which have been harmful for his [*sic*] health
- Patient attempted or committed suicide due to the visit of websites or newsgroups containing suicide instructions
- Other (Database of Adverse Events Related to the Internet n.d.)

Proposed Solutions

Numerous strategies were presented during the first ten years of the web addressing the health information quality problem, along a spectrum from pure human to pure machine. Some writers saw a need for greater physician-patient communication (McLeod 1998); others, for communication between the health care professionals and the public they served (Baur and Deering 2001). Others argued it was most important to understand the patient—and public—in terms of their information behavior (Burkell 2004; Coiera 1998). One early piece obliquely identified librarians as the answer: "there are places where quality is a watchword and professionals play the sorcerer's apprentice" (Makulowich 1996, 93), but consumer educators saw it as a consumer education problem (Greenberg, D'Andrea, and Lorence 2004). One typology of solutions (Childs 2005) continues to be applicable today; the discussion below is organized accordingly.

Principles and Codes of Conduct

The Health on the Net (HON) Foundation in Geneva, Switzerland, was organized and then promulgated its Eight Principles in 1995 (Health on the Net Foundation 2005). Those eight ethical principles are as follows: a website is *Authoritative*; achieves *Complementarity* between physician and patient; respects *Privacy*; does *Attribution*; supports treatments, products, and services with *Justifiability*; observes *Transparency*; practices *Financial Disclosure*; and has an *Advertising Policy*. Sites adhering to these principles are awarded an HONCode seal by volunteer reviewers.

The AMA opinion piece by Silberg et al. (1997) also contained four recommendations for high-quality content: authorship, attribution, disclosure (of financing and overall sponsorship), and currency; these four have survived for decades as a set of quality principles for use in evaluating content.

Checklist/Scoring Instrument

The 2019 systematic review of health information quality studies by Daraz et al. (2019) identified 14 quality assessment tools used in 153 studies. The DISCERN instrument is one of the longest-lived of these tools. DISCERN was developed at Oxford University in 1996 by a multifaceted group of stakeholders as a partnership between the British Library and the UK National Health Service (Charnock et al. 1999). Unusual for the time, DISCERN was designed as much for patients as for their physicians. Users complete an online questionnaire of fifteen items about attributes, ranging from the clarity of presentation to risks and benefits of treatment. Importantly, DISCERN was designed specifically for textual information and continues to be applicable only to information about *treatments*.

Quality Label/Trustmark/Kitemark

These different terms all convey the idea of a seal of approval. By 1997, when the World Wide Web was only three years old, Silberg et al. (1997) and Kennedy (1997) were already referring to the HONCode certification in this way. But the HON Foundation is not the only independent group to attempt this. An early US competitor was Six Senses, a quality rating scheme from a team of health care professionals, marketing and communications in the US Six Senses was named for its six quality criteria: *aesthetics*, *content*, *innovation*, *interactivity*, *freshness*, and *character* ("personality") (FAQ 1999).

Electronically Readable Metadata

The MEDCERTAIN initiative described in detail in Eysenbach et al. (2000) was a European Union project with multiple ambitious goals, including the construction of "an organizational and technical infrastructure which allows individuals and organizations to evaluate information on other websites" (231) by producing evaluative metainformation that could be deployed as filters of search results. Project developers consciously rejected the quality label approach, arguing that since "such awards and logos can be included by webmasters themselves" they were "more suited for marketing purposes . . . than to provide reliable reassurance to consumers" (231).

Gateway/Quality Filter

A trusted web gateway contains only links to websites that have been vetted according to selection criteria. One of the longest-living examples is the National Library of Medicine's MedlinePlus, released on October 22, 1998, and explicitly targeting a consumer readership (Wood et al. 2000). New York Online Access to Health (NOAH) was another gateway produced by a multilibrary type organization in cooperation with voluntary health agencies. NOAH was notable for its bilingual (English/Spanish) content (Voge 1998). One commercial gateway was Medem, short for "medical empowerment," from the American Medical Association and sister physician groups. Launched in 1999, Medem's stated mission was "to combat fears that . . . patients are getting inaccurate and misleading information over the Internet" (Galewitz 1999, 1). Access was free to the public, made possible by advertising and fees paid by physicians. By 2007, Medem had moved on, becoming a physician-patient communication network.

Childs (2005) comments that all the solution types listed above will naturally overlap, since standards can be deployed in different ways in different tools. For example, the HONCode is simultaneously a code of conduct and a trustmark; DISCERN is essentially principles encoded in a checklist. MEDCERTAIN, however, was a third-party automated evaluator that generated useable metadata.

In addition to these strategies, researchers also proposed machine solutions to the health information quality problem. Aguillo (2000) proposed that medical sites could be classified by attributes such as information producer type ("academic and research" and "virtual communities") as well as topic ("diseases and conditions"). These attributes could then be factored into algorithmic determination of search engine results. Other metrical proxies for quality were the number of pages per site and links per page, proportion of self-citations ("inbreeding"), exposure on the web, diversity of disciplines reflected in citations, and "geographical bias" (244). And the evaluators were evaluated. Griffiths and Christensen (2005) found that Google ranking was as strong an indicator of evidence-based content as DISCERN's quality ratings. Machine solutions can also work with integrated, collaborating tools. Kinkead, Allam, and Krauthammer (2020) constructed a dataset of "high-volume medical topics" flagged by Google Trends and built machine learning models based on criteria from DISCERN.

Challenges

The original filters for bad information in print were human beings: first the editors, publishers, and reviewers (Piper 2000), then, post-publication, the librarians and other information intermediaries ensuring that factually problematic material never made it onto the shelf. Authorship, attribution of sources, disclosure of financial relationships, and currency were qualities used as benchmarks and proxies for the quality control exerted during all the stages of the production process. Evaluators of online health information have a different task. They are attempting to understand and describe post-published content that is, in a digital sense, instantly "on the shelf." This means that health information evaluation online has from the beginning presented unique challenges.

Who Evaluates?

Evaluation places strains on human resources. When Eysenbach and Diepgen (1998) proposed an author annotation system for medical webpages, they admitted at the same time that the medical community did not seem to want to help. Six Senses publicized their highly qualified editorial staff and argued that competitors without this inhouse expertise were not as well equipped. Quality took time: Six Senses admitted that, due to high volume, "not all sites may be reviewed" and advertised a forty-five to sixty day wait for ratings" (FAQ 1999). By 2000 Aguillo, in a review of strategies to attack the health information quality problem, stated that "the majority of suggested solutions would require a large amount of human effort" (2000, 141). Alternative medicine researcher Muret addressed this tight coupling of evaluation and expertise. Complaining that alternative medicine content was neglected by evaluation services, he proposed the creation of a virtual team of specialists in alternative practices—homeopaths, acupuncturists—"in order to establish quality criteria, screen, control, and grade" (Muret 2000).

What Gets Evaluated?

In health information evaluation research, content about Western, scientific medicine in the form of text on webpages has typically been the default object of study. However, the content *not* evaluated is worth inspecting. Purcell, Wilson, and Delamothe (2002) made a good case that the nature of this information made it very difficult to evaluate: context was important; the same quality standard could not possibly be applied to personal stories, advice exchanged in patient groups, and peer-reviewed literature. Williams et al. (2002) stressed that a single website had multiple functions besides information dissemination, including entertainment, education, and commerce. Even if a gold standard for quality existed, it would be impossible to use as a benchmark in every context. As research into the question advanced, the list of digital health content excluded from analysis by health information researchers grew longer, which resulted in a constricting definition of "information." For example, the National Quality Health website survey, part of the US Healthy People initiative, excluded *unmoderated* "online forums or groups, or other social media platforms" from analysis to inform their benchmark evaluation tool (Devine et al. 2016). Confining investigation to static text-based media—for example, health information on webpages—also incurs a risk; the evaluation instruments trained on this data will not develop beyond the boundaries of text and will be thus entrapped in the quality standards of the print world. This limits the generalizability of evaluation results:

> The reality is that the web is no longer a vast library of web pages accessed through discrete websites; it is a complex mix of information sources and formats, online interfaces, searching tools and brokers, and participation and management gateways. It is unknown whether similar approaches to evaluation can be used for other types and forms of online information dissemination and exchange. (Tieman and Bradley 2013, 323)

What Instruments Are Used in Evaluation?

The biggest problem for evaluators, apparent early in the web's evolution, was the popularity of evaluation as a research topic. Because so many people recognized evaluation as particularly important in their specialty, scores of instruments were continually being developed. Different clinical domains create different assessment instruments based on the priorities and patient populations of those domains. The health information explosion meant a concomitant explosion of instruments to measure that information. This was recognized early as inevitable because no one instrument—or evaluator—could fit every information need. Silberg et al. (1997) emphasized that they did not argue for "a single centralized review process, institution, or agency . . . the Internet is a decentralized, global medium" (1245), but the appeal of a single checklist, an instrument with which to streamline and structure an opinion, remains very powerful.

Checklists deploy principles; they operationalize quality markers. Researchers who investigate health information quality and propose solutions to the problems they find are very often health care professionals, which enforces and reifies whatever the dominant domain expert perspective is at the time (Childs 2005). This all guarantees that multiple assessment instruments will compete for attention in the same evaluation space.

One effect: while certain instruments (e.g., DISCERN) became popular in the literature, there never emerged a reliable gold standard, or even a consistent standard, with which to evaluate (Eysenbach et al. 2000; Gagliardi and Jadad 2002). Specific elements expressing "quality"—authorship, publisher, sources, and so on—were just as unstandardized—unclear in definition and widely variable in meaning (Risk and Dzenowagis 2001).

Or perhaps there were just too many gold standards to choose from. Two very significant studies from Canadian researchers Jadad and Gagliardi delineate the scope of the problem; in 1998, they identified forty-seven distinct rating instruments for health information, not one of which reported either interobserver reliability or construct validity. In 2002, they replicated the analysis; thirty-eight of the original forty-seven instruments had disappeared, succeeded by fifty-one entire new ones, none of which—again—reported on reliability or validity. Gagliardi and Jadad (2002) concluded plaintively that evaluation was ephemeral: "Is it desirable or necessary to assess the quality of health information on the Internet?" (571). This produced a vicious cycle; because it was very difficult to make comparisons between studies of health information quality (Childs 2005), no single gold standard was able to evolve.

The Rise of the Proxy

Standards, codes and their progeny, checklists, and instruments, all encode shared values about information. However, these tools cannot fulfill individual users' information needs in one critical domain that is central to understanding the misinformation problem online. That is the problem of *accuracy*. Evaluators may intend their seal of quality as a surrogate for accuracy, but accuracy is not in fact being assessed. As machine learning researchers Kinkead et al. (2020) express it:

> These guidelines describe a set of criteria an article must meet to be considered of high quality. It is worth noting that *quality* is distinct from *accuracy*. While these guidelines check for indicators of well written, unbiased and evidence-based articles, they do not attempt to verify the scientific accuracy of the information (a significantly more challenging problem). (2)

The DISCERN project makes the reason for the omission of the accuracy criterion clear both in its handbook (Charnock 1998) and on its website: "DISCERN cannot be used to assess the scientific quality or accuracy of the evidence on which a publication is based, as this would require checking against other sources" (7).

The developers of the HONCode, similarly, valorize evidence and especially the *provision* of evidence by a content creator, but the fact-based nature of that evidence is not *itself* assessed; see Principles 4 and 5 of the Code:

> 4. Attribution.
>
> Where appropriate, information contained on this site will be supported by clear references to source data and, where possible, have specific HTML links to that data . . .
>
> 5. Justifiability
>
> Any claims relating to the benefits/performance of a specific treatment, commercial product or service will be supported by appropriate, balanced evidence in the manner outlined above in Principle 4. (Health on the Net Foundation, n.d.)

No health information evaluation instrument currently available attempts to approach the idea of accuracy for the simple reason that accuracy cannot be established in a contextual vacuum. Instead, an accuracy benchmark is required against which web-based content can be measured. That benchmark itself requires scaffolding: it needs to have been constructed with knowledge contributed by appropriate experts (Fahy et al. 2014), and it must be timely, because the mercurial nature of health information guarantees that it may fall out of date rapidly.

For example, the first published evaluation of health information online focused on webpages about pediatric fever treatment. Impicciatore et al. (1997) noted that "there is no consensus in every aspect of the home management of feverish children" (1877) but nonetheless compared forty-one webpages to the guidelines for fever management in a pediatric textbook; they found only four pages in harmony with the textbook. Wyatt noted that the benchmark itself, representing a consensus opinion, might not have been accurate:

> These investigators compared the information available on each site with statements in a reputable textbook, but such statements often disagree with contemporary systematic reviews of the literature . . . to determine the accuracy of web material we need to compare it with the best evidence, which usually means a meta-analysis of the appropriate kind of evidence. (Wyatt 1997, 1880)

For all these reasons, Burkell (2004) concluded that "for most if not all health information, there exists no gold standard that can be used to determine whether the information is in some absolute sense correct" (502). Eysenbach (2001) argued that even considering a gold standard in the context of web-based information missed the point: "quality is not 'degree of excellence' in relation to some abstract concept, but is seen in relation to (and must be measured against) the needs and preferences of the users of the product or service" (18).

The Proxy Solution: Consumer as Evaluator

Between the difficulty of getting humans to spend the time on the task, the volume of information requiring evaluation, and the absence of a "gold standard" against which to measure in a context of multiple overlapping and competing standards, it is unsurprising that the use of quality proxies has emerged. Characteristics such as accuracy, completeness, and coverage are subjective and difficult to measure directly without the right experts or gold standards. The number of typographical errors on a page or the absence of contact information for a content creator is neither subjective nor difficult (Burkell 2004).

Perhaps the best evidence for the objectivity of proxy indicators is the fact that they can be inverted and remain effective. Consider HealthWyze.com. This is an alternative medicine website run by activists Thomas Corriher and his adopted daughter, conservative commentator ("The Crusader Gal") Sarah Corriher. The Corrihers, who write that they treated themselves for Lyme disease with colloidal silver, have interesting opinions about the HONCode:

> The HONCode certification is listed on mainstream, team-playing health sites from Mayoclinic to WebMD, and even Dr. Andrew Weil's, but it is noticeably absent from all legitimate alternative health sites. There are multiple reasons for this. Not only are the HONCode people only interested in FDA science (as evidenced by their love of pharma-blessed credentials), but most honest web sites actually want nothing to do with them. (Corriher 2010)

The HONCode is clearly serving as an objective marker of a particular brand of health information quality—even for those who are diametrically opposed to the principles of the Health on the Net Foundation.

A focus on proxies is also a focus on the information consumer. Some of the various strategies to solve the problem of health misinformation put the responsibility on content creators, others on publishers, and others on trusted third parties. But still other solutions reposition patients and consumers in the center by visioning them as quality assessors. This awards control to—or places a burden on—the consumer doing the information seeking. For example, Mayer has argued for an information retrieval system that permits users to interact with quality labels when they search and view resource annotations: consumers can express their opinion about both the content and labels and share opinions about what they have found with other members of their online communities (Mayer et al. 2011).

Two of the most prominent and the most long-lasting health information evaluation initiatives educate consumer information seekers on proxies: the HON Foundation and the DISCERN project from Oxford University. Consumers can choose to interpret the presence of the HONCode as a certificate of information quality. In addition, the HON Foundation has developed a consumer-facing tool to help consumers deploy health information quality standards: an HONCode browser extension, the HONCode Toolbar, limits search engine results to HON-certified trustworthy sites. The DISCERN approach is different and comparatively old-fashioned: a handbook including the instrument detailed explanations of each evaluation item.

Is a consumer-facing instrument helpful? As the example of HealthWyze illustrates, it seems to depend on the consumer. Some have argued that the usefulness of these tools will vary with the skill set and the knowledge base of the individual consumer; consumers might make assumptions about the quality criteria and the organizations awarding them. Those assumptions themselves would factor into consumer decision-making—interpretations and misinterpretations—about content on a website (Burkell 2004; Hanif et al. 2009). Adams and de Bont (2007) propose that consumers had to understand not just the HONCode but the entire HONCode certification process, for that certification to have any meaning, because casual use will not help the consumer with quality control: "the lay medical end user either will not notice such a seal at all, or will notice the seal but not understand what it means" (S14). The low health-literate consumer seeking health information online appears particularly at risk of poor interpretation: low health literacy has been found to be statistically negatively associated both with evaluation skills and trust in what the consumer finds when they search (Diviani et al. 2015).

Conclusion

As the brief historical review with which this chapter began makes clear, concerns about medical misinformation recur, reliably, at points in human history when medical content is being made widely available to an audience other than that for which it was written. Checklists and other quality-assessing tools represent attempts by specialists in different fields to solve the problem. By empowering consumers to understand proxies for *likely* accuracy—or at least credibility—health literacy trainers in and out of libraries hope to bridge the gap between consumer expertise and the expertise reflected in the content those consumers desire to access. This is the reason that librarians and patient educators, like the literacy specialists involved in Wisconsin Health Literacy, focus on training consumers to recognize proxy markers of quality online.

References

Adams, Samantha, and Antoinette De Bont. 2007. "More Than Just a Mouse Click: Research into Work Practices Behind the Assignment of Medical Trust Marks on the World Wide Web." *International Journal of Medical Informatics* 76: S14–S20.

Aguillo, Isidro. 2000. "A New Generation of Tools for Search, Recovery and Quality Evaluation of World Wide Web Medical Resources." *Online Information Review* 24, no. 2: 138–143.

Baur, Cynthia, and Mary Jo Deering. 2001. "Commentary to 'Review of Internet Health Information Quality Initiatives.'" *Journal of Medical Internet Research* 3, no. 4. http://dx.doi.org/10.2196/jmir.3.4.e29.

Biermann, J. Sybil, Gregory J. Golladay, Mary Lou V.H. Greenfield, and Laurence H. Baker. 1999. "Evaluation of Cancer Information on the Internet." *Cancer* 86, no. 3: 381–390.

Bopp, Richard E., and Linda C. Smith. 1995. *Reference and Information Services: An Introduction.* Second Edition. Santa Barbara, CA: Libraries Unlimited.

Burkell, Jacquelyn. 2004. "Health Information Seals of Approval: What Do They Signify?" *Information, Communication & Society* 7, no. 4: 491–509.

Charney, Norman. 1982. "Ethical and Legal Questions in Providing Health Information." In *Reference and Information Services: A New Reader,* edited by Bill Katz and Anne Clifford, 97–109. Metuchen, NJ: Scarecrow.

Charnock, Deborah, comp. 1998. *The DISCERN Handbook: Quality Criteria for Consumer Health Information on Treatment Choices.* Radcliffe Medical Press. http://www.discern.org.uk/discern.pdf.

Charnock, Deborah, Sasha Shepperd, Gill Needham, and Robert Gann. 1999. "DISCERN: An Instrument for Judging the Quality of Written Consumer Health Information on Treatment Choices." *Journal of Epidemiology and Community Health* 53, no. 2: 105–111.

Childs, Sue. 2005. "Judging the Quality of Internet-Based Health Information." *Performance Measurement and Metrics* 6, no. 2: 80–96.

Coiera, E. 1998. "Information Epidemics, Economics, and Immunity on the Internet. We Still Know so Little About the Effect of Information on Public Health." *BMJ* 317, no. 7171: 1469–1470. doi:10.1136/bmj.317.7171.1469.

Connor, John M. 1963. "Questionable Medical Literature and the Library: A Symposium: The Medical Society Library." *Bulletin of the Medical Library Association* 51, no. 4: 467–471.

Corriher, Sarah C. 2010. "Why You Should Avoid All HONCode Certified Websites." Accessed February 3, 2022. https://healthwyze.org/reports/403-why-you-should-avoid-all-honcode-certified-websites.

Craan, F., and D. M. Oleske. 2002. "Medical Information and the Internet: Do You Know What You Are Getting?" *Journal of Medical Systems* 26, no. 6: 511–518.

Crocker, Jane Lopes. 1978. "How Much Should We Tell? Some Implications of Medical-Legal Reference." In *Reference and Information Services: A Reader,* edited by Bill Katz and Andrea Tarr, 24–27. Metuchen, NJ: Scarecrow.

Culver, Jean Deason, Frederic Gerr, and Howard Frumkin. 1997. "Medical Information on the Internet: A Study of an Electronic Bulletin Board." *Journal of General Internal Medicine,* 12: 466–470.

Daraz, Lubna, Allison S. Morrow, Oscar J. Ponce, Bradley Beuschel, Magdaleen H. Farah, Abdulrahman Katabi, Mouaz Alsawas et al. 2019. "Can Patients Trust Online Health Information? A Meta-Narrative Systematic Review Addressing the Quality of Health Information on the Internet." *JGIM: Journal of General Internal Medicine* 34, no. 9: 1884–1891.

"Database of Adverse Events Related to the Internet." n.d. On Internet Archive. Accessed December 2, 2021. https://web.archive.org/web/20010814182237/http://www.medcertain.org/daeri/en/form.asp.

Devine, Theresa, Jordan Broderick, Linda M. Harris, Huijuan Wu, and Sandra Williams Hilfiker. 2016. "Making Quality Health Websites a National Public Health Priority: Toward Quality Standards." *Journal of Medical Internet Research* 18, no. 8: e211. doi: 10.2196/jmir.5999.

Diviani, Nicola, Bas van den Putte, Stefano Giani, and Julia Cm van Weert. 2015. "Low Health Literacy and Evaluation of Online Health Information: A Systematic Review of the Literature." *Journal of Medical Internet Research* 17, no. 5:e112. doi: 10.2196/jmir.4018.

Drury, Francis, and Keese Wynkoop. 1930. *Book Selection.* Chicago: American Library Association.

Enoch Pratt Free Library. "Book Selection Policies" (unpublished manuscript, 1963). https://babel.hathitrust.org/cgi/pt?id=umn.31951000954054d&view=1up&seq=3.

Eysenbach, G. 2001. *1st Progress Report MedCERTAIN Project. Vol 1: Quality of Health Information on the Web, version 1.8* [excerpt]. Heidelberg: University of Heidelberg.

Eysenbach, G. 2000. "A Framework for Evaluating e-health: Systematic Review of Studies Assessing the Quality of Health Information and Services for Patients on the Internet." *Journal of Medical Internet Research* 2, supplement 2: e9. doi: 10.2196/jmir.8.2.e9.

Eysenbach, G., and Thomas L. Diepgen. 1998. "Information on the Internet: Evaluation, Labelling, and Filtering of Information." *BMJ* 317, no. 7171: 1496–1500. doi: 10.1136/bmj.317.7171.1496.

Eysenbach, G., G. Yihune, K. Lampe, P. Cross, and D. Brickley. 2000. "MedCERTAIN: Quality Management, Certification and Rating of Health Information on the Net." *Proceedings of the American Medical Informatics Association Symposium* 230–234.

Fahy, Eamon, Rohan Hardikar, Adrian Fox, and Sean Mackay. 2014. "Quality of Patient Health Information on the Internet: Reviewing a Complex and Evolving Landscape." *Australasian Medical Journal* 7, no. 1: 24–28.

"FAQ." 1999. Sixsenses.com. On Internet Archive. Accessed December 2, 2021. http://web.archive.org/web/19991013020857/http://sixsenses.com:80/FAQ.html.

Gagliardi, Anna, and Alejandro R. Jadad. 2002. "Examination of Instruments Used to Rate Quality of Health Information on the Internet: Chronicle of a Voyage with an Unclear Destination." *BMJ* 3247, no. 337: 569–573.

Galewitz, Phil. 1999. "AMA Joins Health Information Internet Game." *The Associated Press,* October 28, 1999.

"Get your Web Site Reviewed for Free." 1996. *Healthcare PR & Marketing News*, April 4, 1996.

Getchell, A.C. 1898. "The Worcester District Medical Library." *Medical Libraries* 1, nos. 5–6: 33–40.

Greenberg, Liza, Guy D'Andrea, and Dan Lorence. 2004. "Setting the Public Agenda for Online Health Search: A White Paper and Action Agenda." *Journal of Medical Internet Research* 6, no. 2. doi: http://dx.doi.org/10.2196/jmir.6.2.e18.

Griffiths, Kathleen M., and Helen Christensen. 2005. "Website Quality Indicators for Consumers." *Journal of Medical Internet Research* 7, no. 5: e55. doi: 10.2196/jmir.7.5.e55.

Haines, Helen E. 1950. *Living with Books: The Art of Book Selection.* Second Edition. New York: Columbia University Press.

Hanif, Faisal, Janet C. Read, John A. Goodacre, Afzal Chaudhry, and Paul Gibbs. 2009. "The Role of Quality Tools in Assessing Reliability of the Internet for Health Information." *Informatics for Health & Social Care* 34, no. 4: 231–243.

Health on the Net Foundation. "About Health on the Net." Last modified 2005. https://www.hon.ch/en/about.html

Health on the Net Foundation. n.d. "Discover the 8 Principles of the HONCode in 35 Languages." Accessed December 2, 2021. https://www.hon.ch/cgi-bin/HONcode/principles.pl?English.

Impicciatore, Piero, Chiara Pandolfini, Nicola Casella, and Maurizio Bonati. 1997. "Reliability of Health Information for the Public on the World Wide Web: Systematic Survey of Advice on Managing Fever in Children at Home." *BMJ* 314, no. 7098: 1875–1879. doi: 10.1136/bmj.314.7098.1875.

Jadad, Alejandro R., and Anna Gagliardi. 1998. "Rating Health Information on the Internet: Navigating to Knowledge or to Babel?" *Journal of the American Medical Association* 279, no. 8: 611–614. doi: 10.1001/jama.279.8.611.

Katz, William A. 1982. *Introduction to Reference Work.* New York: McGraw-Hill.

Kennedy, Shirley Duglin. 1997. "Intelligent Decisions about Information: An Epidemic of Questionable Medical Information Infects Cyberspace." *Information Today* 14, no. 10: 40–41.

Kinkead, Laura, Ahmed Allam, and Michael Krauthammer. 2020. "AutoDiscern: Rating the Quality of Online Health Information with Hierarchical Encoder Attention-Based Neural Networks." *BMC Medical Informatics & Decision Making* 20, no. 1: 1–13.

Köhler, C., and G. Eysenbach. 2002. "DAERI–A Case Database for Adverse Events Related to the Internet." *Proceedings of the AMIA Symposium*: 1066.

Makulowich, John S. 1996. "Net Sitings: Quality Control on the Net." *Database* 19, no. 1: 93.

Mayer, Miguel A., Pythagoras Karampiperis, Antonis Kukurikos, Vangelis Karkaletsis, Kostas Stamatakis, Dagmar Villarroel, and Angela Leis. 2011. "Applying Semantic Web Technologies to Improve the Retrieval, Credibility and Use of Health-Related Web Resources." *Health Informatics Journal* 17, no. 2: 95–115.

McLeod, S.D. 1998. "The Quality of Medical Information on the Internet: A New Public Health Concern." *Archives of Ophthalmology* 116: 1663–1665.

Muret, Marc. 2000. "Alternative Medicine on the Internet." *Journal of Medical Internet Research* 2, supplement 2: e6. doi: 10.2196/jmir.2.suppl2.e6.

National Library of Medicine. 2020. "Evaluating Internet Health Information: A Tutorial from the National Library of Medicine." Accessed February 3, 2022. https://medlineplus.gov/webeval/webeval.html.

Piper, Paul S. 2000. "Better Read That Again: Web Hoaxes and Misinformation." *Searcher* 8, no. 8. pp. 40–49.

Purcell, Gretchen P., Petra Wilson, and Tony Delamothe. 2002. "The Quality of Health Information on the Internet." *BMJ* 324, no. 7337: 557–558. doi: 10.1136/bmj.324.7337.557.

Radmacher, Mary. 1963. "Questionable Medical Literature and the Library: A Symposium: The Public Library." *Bulletin of the Medical Library Association* 51, no. 4: 463–466.

References Adult Services Division, American Library Association. 1992. *Reference Collection Development: A Manual.* RASD Occasional Papers, No. 13. Chicago: American Library Association.

Risk, Ahmad, and Joan Dzenowagis. 2001. "Review of Internet Health Information Quality Initiatives." *Journal of Medical Internet Research* 3, no. 4, E28. doi: 10.2196/jmir.3.4.e28.

Severns, Hannah. 1962. *Reference Services in a Small Public Library.* Chicago: American Library Association.

Silberg, William M., George D. Lundberg, and Robert A. Musacchio. 1997. "Assessing, Controlling, and Assuring the Quality of Medical Information on the Internet: Caveant Lector et Viewor—Let the Reader and Viewer Beware." *Journal of the American Medical Association* 277, no. 15: 1244–1245.

Smith, Catherine Arnott. 2015. "Medical Information for the Consumer before the World Wide Web." In *Meeting Health Information Needs Outside of Healthcare: Opportunities and Challenges,* edited by Catherine Arnott Smith and Alla Keselman, 41–76. Cambridge, England: Chandos Publishing.

Tieman, Jennifer, and Sandra L. Bradley. 2013. "Systematic Review of the Types of Methods and Approaches used to Assess the Effectiveness of Healthcare Information Websites." *Australian Journal of Primary Health* 19, no. 4: 319–324. doi: 10.1071/PY13030.

Trochim, William. 1996. "Evaluating Websites." Paper presented at the Annual Conference of the American Evaluation Association, Atlanta, GA, November. http://www.billtrochim.net/research/research.htm.

Voge, S. 1998. "NOAH—New York Online Access to Health: Library Collaboration for Bilingual Consumer Health Information on the Internet." *Bulletin of the Medical Library Association* 86, no. 3: 326–334.

Wang, Yuxi, Martin McKee, Aleksandra Torbica, and David Stuckler. 2019. "Systematic Literature Review on the Spread of Health-related Misinformation on Social Media." *Social Science & Medicine* 240: 112552.

Wannarka, M. 1968. "Medical Collections in Public Libraries of the United States: A Brief Historical Study." *Bulletin of the Medical Library Association* 56, no. 1: 1–14.

Williams, P., D. Nicholas, P. Huntington, and F. McLean. 2002. "Surfing for Health: User Evaluation of a Health Information Website. Part One: Background and Literature Review." *Health Information and Libraries Journal* 19, no. 2: 98–108.

Wisconsin Health Literacy. 2021. "Health Literacy Services." Accessed February 3, 2022. https://wisconsinliteracy.org/health-literacy/services/.

Wisconsin Health Literacy. n.d. "Health Online Handout 1 with Checklist." Accessed February 3, 2022. https://wisconsinliteracy.org/health-literacy/programs/wisconsin-health-literacy-resources---community-projects.html.

Wisconsin Literacy. 2021. "Wisconsin Literacy Received a COVID-19 Community Outreach Grant from the Wisconsin Department of Health Services." Accessed February 3, 2022. https://wisconsinliteracy.org/about/our-news.html/article/2021/04/06/wisconsin-literacy-received-a-covid-19-community-outreach-grant-from-the-wisconsin-department-of-health-services.

Wood, Fred B., Becky Lyon, Mary Beth Schell, Paula Kitendaugh, Victor H. Cid, and Elliot R. Siegel. 2000. "Public Library Consumer Health Information Pilot Project: Results of a National Library of Medicine Evaluation." *Bulletin of the Medical Library Association* 88, no. 4: 314–322.

Wyatt, Jeremy C. 1997. "Commentary: Measuring Quality and Impact of the World Wide Web." *BMJ 314*, no. 7098: 1879–1881. doi: 10.1136/bmj.314.7098.1879.

Yellott, Lynn, and Robert Barrier. 1986. "Evaluation of a Public Library's Health Information Service." In *Reference and Information Services: A Reader for Today,* edited by Bill Katz, 111–123. Metuchen, NJ: Scarecrow.

Zhang, Yan, Yalin Sun, and Bo Xie. 2015. "Quality of Health Information for Consumers on the Web: A Systematic Review of Indicators, Criteria, Tools, and Evaluation Results." *Journal of the Association for Information Science & Technology* 66, no. 10: 2071–2084.

6

Preventing Health Number Confusion through Clear Communication Design

Brian J. Zikmund-Fisher and Jessica S. Ancker

It is axiomatic that we can lie with statistics (Huff 1954). However, even when we do our best to provide accurate and relevant numbers, the public often still takes away an inaccurate or incomplete understanding. In other words, the major problem with number communications tends to be less about deliberate misinformation and more about misunderstanding and misinterpretation, leading to mistrust and misuse (or nonuse altogether). To combat this problem, both communicators (experts, librarians, journalists) and audiences (including both the public and their representatives) need to become critical consumers of numbers, able to recognize what a number is and is not representing, and to seek out and use contextual information to determine not just what the number is but what it means for them.

The Three Main Types of Health Number Communications to the Public

While in theory, there are many types of communications from experts or the media to the public, in practice, these types of communication tend to fall into one of three categories, which we will describe as *counts*, *levels*, and *risks*.

Counts are the bread and butter of journalism and of public health. Any number that answers the question "How many?" generally falls in this category. For example, how many people have been affected by this disease, how many died in this event, and how many people live in this location? Note that count communications sometimes focus on negative outcomes (e.g., disease cases, deaths, people exposed, and jobs lost), but they are also commonly used to show positive outcomes such as the number of people vaccinated or graduating college or starting a new job.

Counts are usually communicated because they represent what is known and directly observed. Public safety officials might record three reported homicides and fifteen reported robberies. Public health officials might record 173 cases of a particular disease in the last week or month. Economists might report that the country recorded 500,000 new jobs last month.

Levels differ from counts in that they usually represent some form of scientific measurement, something that is often not intrinsically numerical until it is measured. One of the most common types of level communication in public and media contexts is environmental measurements (e.g., daily temperatures, monthly rainfall, air quality index levels, or global temperature levels as a measure of climate change). The public also interacts with many types of chemical levels, such as vitamin or nutrient levels provided in nutrition communications. People are also frequently presented with what we might term biomonitoring readings, which include measures from the human body (e.g., body weight, blood levels of biological compounds like cholesterol, blood glucose, or antibodies) and measures of things that are relevant to human health (e.g., levels of contaminants like lead, arsenic, or per- and polyfluoroalkyl substances [PFAS] found in our environment or our food).

Numerical *risks* differ from both counts and levels in that they describe the chance that something might happen. Sometimes risks are described qualitatively (e.g., people are "at risk" or have a "high risk" of getting sick). When risks are described in numbers, they tend to come in one of three major forms:

- *Absolute chances* (e.g., an analysis of cancer statistics might note that the average person has a 6 percent chance of developing a particular type of cancer at some point in their life).
- *Absolute differences in chances.* These can be presented either as side-by-side numbers (e.g., people with a particular genetic marker have a 9 percent chance of developing cancer, as compared to the 6 percent chance of the average person) or as absolute risk differences (e.g., three more people out of one hundred develop this type of cancer if they have the genetic marker versus if they do not). Note that absolute differences can be used to represent differences across populations or differences in risk in a single individual or population with or without another factor.
- *Relative risk reductions or increases.* When risks for an individual or single population are changed by the presence or absence of risk factors, the influence of preventive actions, or the effect of treatment, they can sometimes be communicated using relative risk reduction or increased statistics. Relative risk calculations create a ratio by dividing two absolute chances. Using the above example, having the genetic marker increases people's risk of getting this type of cancer by 50 percent ([9–6 percent]/6 percent = 50 percent relative risk increase).

A key challenge in understanding risks is that it is a population construct being applied to an individual. When a story says that one group reports data showing that more people in Group X developed a disease than did people in Group Y, it is simultaneously true that (a) the overall disease burden is higher in Group X than Group Y; (b) that the per capita disease rate in Group X might be higher, lower, or equal to the rate in Group Y, depending on the groups' relative size; and (c) that both groups contain people who will get sick and people who will not. Risk statistics communicate the chance of something happening, and, as a result, they are often used to motivate people to change something (e.g., their behavior, their environment, and their policy) to try to prevent the feared negative outcome for which they are at risk.

When Numbers Are Meaningful

Regardless of whether the number in question is a count, a level, or a risk, numerical communications provide value if three conditions are met:

1. Users must actually notice and attend to the numbers,
2. Users must accurately determine what the numbers represent, and

3. Users must understand how the numbers relate to things that they care about (i.e., what the numbers mean for them).

Still, number communications often fail to meet these criteria. Many people have poor number skills, and these people tend to avoid reading or thinking about numbers, violating condition 1. The use of confusing number formats can make it difficult for people to interpret numbers, violating condition 2. Finally, failures to contextualize numbers can often lead recipients to be confused about what numbers mean for them, even when they know exactly what the numbers are, violating condition 3. In the rest of this chapter, we discuss the specific number communication problems that most often lead to misunderstanding, misinterpretation, mistrust, and misuse of numerical data. We also provide a checklist for identifying high-quality number communications to enable both communicators and users to become critical consumers of the quality of the health data communications they interact with in the media, in health and science communications, and in everyday life.

Problem #1: Low Numeracy Skills

The first challenge is low numeracy, which is prevalent in almost all parts of society, even in industrialized countries such as the United States or Germany (Galesic and Garcia-Retamero 2010). Just as weak health literacy skills are a huge barrier to the public's comprehension and use of textual health and science information (Institute of Medicine and National Academies of Sciences, Engineering, and Medicine 2015), so too the limitations in people's quantitative skill sets inhibit their use of health and science numbers. Low numeracy has a huge impact on people's ability to recognize, think about, or apply the numbers that they face in daily life. While many others have reviewed the effects of low numeracy (Ancker and Kaufman 2007; Institute of Medicine 2014; Nelson et al. 2008; Peters et al. 2007; Peters 2012), here we highlight some of the specific challenges that people with low numeracy face when presented with health or science numbers in the news or social media or in their doctor's offices.

People with low numeracy are less likely to look for, attend to, apply, or recognize numerical data as relevant to a decision. They find it harder to identify relevant numbers out of larger sets of data (e.g., to find how many cases have occurred in their location or to identify the risk faced by people of their age and gender). They also find it harder to translate numbers between different formats (e.g., recognizing that 10 percent risk, a 1 in 10 chance, and 100,000 people per 1 million ratio all describe exactly the same information).

Practically, what this means is that when experts, product labels, news stories, or social media postings present numerical data, people with lower numeracy skills are less likely to see the number as providing useful information, less likely to comprehend its meaning accurately, and less likely to change their perceptions or decisions based on the numbers.

Solution #1: Universal Precautions Approaches to Number Communications

Although individuals with low numeracy are disproportionately likely to misinterpret numbers, in practice these individuals are difficult to identify. There are many numeracy screening tools available, but they are not routinely applied to either patients or members of the public. We cannot rely on what the user looks like or how well they are educated because even college-educated populations have substantial numbers of people with low numeracy (Lipkus, Samsa, and Rimer 2001). In addition, even the most highly numerate users can sometimes face difficulties with numbers. These facts mean that in practice, it is very difficult to stratify communication interventions and target some of them specifically at users with low numeracy.

Instead, we recommend a "universal precautions" approach to communication (DeWalt et al. 2010). Under this approach, the communicator assumes that *any* user may encounter difficulty in using numerical information. Ease of comprehension for all audiences is the goal.

Specifically, we encourage communicators to focus on the user's needs (Zikmund-Fisher 2013). The right question is this: what form and format of numbers will make it easiest for the intended recipient (regardless of their numeracy skills) to use those numbers to meet *their needs*? The critical insight is that "understanding" numbers is not one thing but many, and communicators may be using numbers to try to achieve many different outcomes (Ancker et al. 2022). Does someone need to remember their particular number (recall)? Do they need to recognize that they fall into a particular category (e.g., high risk or low risk)? Do they need a precise understanding of how much risk is increased by a particular characteristic or decreased by an intervention, or is it sufficient to know that risk is either increased or decreased by these factors?

By focusing on people's needs for numerical information, communicators can avoid two common errors in number communications that often lead to misunderstanding and misinformation. First, many number communications simply provide the available data, in whatever format it was originally created. That can be acceptable for communications between experts, who likely share common training, background knowledge, and needs for the data. However, it is often highly problematic when health numbers are provided to patients, the public, and/or policymakers, each of whom have different perspectives and needs. Second, focusing on user needs helps people recognize that (a) different people need different things and (b) even the same person may have different needs at different points in time or in different situations.

Problem #2: Numbers Can Be Difficult to Work With

Most people—even highly numerate people—find it somewhat effortful to interpret numbers. The more effortful it is, the more likely it is that people will misinterpret the number, make a (possibly erroneous) guess about what it means, or even give up and ignore it. Fortunately, the same number can be presented in different ways, and some ways are easier to use than others. That insight provides the solutions we discuss here.

Solution #2: Use Number Formats that Reduce Ambiguity and Minimize User Work

Effective number communications (i.e., those that minimize confusion and maximize usability) are those that minimize the degree that the message recipient or user has to do work to get the information they need and to know what the numbers represent.

To minimize audience's effort, health and science data communications should follow several key principles:

- *Provide units.* Units are essential for all levels of communication. For example, is a lead measured in parts per million (ppm) or parts per billion (ppb)? Both rate and risk communications have similar issues regarding clear denominators (e.g., cases per 100,000 people vs. per 1 million, percentage out of 100 vs. out of 1,000).

- *Be consistent with units and denominators.* Whatever units, denominators, or formats are used, the format must remain consistent. People derive meaning from numbers by making comparisons, and unit or denominator inconsistency guarantees confusion. In particular, for risk communications, both experimental evidence and expert guidance argue strongly against the use of 1-in-X formats, which change the denominator (i.e., the risk unit) rather than the numerator (Bonner et al. 2021; Sirota, Juanchich, and Bonnefon 2018; Zikmund-Fisher 2011).
- *Define the reference class.* The reference class of a statistic is the population from which the data derive. It always needs to be clear what group of people or locations are included or excluded. For example, the prevalence rate of diabetes in Michigan adults over age fifty is not the same as the rate of diabetes in the full US adult population.
- *Define the time interval.* What day, month, year, or interval is represented? This is particularly important for risk communications since many risks accumulate over time. For example, a 2 percent risk of developing breast cancer over five years is not the same as a 2 percent risk over fifteen years or over the woman's lifetime.
- *Use round numbers and avoid decimals when possible.* Round numbers are easier to remember and may be trusted more (Witteman et al. 2011). The right question is what level of precision is necessary for the user to accomplish their goals. In effect, communications should endeavor to embody the idea often attributed to Albert Einstein that everything should be made as simple as possible, but no simpler.
- *Present absolute differences, not relative risk reductions or increases.* Describing the change from 3 percent to 2 percent as a 50 percent relative risk reduction makes it look much bigger than describing it as changing the outcome for 1 in 100 people (Akl et al. 2011; Malenka et al. 1993). In addition to the absolute difference, the baseline risk should always be presented, although relative risk reduction is often perceived as more effective than absolute risk reduction even when the baseline risk information is explicitly reported (Marcatto, Rolison, and Ferrante 2013). If the change in risk is a 1 percent absolute increase (often described as one percentage point), then the reader should be told whether this is a 1 percent increase from a baseline of 2 percent or a 1 percent increase from a baseline of 95 percent. The psychological impact of the relative difference is why advertisements for health interventions tend to present benefits in relative terms (e.g., a 50 percent risk reduction) while presenting side effect risks in absolute terms (e.g., a 2 percent risk of headaches). Disturbingly, asymmetric presentations of benefit and risk also appear in the scientific evidence used to support medical guidelines (Caverly et al. 2016).
- *Perform all calculations for the reader.* Perhaps most importantly, never force the reader to subtract, multiply, or divide numbers to determine the important information they need (Baur and Prue 2014). For example, when presenting the benefits and drawbacks of tamoxifen as chemoprevention, it is not sufficient to tell a patient that tamoxifen reduces the risk of breast cancer by X percent while raising the risk of endometrial cancer by Y percent. This presentation would require a patient to perform a series of calculations to determine the impact on her risk of breast and endometrial cancers. Instead, calculations should be performed for the patient.

One strategy that is often used to help make health and science numbers easier to understand is to use data graphics. Data graphics represent the data in visual structures such as height, position, or area, which makes the quantities represented more concrete in a way that can be particularly helpful for people with lower numeracy skills. For example, a bar chart allows the comparison of two different case counts or level measurements using visual perception rather than mental representations of the numbers themselves.

Data graphics have proven to be particularly valuable in communicating risks. A key finding from the literature is that visual displays of risk should always show the part-to-whole relationship (Ancker et al. 2006), as graphics that only display the numerator tend to increase risk perceptions (Stone et al. 2017). Thus, stacked bar charts (which show multiple outcomes in a single vertical or horizontal bar) that visualize the entire population are preferred to separate bars for events and nonevents. Note that pie charts, while also representing the part-whole relationship, are generally not recommended, as people find them difficult to read precisely. Instead, research has supported the use of icon arrays, which use an array of people figures or abstract symbols to represent the entire population and then use color cues to indicate how many or what proportion are affected by the risk (Galesic, Garcia-Retamero, and Gigerenzer 2009; Hawley et al. 2008; Zikmund-Fisher, Fagerlin, and Ubel 2008).

As with numerical communications, there are some basic design principles that minimize the chance that a visual display will create confusion or distort people's perceptions of the underlying data. These include the following:

- *Use complete axis scaling.* Clear data graphics should use axis scaling that displays (a) the full range of potential values and (b) is not interrupted. Using narrower axes (e.g., only showing values from fifty to eighty instead of from zero to eighty) is one of the simplest ways to distort people's perceptions, making any visual differences displayed seem larger than they are. Even if complete, the choice of axis scale exerts a strong influence on perceptions: for example (Figure 6.1), a change from twenty to thirty looks a lot smaller on a graphic that is scaled from zero to one hundred than it does on a graph scaled from zero to thirty-five.
- *Use linear scaling.* Most people, including experts, find it difficult to process exponential growth of any quantity. While scientific communications often use logarithmic scaling to represent wide ranges of data, doing so tends to minimize people's perceptions of what are in fact enormous differences.
- *Choose the graphic type to highlight the type of outcome that is most important to the user.* Data graphics show multiple data points at one time, and, as a result, they can represent

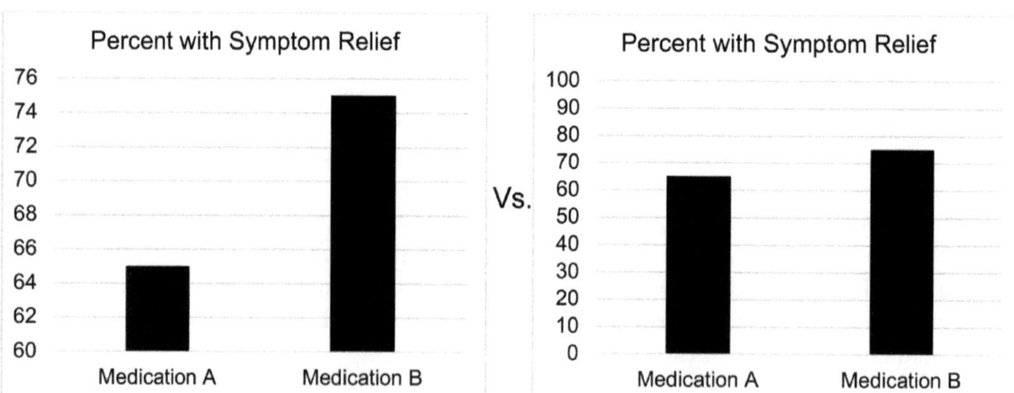

FIGURE 6.1
The Visual Impact of Excessively Narrow Axis Scaling (Left) versus Complete Axis Scaling (Right).

multiple numerical concepts simultaneously, but no data graphic is perfect for every task. Do users need to understand the level of the quantity or its trend over time or in comparison to other data points? Do they need to find one data point that is relevant to them, or do they need to understand the holistic picture of all the data? Good data graphics are designed to present one primary message to the reader.

Problem #3: Numbers without Context Are Meaningless

Regardless of their scientific accuracy, single data points are not intrinsically meaningful. Put another way, knowing what the number is does not ensure that someone knows what the number means. People don't care about the level or the count or the risk per se; we care about the implications of that information on our health, our safety, our world, and our actions. Is the 10 percent cancer risk something that should be seen as high or low? Concerning or relieving? Requiring action or good enough? Is the 7 ppb lead measurement a signal that a homeowner needs to buy a filter or the water system needs to change procedures, or should the level be taken as a marker of acceptable water quality? If you're not an expert in cancer or water quality, you probably can't answer these questions, and if they are not answered in the number communication, that represents a fundamental failure of communication.

The scientific term for this problem is information evaluability (Hsee 1996; Hsee and Zhang 2010; Zikmund-Fisher, Fagerlin, and Ubel 2004). Some information is easy to evaluate; that is, we immediately know whether it is good or bad. However, most health and science data are hard to evaluate. Lacking the topic-specific contextual knowledge that experts have, nonexperts like patients or community members often struggle to translate the numbers they are given into any type of meaningful gist. In fact, research shows that when people are presented with hard-to-evaluate numbers, they ignore them in making decisions. Regardless of our number skills, we need context (e.g., comparison standards) to make sense of the numbers that we receive. In the absence of context, the data provided is meaningless.

Thus, many "misinformed" consumers are not actually misinformed but simply struggling to make sense of information for which they lack relevant context. For example, the public often struggles to understand measures of climate change. Despite having the same units (Centigrade or Fahrenheit) as daily temperatures, global average temperatures have a vastly narrower range of potential variability. Thus, while a 1°C change in daily temperature is barely noticeable, a 1°C change in global average temperature represents a huge change. Another good example is disease case counts. Whether a count of one hundred or ten thousand disease cases implies a good or bad outcome depends on context (e.g., How many people get other diseases [in the same area and over the same time interval]?). Note that the relevant comparison likely differs based on disease severity or characteristics: Comparing strokes to heart attacks makes more sense than comparing them to sunburns.

Solution #3: Provide Use-Relevant Context for Every Number

Although the problem of meaningless numbers is widespread, there are many potential approaches to increase information evaluability and meaningfulness. Zikmund-Fisher (2019) provides a detailed discussion of these issues in science communications, while Heath and Starr's book, *Making Numbers Count* (2022), describes many useful ways to convert unfamiliar and abstract numerical statistics into comparisons that people can more intuitively grasp. From our perspective, some of the most useful strategies include the following:

- *Provide action or relief thresholds.* In other words, give people a clear signal as to whether they do, or do not, need to act.
- *Provide evaluative categories.* The number, type, and labeling of categories ideally should align with user needs. For example, categorizing a value as "high" or "concerning" is likely to evoke a stronger reaction than "above average" or "Tier 2."
- *Provide comparison values* that the audience is already familiar with (e.g., case counts for the 2009 H1N1 influenza pandemic were more interpretable when compared to seasonal influenza case counts).
- *Define the possible range* by providing the extreme values and their evaluative meaning. For example, inform people that a water quality scale runs from 0 (indicating no bacterial contamination) to 10 (indicating high levels of contamination).
- *Make directionality clear.* Directionality information is often so obvious to experts that they fail to realize how nonobvious it is to members of the public. Do higher values represent better outcomes, worse outcomes, or is there a target range? For example, a pain scale might use higher numbers to represent worse pain, while a sleep scale may be reversed so that higher numbers indicate better sleep quality. Note that clearly defining what extreme values mean is a solution to this problem.
- *Clarify practically significant differences.* How much change is needed to be worthy of attention?
- *When appropriate, translate the number into something more familiar, concrete, and human scale.* Heath and Starr (2022) give many examples of this approach, including making comparisons to things people are familiar with (e.g., a 3-cm tumor is the size of a grape) and translating large numbers into rates per person or per time (e.g., 800,000 US COVID-19 deaths over two years means that on average more than 1,000 people died each day for 2 years). Note, however, that these techniques can amplify reactions to numbers and hence should be used in an intentional way.
- *If using data graphics, visualize these important contextual elements.* Avoid requiring the reader to look away to learn what the graphic means. Visually showing action thresholds, interpretive categories, and relevant comparisons allows people to see how close their data are to these anchor points.
- *Consider whether the number is important to show at all.* In general, numbers allow more precise judgment of how big or small something is and also lend credibility to communications. However, in some situations, it may be sufficient to communicate the gist (e.g., whether the value is high enough that the user should take some action) instead of the precise number (Zikmund-Fisher 2013).

Note that the above strategies are all subjective to at least some degree. Experts may disagree about where an action threshold should fall or even if there is a universal action threshold or categorization scheme. However, the uncertainty inherent in expert opinion should never prevent health and science communicators from attempting to convey contextual knowledge. For the public to understand the health data they are given, they need a window into the way that experts' knowledge and experience color their understanding and interpretation, even if there is scientific uncertainty.

Note also that simply providing more and more context is not generally helpful. What people need is the *specific* contextual information that is *most relevant* to their needs (Scherer et al. 2018). For example, if what a communication audience most needs to know is whether a number is getting better or worse over time, then the most relevant contextual information is the past measurements or estimates. Providing detailed category information in addition to past values may cause confusion, even if such information might be valuable to inform a different communication whose goal was to help people know whether the values imply high or low risk.

Problems and Solutions in Practice: The Case of COVID-19

Perhaps no other event in recent memory has generated more health number communications to the public than the COVID-19 pandemic.

Case counts. From the very start of the pandemic, the public has been bombarded with ever-changing case counts (both disease cases and disease-related deaths), broken down by time, by location, by demographic characteristics, and so on. These counts are uninterpretable without a clear statement of the reference class and time interval. As a result, maps and time trend displays of COVID-19 case data have been commonplace. However, count data are not helpful for estimating personal risk, which depends both on the total population (which most people won't know) and on patterns of behavior and interaction (which vary widely). Furthermore, it is easy to create misleading comparisons by obscuring differences in the reference class. For example, a consumer who is trying to compare the counts of COVID-19 deaths among people who were vaccinated versus unvaccinated will end up with a distorted picture of the degree of protection provided by COVID-19 vaccines if they do not adjust for the relative numbers of vaccinated versus unvaccinated people in the population.

Even the visual maps of COVID-19 case counts can create confusion by the way that color or other cues are used to categorize the data. For example, many map graphics have used color gradients (e.g., light to dark red) to represent areas with higher versus lower case counts. However, the range in case counts early in the pandemic (e.g., April 2020) was vastly smaller than the range a year later. As a result, many news organizations have rescaled their color-coding categorization multiple times. However, it means that a consumer seeing their state going from dark red in April 2020 to light red in August 2021 probably won't realize that the number of cases might actually be much higher at a later time point. While such scale adjustments are acceptable to allow continued accurate communication of relative geographic status (i.e., this location vs. that one at one point in time), they hide the magnitude of the growth in cases that occurred over time.

Case or mortality rates. Many COVID-19 communications have converted case counts into case or mortality rates to allow comparisons between locations with varying population density. However, rates are easy to compare only if both the ratio denominator and the time interval are consistent. Unfortunately, different news and governmental organizations have calculated COVID-19 case rates per one hundred thousand people or per million people, and both daily and weekly rates are commonly provided. This inconsistency has created many opportunities for confusion.

Vaccine risks. Although the COVID-19 vaccines have proven to be extremely safe, monitoring of outcomes has identified certain rare risks (e.g., thrombosis with thrombocytopenia syndrome or myocarditis/pericarditis) associated with different vaccines (See et al. 2021). As with

COVID-19 illness, the challenge has been translating the counts of adverse events recorded into approximations of individual risk. Some have tried to compare the risk of blood clots from the Johnson & Johnson vaccine to the risk of (different) blood clots from hormonal birth control pills, but the lack of consistent reference class, time intervals, and outcome severity makes such comparisons confusing at best and inappropriate at worst.

In addition, it is essentially impossible to compare risks of vaccine administration to risks of COVID exposure at the individual level, because disease risk is determined by uncontrolled variables like exposure, whereas vaccine exposure is guaranteed with vaccination. In short, the data are not well aligned to the needs of the individual making decisions about their own protective actions. For an audience of policymakers, however, the data can easily be interpreted to show that the total vaccine-related events in a community are vastly fewer than the risks associated with community members remaining unprotected from the disease.

Vaccine effectiveness. The concept of vaccine effectiveness is difficult to communicate. What is reported is the proportion of cases in a study of unvaccinated versus vaccinated participants, not the proportion of vaccinated or unvaccinated people who get sick. In addition, it's important to ask, "Effectiveness against what?" The various COVID-19 vaccine trials have focused on different outcomes (e.g., moderate to severe infections vs. symptomatic illness) and were conducted at different times (e.g., before vs. after more infectious variants were present). Note that this is a reference class problem: absent clear labeling, most people misunderstand what is meant by the published percentage.

Even once one understands what is measured, how effective is good enough? This evaluability question became very salient when the initial COVID-19 vaccine effectiveness rates ranged from 66 percent to 95 percent. This difference made certain vaccines seem better, so much so that the mayor of the city of Detroit initially refused a vaccine allocation on the grounds that he wanted "to make sure the residents of the city of Detroit get the best" (Setty 2021). Yet, even 66 percent of effectiveness looks good when compared instead to the effectiveness of seasonal influenza vaccines, which have varied from 19 percent to 60 percent from 2010 through 2019 (Centers for Disease Control and Prevention 2021).

Final Thoughts on Avoiding Number Confusion and Number Manipulation

Numbers are essential to communication about health and medical concepts but can be difficult to communicate clearly. Poor communication of numbers, even by the best-intentioned communicators, can result in misinformation. In fact, many apparently misinformed members of the public are simply struggling to make sense of the information presented without sufficient attention to their goals, needs, and abilities.

We recommend assisting the public by applying a universal precautions approach to communication by assuming that all readers may have low numeracy, using numerical formats that minimize cognitive work (e.g., performing necessary calculations and providing essential reference information such as units), and providing user-specific context to help the user evaluate the meaning of the number (e.g., whether it is high or low, or concerning or reassuring). Some of our most important specific recommendations are listed in Box 6.1.

However, it should come to no one's surprise that the more we have learned about how to design clear number communications, the more we have also learned how to intentionally design number communications to change their perception and their meaning. Whether one

BOX 6.1
Recommendations for Clear Communication of Health Numbers

1. Take a universal precautions approach
   - Assume all readers may have low numeracy
   - Focus on the user's needs for information
2. Reduce cognitive work and guesswork
   - Provide units of measure for any quantities
   - Use the same units or denominators for all numbers in a communication
   - Clearly state the reference class and/or time interval
   - Use round numbers when possible
   - Present absolute differences (not relative risk reductions or increases)
   - Do the math for readers
   - Use complete, linear scaling in graphics
   - Choose graphic formats to clarify the primary message
3. Provide user-relevant context for every number
   - Provide the action thresholds, evaluative categories, or comparison values that most align with the user's needs
   - Make directionality clear (i.e., is "more" good or bad?)
   - Clarify practically significant differences
   - When appropriate, translate the number into something more familiar, concrete, and human scale
   - Consider whether the number is important to show at all

calls such actions health marketing tools or deceptive practices depends on whether those actions create desired or undesired outcomes from your perspective.

Fortunately, clarity is a vaccine against manipulation. Put simply, any guide to creating clear numerical communication is also a guide to identifying and preventing numerical manipulation. However, prevention of misunderstandings (whether accidental or intentional) can only occur if communicators both recognize that their current communications are suboptimal and are given exposure to better, evidence-based approaches. Preparing communicators to apply these principles can help in the battle against health and medical misinformation.

References

Akl, Elie A., Andrew D. Oxman, Jeph Herrin, Gunn E. Vist, Irene Terrenato, Francesca Sperati, Cecelia Costiniuk, Diana Blank, and Holger J Schünemann. 2011. "Using Alternative Statistical Formats for Presenting Risks and Risk Reductions." *Cochrane Database of Systematic Reviews*, no. 3. https://doi.org/10.1002/14651858.CD006776.pub2.

Ancker, Jessica S., and David Kaufman. 2007. "Rethinking Health Numeracy: A Multidisciplinary Literature Review." *Journal of the American Medical Informatics Association: JAMIA* 14 (6): 713–21. https://doi.org/10.1197/jamia.M2464.

Ancker, Jessica S., Yalini Senathirajah, Rita Kukafka, and Justin B. Starren. 2006. "Design Features of Graphs in Health Risk Communication: A Systematic Review." *Journal of the American Medical Informatics Association: JAMIA* 13 (6): 608–18. https://doi.org/10.1197/jamia.M2115.

Ancker, Jessica S., Natalie C. Benda, Mohit M. Sharma, Stephen B. Johnson, Stephanie Weiner, and Brian J. Zikmund-Fisher. "Taxonomies for Synthesizing the Evidence on Communicating Numbers in Health." *Risk Analysis.* Published online ahead of print, January 2022.

Baur, Cynthia, and Christine Prue. 2014. "The CDC Clear Communication Index Is a New Evidence-Based Tool to Prepare and Review Health Information." *Health Promotion Practice* 15 (5): 629–37. https://doi.org/10.1177/1524839914538969.

Bonner, Carissa, Lyndal J. Trevena, Wolfgang Gaissmaier, Paul K. J. Han, Yasmina Okan, Elissa Ozanne, Ellen Peters, Daniëlle Timmermans, and Brian J. Zikmund-Fisher. 2021. "Current Best Practice for Presenting Probabilities in Patient Decision Aids: Fundamental Principles." *Medical Decision Making* 41 (7): 821–33. https://doi.org/10.1177/0272989X21996328.

Caverly, Tanner J., Rodney A. Hayward, Elyse Reamer, Brian J. Zikmund-Fisher, Daniel Connochie, Michele Heisler, and Angela Fagerlin. 2016. "Presentation of Benefits and Harms in US Cancer Screening and Prevention Guidelines: Systematic Review." *Journal of the National Cancer Institute* 108 (6): djv436. https://doi.org/10.1093/jnci/djv436.

Centers for Disease Control and Prevention. 2021. "Past Seasons Vaccine Effectiveness Estimates." https://www.cdc.gov/flu/vaccines-work/past-seasons-estimates.html.

DeWalt, Darren A., Leigh F. Callahan, Victoria H. Hawk, Kimberly A. Broucksou, Ashley Hink, Rima E. Rudd, and Cindy Brach. 2010. "Health Literacy Universal Precautions Toolkit." AHRQ Publication No. 10-0046-EF. Rockville, MD: Agency for Healthcare Research and Quality.

Galesic, Mirta, and Rocio Garcia-Retamero. 2010. "Statistical Numeracy for Health: A Cross-Cultural Comparison with Probabilistic National Samples." *Archives of Internal Medicine* 170 (5): 462–68. https://doi.org/10.1001/archinternmed.2009.481.

Galesic, Mirta, Rocio Garcia-Retamero, and Gerd Gigerenzer. 2009. "Using Icon Arrays to Communicate Medical Risks: Overcoming Low Numeracy." *Health Psychology* 28 (2): 210–16. https://doi.org/10.1037/a0014474.

Hawley, Sarah T., Brian Zikmund-Fisher, Peter Ubel, Aleksandra Jancovic, Todd Lucas, and Angela Fagerlin. 2008. "The Impact of the Format of Graphical Presentation on Health-Related Knowledge and Treatment Choices." *Patient Education and Counseling* 73 (3): 448–55. https://doi.org/10.1016/j.pec.2008.07.023.

Heath, Chip, and Karla Starr. 2022. *Making Numbers Count: The Art and Science of Communicating Numbers.* New York: Avid Reader Press.

Hsee, Christopher K. 1996. "The Evaluability Hypothesis: An Explanation for Preference Reversals between Joint and Separate Evaluations of Alternatives." *Organizational Behavior and Human Decision Processes* 67 (3): 247–57. https://doi.org/10.1006/obhd.1996.0077.

Hsee, Christopher K., and Jiao Zhang. 2010. "General Evaluability Theory." *Perspectives on Psychological Science* 5 (4): 343–55. https://doi.org/10.1177/1745691610374586.

Huff, Darrell. 1954. *How to Lie with Statistics.* New York: Norton.

Institute of Medicine. 2014. *Health Literacy and Numeracy: Workshop Summary.* Washington, DC: The National Academies Press.

Institute of Medicine and National Academies of Sciences, Engineering, and Medicine. 2015. *Health Literacy: Past, Present, and Future: Workshop Summary.* Washington, DC: The National Academies Press.

Lipkus, Isaac M., Greg Samsa, and Barbara K. Rimer. 2001. "General Performance on a Numeracy Scale among Highly Educated Samples." *Medical Decision Making* 21 (1): 37–44. https://doi.org/10.1177/0272989X0102100105.

Malenka, David J., John A. Baron, Sarah Johansen, Jon W. Wahrenberger, and Jonathan M. Ross. 1993. "The Framing Effect of Relative and Absolute Risk." *Journal of General Internal Medicine* 8 (10): 543–48.

Marcatto, Francesco, Jonathan J. Rolison, and Donatella Ferrante. 2013. "Communicating Clinical Trial Outcomes: Effects of Presentation Method on Physicians' Evaluations of New Treatments." *Judgment and Decision Making* 8 (1): 29–33.

Nelson, W., V. F. Reyna, A. Fagerlin, I. M. Lipkus, and E. Peters. 2008. "Clinical Implications of Numeracy: Theory and Practice." *Annals of Behavioral Medicine* 35 (3): 261–74. https://doi.org/10.1007/s12160-008-9037-8.

Peters, Ellen. 2012. "Beyond Comprehension: The Role of Numeracy in Judgments and Decisions." *Current Directions in Psychological Science* 21 (1): 31–35. https://doi.org/10.1177/0963721411429960.

Peters, Ellen, Judith Hibbard, Paul Slovic, and Nathan Dieckmann. 2007. "Numeracy Skill and the Communication, Comprehension, and Use of Risk-Benefit Information." *Health Affairs* 26 (3): 741–48. https://doi.org/10.1377/hlthaff.26.3.741.

Scherer, Aaron M., Holly O. Witteman, Jacob B. Solomon, Nicole L. Exe, Angela Fagerlin, and Brian J. Zikmund-Fisher. 2018. "Improving Understanding of Test Results by Substituting (Not Adding) Goal Ranges: Experimental Study." *Journal of Medical Internet Research* 20 (10): e11027. https://doi.org/10.2196/11027.

See, Isaac, John R. Su, Allison Lale, Emily Jane Woo, Alice Y. Guh, Tom T. Shimabukuro, Michael B. Streiff et al. 2021. "US Case Reports of Cerebral Venous Sinus Thrombosis With Thrombocytopenia After Ad26.COV2.S Vaccination, March 2 to April 21, 2021." *JAMA* 325 (24): 2448–56. https://doi.org/10.1001/jama.2021.7517.

Setty, Ganesh. 2021. "Detroit Mayor Declines Johnson & Johnson Allotment, Saying the Other Vaccines Are Better." CNN, March 5, 2021. https://www.cnn.com/2021/03/04/health/detroit-mayor-johnson-and-johnson-vaccine/index.html.

Sirota, Miroslav, Marie Juanchich, and Jean-Francois Bonnefon. 2018. "'1-in-X' Bias: '1-in-X' Format Causes Overestimation of Health-Related Risks." *Journal of Experimental Psychology: Applied* 24 (4): 431–39. https://doi.org/10.1037/xap0000190.

Stone, Eric R., Wändi Bruine de Bruin, Abigail M. Wilkins, Emily M. Boker, and Jacqueline MacDonald Gibson. 2017. "Designing Graphs to Communicate Risks: Understanding How the Choice of Graphical Format Influences Decision Making." *Risk Analysis* 37 (4): 612–28. https://doi.org/10.1111/risa.12660.

Witteman, Holly O., Brian J. Zikmund-Fisher, Erika A. Waters, Teresa Gavaruzzi, and Angela Fagerlin. 2011. "Risk Estimates from an Online Risk Calculator Are More Believable and Recalled Better When Expressed as Integers." *Journal of Medical Internet Research* 13 (3): e54. https://doi.org/10.2196/jmir.1656.

Zikmund-Fisher, Brian J. 2011. "Time to Retire the 1-in-X Risk Format." *Medical Decision Making* 31 (5): 703–4. https://doi.org/10.1177/0272989X11418238.

Zikmund-Fisher, Brian J. 2013. "The Right Tool Is What They Need, Not What We Have: A Taxonomy of Appropriate Levels of Precision in Patient Risk Communication." *Medical Care Research and Review* 70 (1 suppl): 37S–49S. https://doi.org/10.1177/1077558712458541.

Zikmund-Fisher, Brian J. 2019. "Helping People Know Whether Measurements Have Good or Bad Implications: Increasing the Evaluability of Health and Science Data Communications." *Policy Insights from the Behavioral and Brain Sciences* 6 (1): 29–37. https://doi.org/10.1177/2372732218813377.

Zikmund-Fisher, Brian J., Angela Fagerlin, and Peter A. Ubel. 2004. "'Is 28% Good or Bad?' Evaluability and Preference Reversals in Health Care Decisions." *Medical Decision Making* 24 (2): 142–48.

Zikmund-Fisher, Brian J., Angela Fagerlin, and Peter A. Ubel. 2008. "Improving Understanding of Adjuvant Therapy Options by Using Simpler Risk Graphics." *Cancer* 113 (12): 3382–90. https://doi.org/10.1002/cncr.23959.

7

The Case of Everyday Science

Science Literacy and Resilience against Health Misinformation

Alla Keselman

Disclaimer: The opinions expressed by the author are her own and this material should not be interpreted as representing the official viewpoint of the US Department of Health and Human Services, the National Institutes of Health, or the National Library of Medicine.

The Problem of Health Misinformation

TODAY, PEOPLE ARE BOMBARDED by health misinformation, or claims that are not grounded in scientific evidence. What science-related knowledge do they need to have to be skeptical about these claims? The concern about health misinformation is both new and old. It is new because medicine, the way it is practiced today, is a relatively new field. Until the adoption of the germ theory of disease at the end of the nineteenth century (Bantock 1899), medicine had a rather tenuous relationship with science. Doctors were not highly regarded professionals, and there was no clear separation between professional and other kinds of healing-related knowledge (e.g., knowledge of traditional healers or experienced community members) (Roberts 1999). The second half of the twentieth century was marked by the growing emphasis on research as the foundation of standard of care. In the early 1990s, Gordon Guyatt coined the term "evidence-based medicine" or EBM (Guyatt 1991). According to an authoritative definition, EBM is "the conscientious, explicit and judicious use of current best [research-based] evidence in making decisions about the care of individual patients" (Sackett et al. 1996).

At the same time, the problem of health misinformation predates by far both the internet and terminologies like "infodemic" and "fake news." The United States did not introduce federal regulation of drugs' safety and effectiveness until 1906 (US Food and Drug Administration, n.d.), and many newspaper advertisements and traveling salesmen touted dubious remedies as panaceas. One such remedy, "snake oil," became synonymous with fraud, entering English-language dictionaries. The remedy was made infamous by Clark Stanley, an entrepreneur who, in the late 1800s, marketed his Stanley's Snake Oil as a purported cure for many ailments with great flair. In 1917, federal investigators caught up with Stanley. The investigation showed not only that the concoction was not effective against what it claimed to cure but that it also did not actually contain snake oil. Clark Stanley had to pay a small fine for his transgressions (Gandhi 2013).

Today, medicine is very different from what it used to be before the second half of the twentieth century. Professional medical societies issue evidence-based practice guidelines based on systematic reviews of biomedical research findings (American Medical Association, n.d.). Federal agencies regulate testing, manufacturing, and marketing of drugs and medical devices, focusing on their safety and effectiveness. Yet, the presence of nonevidence-based treatments and health beliefs is not going away. If anything, it is getting bigger. The internet and social media provide channels for easy spread. Nonevidence-based health messages differ in intent, with some authors distinguishing between intentionally deceitful "disinformation" and unintentional "misinformation" (see chapter 1, "Defining Health Misinformation," in this book). Misinformation and disinformation also differ in their relationships to evidence, ranging from omissions and exaggerations to contradictions and unsupported claims. For the purpose of this chapter, we define health "misinformation" as claims that are not supported by conventional scientific evidence, regardless of their intent. Generally, these claims warn about the supposed dangers of established conventional approaches or promise the hope of alternative solutions to serious health problems.

Examples abound. While the biomedical establishment expresses an evidence-based consensus that childhood vaccines and vaccine ingredients do not cause autism (Institute of Medicine 2004; Zhukivska and Lambert 2021), many members of the public remain concerned. Tomeny et al. (2017) coded a large body of tweets that contained vaccine-related and autism-spectrum-disorder-related keywords. Fifty percent of those tweets expressed negative beliefs about vaccines. Dhaliwal and Mannion (2020) show how antivaccination campaigns use social media to spread myths about vaccines (e.g., vaccines overstimulate the immune system; adjuvants in vaccines cause cancer, infertility, Alzheimer's, and autism). Various self-proclaimed experts promote alternative cures where conventional medical best practices cannot provide them. For example, best-selling *New Age* book author Gregg Braden uploaded a video to YouTube titled "Bladder Cancer Dissolves in Less than 3 Minutes Using the Language of Emotion," which espouses a view that positive emotions can cure cancer by affecting DNA. By October 14, 2021, the YouTube video had been viewed 259,641 times, generating 1,700 thumbs up and 87 thumbs down reactions (Braden 2011). In a study of the top search results for the query "diabetes, reversal, natural," Keselman et al. (2019) found that fourteen of twenty-five analyzed sites "either promised complete recovery [from type 2 diabetes] or strongly implied that it was highly possible," with eleven promising cures within a period from eleven days to three months. In the meantime, health authority exemplified by the American Diabetes Association maintains that while type 2 diabetes can be put into remission, except in rare cases, it cannot be permanently reversed or cured (Riddle et al. 2021). The majority of cures proposed by participants in Keselman et al. (2019) involved dietary supplements.

Why do people hold beliefs that contradict the scientific consensus? Can science education and engagement with science make a difference? When people make decisions that do not align with recommendations that are based on scientific evidence, do they do it because they "reject science?" We have to remember that the edges of the misinformation phenomenon are fuzzy, because scientific evidence is complex, works in complex contexts, and is often a work in progress. Moreover, science is a debate, with scientists disagreeing about what constitutes good evidence, especially regarding novel issues. Promises of unrealistic remedies often emerge not to spite science but because science does not provide all the answers, so other parties rush in to fill the gap left by scientific imperfections, looking to make profit or ease despair.

In the House of Commons in 1947, Winston Churchill famously said, "No one pretends that democracy is perfect or all-wise. Indeed, it has been said that democracy is the worst form of Government except for all those other forms that have been tried from time to time." A similar thing can be said about science as a foundation for health care standards. While not perfect, it is the most reliable method humans have developed for learning and answering questions about the natural world. There are many important questions that cannot be answered by science alone because they involve personal and group values and priorities. For example, it does not answer the question "Should I visit my unvaccinated grandchildren for Christmas during the pandemic, given that I am vaccinated but immunocompromised, and they are not?" Science is, however, the most effective way of answering "Are COVID-19 vaccines effective against COVID?"

This chapter focuses on science literacy as a barrier against health misinformation, challenges to science literacy as a solution, and ways to enhance science literacy in a way that supports dealing with health information in the real world.

How Do Laypeople Use Science?

Science is both a profession that requires many years of specialized study and an area of important social application. Science educators have long claimed that all people, regardless of their future profession, benefit from learning some science (Jenkins 2000). One of their claims was that knowing science improves daily life, leading to better decisions. However, ironically, this claim is much more often expressed as a conviction than an empirically based assertion.

Is some grasp of science helpful in recognizing misinformation for what it is? How can science be used? Let's look at two hypothetical examples:

Parents of an eleven-year-old girl are concerned. Their pediatrician recently recommended that their daughter receive the HPV vaccine that prevents cervical cancer. HPV vaccination at this age is also supported by the recommendation of the Centers for Disease Control and Prevention (CDC). However, a family member recently sent them a link to a website that says that in some cases HPV vaccine actually causes cervical cancer. The parents are not sure what to do.

What kind of information can reassure this family that the HPV vaccine is likely to be safe for their daughter? The parents may read several articles about the HPV vaccine and be reassured that it does not contain a live virus. This information may alleviate parental concern if they have a basic understanding of how viruses cause diseases. This is not the only way to go about thinking through the situation. Parents may, for example, do a search about HPV vaccine safety in the PubMed database of peer-reviewed biomedical literature and feel reassured by the number of publications that claim safety, the authority of the journals, and the sample sizes reported in the publications. Alternatively, without referring to any additional sources, the parents may prefer to go with their pediatrician's advice because they trust their pediatrician's knowledge and its sources.

Let's consider a different situation:

Expectant parents are concerned. They know that the American Academy of Pediatrics recommends many vaccines in their child's infant and toddler years. However, several members of online parenting forums caution that childhood vaccines cause autism. They support their posts with links to websites telling stories of families whose children were harmed by vaccines. The parents are not sure what to do.

The difference compared to the previous situation is a much greater conceptual complexity of the implicated biological mechanism. A high school biology course provides sufficient foundation for understanding the difference between a live virus that can reproduce and cause disease and the nonreproducing material in the HPV vaccine that can stimulate the immune response, but not cause the disease. However, when it comes to autism, its causes are currently uncertain, and the evidence about the lack of connection between vaccination and autism is epidemiological. To accept the recommendation to vaccinate, parents will have no alternative to relying on their trust in scientific and medical authority.

Whatever the parents do, the situation calls for thinking about science and scientists. Research studies of how people think through making such decisions would help us identify components of science-related knowledge and science-related concerns that are relevant to individuals' decision-making. This information, then, could help us address the issues in the classroom, reaching students before they become adult decision-makers, and in other educational settings.

Unfortunately, the body of research that focuses on how knowledge is used in forming health beliefs and evaluating information is very small. Sivaramakrishnan and Patel (1993) showed that limited understanding of biological mechanisms made Indian and Indian Canadian parents susceptible to non-normative health beliefs despite their superficial acceptance of normative facts inconsistent with those beliefs. Keselman, Kaufman, and Patel (2004) conducted a study that looked at how adolescents' conceptual understanding of the biological basis of HIV affected their reasoning about HIV myths. The study found that students who were able to draw on cellular-level biological concepts were more likely to reject the myths. At the same time, knowledge of basic facts about HIV in the absence of a deeper conceptual understanding of HIV biology did not protect adolescents from accepting the myths that were inconsistent with their factual knowledge. For example, a student could answer "no" when asked whether there was a cure for HIV but then read a vignette in which someone claimed that HIV could be expelled from the body with sweat and agree that this could possibly be true.

The findings by Sivaramakrishnan and Patel (1993) and Keselman, Kaufman, and Patel (2004) come from laboratory studies. Little research investigates how beliefs are formed and how science is used in daily life. Such studies are difficult to conduct, because it is difficult to foresee real-life situations that call for the use of science-related knowledge—and to identify what responses constitute applications of science-based knowledge. Indirect evidence suggests that education and health literacy positively correlate with medication adherence, more effective utilization of care, and better health status (Baker et al. 2004; Davis et al. 2006; Lee et al. 2009; White et al. 2008). Yet very few studies tease out the role played by science-related knowledge in those domains, and many studies show reasoning that is primarily driven by social, rather than scientific, factors. For example, Layton et al. (1993) conducted case studies of scenarios in which the public could potentially draw on science: older adults planning their heating budgets, a town managing methane from local landfill sites, and parents raising children with Down Syndrome. The authors found that people facing these challenges rarely framed their concerns in scientific terms. For example, the older adults did not discuss the efficiency of their windows' insulation. Rather, they talked about the comfort of glowing space heaters and the social importance of well-heated homes. For people to draw on science when solving a real-life problem, the problem needs to be viewed as primarily scientific, but real-life problems involve many factors and considerations of a non-scientific nature (e.g., social, emotional, and logistical).

Even in health-related situations when scientific framing appears unavoidable, understanding mechanisms does not tell the full story of behaviors. The author is writing this chapter in the second year of the COVID-19 pandemic, at a time when vaccine hesitancy presents a major public health challenge in the United States and many European countries. Individuals who are reluctant to receive vaccines usually express their hesitancy in the language of science, stating concerns about vaccines' safety, efficacy, rapid development, and short duration of testing (Moore et al. 2021; Pogue et al. 2020; Zahid and Alsayb 2021). Will addressing these concerns by providing scientific explanations of vaccine development and mechanism increase vaccine uptake? At this time, we do not have empirical data speaking to the issue. We hope that a better understanding of how vaccines work will increase their acceptance. However, a *New York Times* podcast titled "Rural Tennessee's Vaccine Hesitators" highlights the limitations of the power of science knowledge (Herndon 2021).

The podcast, aired on May 10, 2021, focused on a rural Tennessee community in a county with a rate of vaccinations significantly below the national average, with only 31 percent of the residents having received at least one dose. The podcast features Dr. Daniel Lewis, a family medicine doctor who was both a trusted, much-loved community member and a survivor of a very serious COVID-19 experience. Dr. Lewis made it his mission to try to promote COVID-19 vaccination in his community. In the episode, the podcast producers are granted permission to be present during Dr. Lewis's conversation with his patients, a married couple in their seventies, Jim and Rita Fletcher. Jim and Rita took COVID very seriously, explaining that they had lost at least eleven people in their circle to this disease. They also were not generally anti-vaccine—both they and their children had received other recommended vaccines. Yet, they had many worries about the COVID-19 vaccine.

One of their concerns was about the possibility of the vaccine containing microchips. In a thoughtful, attentive conversation, Dr. Lewis addressed this concern:

> Well, I would say this. When you get the injection, it comes with a needle that's got an opening about that wide . . . we don't make [microchips] that small. You know, it's, I mean—there has to be some degree, I think, just of faith, I guess, in that regard. But there's no way to introduce a chip through a needle at this point. Or else, we'd do it to dogs and everything else. When you have a dog, it gets microchipped, for example. There's a surgery done, right? They don't inject it into a dog. (Herndon 2021)

At this point, Mr. Fletcher acknowledges that, as a retired engineer, he is aware that a microchip is the size of a grain of rice, too large to be injected with a needle. The couple also asks questions and listens to detailed answers about the possibility of the vaccine altering their DNA. Yet, after taking some time to think about the conversation with the doctor, Mr. and Mrs. Fletcher decide not to get vaccinated.

What is happening here? Is Mr. Fletcher not understanding the scientific explanation given to him? His responses to the doctor do not support this hypothesis. And yet, this episode seems to illustrate the limitations of the power of conceptual knowledge. Mr. Fletcher is a member of a politically conservative, deeply religious community where the COVID-19 vaccination campaign is perceived as something brought by outsiders with different social and political values. Put plainly, it is brought by the forces he does not trust. Concerns about the DNA and microchips may be consequences, rather than causes of the mistrust. If science education or science literacy initiatives are to change these conditions, they need to deliver a lot more than conceptual knowledge of DNA and the immune system.

Science Literacy

The title of this chapter invokes science literacy. Yet, so far in this chapter, when discussing laypeople's reasoning about situations in which professionals derive their guidelines and standards from research, I have been using the term "science-related knowledge." I do this because the knowledge and skills employed in either accepting or rejecting evidence from scientific sources are multifaceted and complex. To answer the question about what the lay public needs to know science-wise, the field of science education has put forward the concept of science literacy as composed of several components (Bybee et al. 2006; OECD 2019). This conceptualization is consistent with that of the National Academies of Sciences, Engineering, and Medicine (2016). These components of science literacy can be represented as follows:

1. Knowledge *of* science (knowledge of facts, laws, and theories)
2. Knowledge *about* science (knowledge about scientific methods)
3. Attitudes *toward* science (attitudes toward the role of science in society and about the scientists' intentions).

The assumption is that, jointly, these competencies provide the full picture of the scientific enterprise, giving not only the "what" but the "how" and, ultimately, the "why" science is the most reliable method of knowing.

Let's consider these three components in turn.

Knowledge of Science

Knowledge of science is the most traditional and the oldest area of K–12 school science education. Students receive the outcomes of the scientific enterprise in the form of facts, concepts, laws, and theories. They learn what molecules and viruses are, why water freezes, how hemoglobin molecules transport oxygen, and how antigens cause the immune system to produce antibodies. People who have very little formal knowledge of science are vulnerable to beliefs that may lead to suboptimal decisions and outcomes. The person with very little knowledge has no reason to prefer biological explanations of health and disease. For example, Bell et al. (2020) interviewed pregnant women and new mothers in Ghana who were hospitalized for life-threatening complications to themselves or their infants. They found that about a third of the interviewed women believed that the illness was caused by the evil eye and that treatment required traditional remedies, usually provided by spiritual healers (e.g., in the form of prayer). Some of the women emphasized that traditional treatment had to be combined with conventional allopathic treatment; others did not. In societies and communities where traditional healing practices are strong, people may forgo or delay turning to conventional medicine for help.

Traditional healing practices are complex and grounded in profound belief systems and sociocultural institutions. While their safety and effectiveness need to be assessed on a case-by-case basis, they undoubtedly provide social and emotional support to their recipients and support societal structures. Battling these institutions is not the mission of science education. However, people often hold multiple, sometimes incompatible, belief systems, that they can call upon when circumstances require (Sivaramakrishnan and Patel 1993). Having science education and the resulting understanding of concepts like the germ theory of diseases will likely increase the probability of utilization of conventional medicine—quite possibly alongside traditional treatments.

In the Western world, the vast majority of people have had exposure to K–12 (pre-college) school science. Research focusing on the knowledge of science education emphasizes the importance of conceptual knowledge or developing an understanding of interrelated facts, their relationships, and domain-underlying principles (Vosniadou 2019). Conceptual understanding is more than just knowledge of facts. It has depth and allows flexibility for thinking critically about specific situations that were not addressed in the classroom. It, thus, provides tools that mere knowledge of facts does not provide. I had previously mentioned a study in which adolescents exposed to basic factual knowledge of HIV (e.g., incurable) still accepted superficially plausible myths of HIV cures (e.g., that it can be expelled from the body via bodily fluids, such as urine and sweat). However, understanding that HIV is a virus that enters cells of the immune system did provide a barrier against the myth (Keselman, Kaufman, and Patel 2004). In the COVID-19 era, some concerns laypeople have about HIV vaccines have to do with the ability of the vaccine to alter their DNA. While the CDC assures the public that "the [vaccine] material never enters the nucleus of the cell, which is where our DNA is kept," one is probably more likely to accept this explanation if they know the structure of a cell and what the nucleus does (Centers for Disease Control and Prevention 2021).

Unfortunately, nonevidence-based beliefs that can be refuted on the basis of high school biology are just the tip of the misinformation iceberg. Theoretical underpinnings of modern medicine are very complex. Mechanisms that underlie most treatments are well outside the scope of high school biology. In fact, they are often outside the knowledge of health practitioners who prescribe them. In some cases, scientists who develop and test disease-modifying drugs do so without fully understanding their mechanism of action. For example, although dimethyl fumarate medication is the approved standard of care therapy for reducing the progression of relapsing multiple sclerosis with established effectiveness, its mechanism of action is still being elucidated (Murri 2021). This example illustrates how, in medicine, it is not unusual to accept evidence of outcomes without a full biological understanding of mechanisms. At the same time, nonevidence-based claims are often presented with detailed descriptions of supposed underlying mechanisms that are too complex for laypeople to evaluate. For example, Keselman et al. (2019) reviewed websites that promoted nonevidence-based remedies for type 2 diabetes and found that many of the sites included complex explanations of treatment mechanisms, evaluating which required knowledge well outside high school biology. Evaluating the plausibility of statements about disease and treatment mechanisms is rarely easy, and, moreover, plausibility is not veracity. The paucity of studies supporting the lay use of scientific concepts in daily life decisions underscores the complexity of using conceptual knowledge to evaluate health information.

Knowledge about Science

Knowledge about science refers to understanding science as a process and familiarity with the tools, methods, and principles that science uses to generate knowledge. The Program for International Student Assessment (PISA), maintained by the Organisation for Economic Cooperation and Development (OECD), distinguishes two areas of knowledge about science: scientific inquiry and scientific explanation (OECD 2019). Scientific inquiry has to do with skills in gathering data, such as designing experiments or planning observations and collecting measurements. In gaining expertise in scientific inquiry, students learn about concepts such as sampling techniques, sample size, measurement precision, and control of variables. Scientific explanation is about coordinating evidence (data gathered via the inquiry process) with prior knowledge and then drawing conclusions. This is the step of using the results of the inquiry in order to reach the goals of scientific investigations.

Another aspect of knowledge about science, increasingly emphasized in science education, is understanding the nature of science (NOS) as an enterprise. The Next Generation Science Standards, a consortium effort among twenty-six US states, the National Science Teachers Association, the American Association for the Advancement of Science, and the National Research Council, put forward a set of principles of science that students should understand (Next Generation Science Standards Lead States 2013). These principles involve understanding that science is a human endeavor of obtaining knowledge about natural phenomena. This endeavor is based on empirical evidence and generates knowledge that is dynamic and self-correcting, open to revisions on the basis of new emerging evidence.

In the past couple of decades, schools around the world have been placing growing emphasis on knowledge about science. Laboratory experimentation has become part of school science curricula for all age groups starting with very young children. Elementary school students test different models of pasta bridges for strength, and high school students extract DNA from strawberries (Education.com 2014). They are taught to generate hypotheses and evaluate their hypotheses in the light of their data. There is also much emphasis on engineering or using scientific knowledge to design processes and structures that help people accomplish tasks (Next Generation Science Standards Lead States 2013).

Does learning about science help people recognize health misinformation? The internet, which features health-related claims supported by "research" that violates methodological principles covered in school biology, is a fertile field for considering this question. A case in point is an online article titled "Circumcision Permanently Alters the Brain," allegedly authored by Paul D. Tinari, PhD. The author describes a situation in which he, as a graduate student "working in the Dept. of Epidemiology," was approached by a group of hospital nurses who "needed some scientific support for their [anti-circumcision] position" (Tinari). Though not claiming to be a health professional, the narrating author alleges to have performed an MRI study recording the brain's response to the circumcision procedure performed on a nurse's infant son. In the words of the narrator, "The operator of the MRI machine in the hospital was a friend of mine, and he agreed to allow us to use the machine for research after normal operational hours" (Tinari). A neurologist, supposedly, later reviewed the data and established that the "circumcision affected most intensely the portions of the victim's brain associated with reasoning, perception and emotions" (Tinari). Although the story, featured on the Circumcision Resource Center website, has its sympathetic audience, a sizable percentage of science-literate readers are unlikely to find the report of a "study" performed on a single infant compelling (there are many more additional problems with this "study," including conducting it without an ethics board review).

However, while the circumcision brain impact story reports a farcically ridiculous study design, most methodological research imperfections, whether in real or confabulated studies, are not nearly as egregious. More often, the flaws are too nuanced for the unprofessional eye to see. In many cases, statements of faulty claims cite legitimate well-designed and executed research studies, and the misinformation lies in overgeneralizing or stretching the implications of findings (e.g., by extending the effect of animal studies to humans).

Unfortunately, when knowledge about science is taught at schools, it is often done via models and content domains that are much too simplistic, while real-world science is complex. Science educator Peter Fensham (2012) used the Cynefin framework adopted from decision analysis (Snowden and Boone 2007) to understand the correspondence between the complexity of school science and real-world science. The framework distinguishes four levels of complexity inherent in systems or problems (Fensham 2012; Zeyer 2021):

- simple (stable and characterized by well-understood, simple cause-and-effect relationships)
- complicated (still stable but characterized by more complicated cause-and-effect relationships)
- complex (constantly changing, not fully understood, difficult to predict, and involving a high degree of risk)
- chaotic (very dynamic, impossible to describe by known cause-and-effect relationships, risky, and unpredictable)

While the most pressing socio-scientific dilemmas of the century pertain to complex and chaotic contexts (e.g., climate change and management of pandemics), the vast majority (90+ percent) of school science education is demonstrated via simple and, very occasionally, complicated models (Fensham 2012; Zeyer 2021). Such education presents an idealized, almost mythical portrayal of science as always successful, fully in control, and having perfect predictive power. This image inevitably collides with the real-world science that is complex, not immune to errors, affected by scientists' biases, and often does not provide full explanations or satisfactory solutions. Thus, people become disillusioned and seek answers elsewhere. Johnson and Slovic (1995) show that when people are given the information about the uncertainty inherent in the science of environmental hazards, they perceive environmental agencies reporting risk information as less competent.

Attitudes toward Science

Discussions of attitudes toward science often focus on the concept of trust in science, composed of trust in the relative effectiveness of the scientific method and the resulting trust in science as a human enterprise (see chapter 8, "An Examination of the Multiple Dimensions of Public Trust in Science as Health Misinformation Roadblocks," in this volume).

At the beginning of this chapter, I made the claim that science, while imperfect, is the preferred method for answering certain kinds of questions over other tried alternatives. Accepting this requires some knowledge about science, understanding that science has developed a method for attempting to control bias and reduce subjectivity, as well as for seeking generalizability. For example, without understanding research principles of randomizations and blind assignment of participants to conditions, there is no reason to believe that the results of a clinical trial are more generalizable than one personal encounter.

At the same time, as discussed above, when knowledge about science is taught through simplified and idealized models, encounters with "real-world" science may lead to disillusionment and loss of trust. People conclude that if science cannot provide certainty, it does not have much value. For example, if science cannot develop medications that work for 100 percent of the recipients or predict who will respond, then "everyone is different," and untested remedies are as worthy of consideration as the best currently known treatment. Students are also not taught that, because of complexity and uncertainty, dissent is a normal part of the scientific process, nor are they taught how the discourse of legitimate dissent is different from scientific denialism (Solomon 2021).

Methodological imperfections of real-world science produce an effect that can be much more disconcerting than imperfect predictions. There is a growing concern in biomedicine and social sciences about the replication crisis, the phenomenon where the results of many published studies cannot be reproduced (Baker 2016; Ioannidis 2005). These studies are not fraudulent. While the problem is largely methodological, the methodological weaknesses are nuanced and not always reported (e.g., ending data collection as soon as significance is reached, and, thus, increasing the likelihood of a false positive). Understanding the causes of the replication crisis phenomenon and the scientific community's efforts to mitigate it require knowledge about science that could potentially be addressed at school but usually isn't (Fensham 2012; Solomon 2021; Zeyer 2021). Scientists are justifiably concerned about the potential impact of the public's awareness of the replication problem on trust in science (Hendriks et al. 2020).

While some studies treat trust in science as a single concept (see chapter 8, "An Examination of the Multiple Dimensions of Public Trust in Science as Health Misinformation Roadblocks," in this volume), others differentiate trust in the scientific method from trust in scientists and science as a social enterprise. Trust in scientists has to do with beliefs about individuals' honesty and goodwill, as well as beliefs about societal forces that fund, support, and promote science. School science education rarely presents science as an enterprise that is affected by money and power. In the real world, funding decisions drive the rate of discoveries and the degree to which different population groups are intended to benefit. Pharmaceutical lobbies are powerful. Scientists work in the "publish or perish" climate, and so choose questions and designs that are likely to produce positive results. Negative results don't get published, which increases the likelihood of false positives and contributes to the replication crisis. As with complexity and uncertainty (Johnson and Slovic 1995), loss of trust is possible when the public becomes aware of these issues.

At present, there are not many studies that demonstrate how people use science in daily life. There is also evidence that when it comes to people's attitudes toward science, especially as it pertains to socially controversial issues such as climate change and vaccination, political ideology may exert a stronger influence than science education (Gauchat 2012). Liberals are much more likely than conservatives to trust scientists, and the gap grows with education level (Gauchat 2012; Funk et al. 2020). At the same time, if people don't apply their science education to evaluate misinformation, it may not be because science literacy isn't useful in daily life, but because the way science is currently taught in schools does not prepare them for such engagement.

Science Literacy or Information Literacy?

In everyday life, most people encounter scientific information and misinformation in secondary sources. Feinstein et al. (2013) point out that in school science classes, unlike later in life, students are introduced to science from the "insider perspective" of professional scientists conducting science (e.g., modeling and arguing from evidence). While critical to science, these practices do not have direct application in the daily life of nonscientists. There are, however, other skills that are important to nonscientists:

> Studies show that competent outsiders make sophisticated judgments about the credibility of scientific claims based on cues like professional reputation, publication venue, institutional affiliation, and potential conflicts of interest, even when they do not understand technical nuances of experimental design or laboratory technique. (Feinstein et al. 2013)

Science educators do not call this competency of evaluating "credibility of claims based on cues" by a specific name. Library and information professionals are very familiar with this as information literacy, or "a set of aptitudes to locate, handle, evaluate and use information efficiently for a wide variety of purposes, generating competent citizens who are better able to perform their activities in the new society" (Pinto, Cordon, and Gomez Diaz 2010).

Science literacy and information literacy may be interconnected. For example, Keselman et al. (2021) found that higher scores on knowledge about science test were associated with an unwillingness to share nonevidence-based YouTube videos promoting dietary supplements as a cure for colds. Knowledge about science appeared to affect information behavior via information literacy as a mediator variable: knowledge about science affected information literacy, which, in turn, influenced the decision to share or not to share the video. More research is needed to characterize the relationship between science literacy and information literacy.

Beyond Science: Other Decision-Influencing Factors

Misinformation is a concern because it can lead people to suboptimal decisions when it comes to their health and well-being. However, as we engage in education and information outreach, we should remember that information derived from scientific evidence is only one of many factors that people bring to decision-making. Some of these factors are unique to the individual and not generalizable. For example, people have different values, circumstances, and quality of life considerations. American College of Physicians (2022) points out that care plans, while built on scientific evidence from biomedical research, should align with people's preferences, as some may be "less concerned about what might happen to them in the future and more focused on how they will feel tomorrow and next week." Some may forgo aggressive life-extending treatments with difficult side effects to enjoy remaining time with friends and family.

Besides the quality of life, people may value hope (which contributes to the quality of life), want to do socially acceptable things that keep them connected to their communities, and differ in how much risk they are willing to accept. Helping people understand and accept scientific evidence does not necessarily result in them taking a specific action recommended by health professionals or endorsed by public health authorities. Educators and information promoters should act as culture brokers who understand the strength and limitations of their culture, while being respectful of other cultures. This does not mean treating facts as relative and quality of evidence as unimportant but involves understanding that opinion change is hard, and behaviors have deep roots that need to be respected.

Final Practitioner Takeaways

More research is needed to understand how various aspects of science literacy enable the public to engage with science. At the present time, these are the practical recommendations I'd like to make to those who promote evidence-based health information and wrangle with misinformation:

- Recognize and acknowledge that science isn't "perfect."
- Promote understanding of uncertainty and complexity as inherent, unavoidable parts of science.
- Foster understanding of the mechanisms that make science self-correcting, conspiracy resistant, and a preferred way of building knowledge about the natural world (e.g., control of variables, random assignment, peer review, meta-science, consensus building).
- Explain the difference between legitimate dissent and denialism in science and medicine.
- Foster information literacy as it pertains to science and health/medicine questions.

- Connect information literacy initiatives to school science education.
- Support the public's engagement with science and scientists.
- Acknowledge the social and financial contexts of science.
- Understand concerns, be respectful, and understand that decisions will (and should) always involve subjective value components.

Acknowledgment

This work was carried out by the staff of the National Library of Medicine (NLM), National Institutes of Health, with support from NLM.

References

American College of Physicians. 2022. "Patient Priorities Care: Aligning Care with What Matters to Patients." *ACP Online*, February 2, 2022. ethosce.acponline.org/patient-priorities-care.

American Medical Association. n.d. "Guideline Central: My Library." Accessed February 14, 2022. https://www.guidelinecentral.com/library.

Baker, D. W., J. A. Gazmararian, M. V. Williams, T. Scott, R. M. Parker, D. Green, J. Ren, and J. Peel. 2004. "Health Literacy and Use of Outpatient Physician Services by Medicare Managed Care Enrollees." *Journal of General Internal Medicine* 19, no. 3: 215–20. https://doi.org/10.1111/j.1525-1497.2004.21130.x.

Baker, M. 2016. "1,500 Scientists Lift the Lid on Reproducibility." *Nature* 533, no. 7604: 452–54. https://doi.org/10.1038/533452a.

Bantock, G. G. 1899. "The Modern Doctrine of Bacteriology, or the Germ Theory of Disease." *British Medical Journal* 1, no. 1997: 846–48. https://doi.org/10.1136/bmj.1.1997.846.

Bell, A. J., Z. Arku, A. Bakari, S. A. Oppong, J. Youngblood, R. M. Adanu, and C. A. Moyer. 2020. "'This Sickness Is Not Hospital Sickness': A Qualitative Study of the Evil Eye as a Source of Neonatal Illness in Ghana." *Journal of Biosocial Science* 52, no. 2: 159–67. https://doi.org/10.1017/S0021932019000312.

Braden, G. "Bladder Cancer Dissolves in Less than 3 Minutes Using The Language of Emotion." Uploaded on May 31, 2011, YouTube video, 14:38. https://www.youtube.com/watch?app=desktop&v=GUbEgg6GklU.

Bybee, R., B. McCrae, and R. Laurie. 2009. "PISA 2006: An Assessment of Scientific Literacy." *Journal of Research in Science Teaching* 46, no. 8: 865–83.

Centers for Disease Control and Prevention. 2021. "Myths and Facts about COVID-19 Vaccines." Last modified December 15, 2021. https://www.cdc.gov/coronavirus/2019-ncov/vaccines/facts.html.

Churchill, Winston. 1947. "Speech at the House of Commons." Accessed February 10, 2022. https://api.parliament.uk/historic-hansard/commons/1947/nov/11/parliament-bill#S5CV0444P0_19471111_HOC_292.

Davis, T. C., M. S. Wolf, P. F. Bass, III, J. A. Thompson, H. H. Tilson, M. Neuberger, and R. M. Parker. 2006. "Literacy and Misunderstanding Prescription Drug Labels." *Annals of Internal Medicine* 145, no. 12: 887–94. https://doi.org/10.7326/0003-4819-145-12-200612190-00144.

Dhaliwal, D., and C. Mannion. 2020. "Antivaccine Messages on Facebook: Preliminary Audit." *Journal of Medical Internet Research Public Health Surveillance* 6, no. 4: e18878. https://doi.org/10.2196/18878; https://www.ncbi.nlm.nih.gov/pubmed/33079072.

Education.com. 2014. "Science Labs in Elementary School?" Accessed February 10, 2022. https://www.education.com/magazine/article/Science_Labs_Elementary_School.

Feinstein, N. W., S. Allen, and E. Jenkins. 2013. "Outside the Pipeline: Reimagining Science Education for Nonscientists." *Science* 340, no. 6130: 314–17. https://doi.org/10.1126/science.1230855.

Fensham, P. J. 2012. "Preparing Citizens for a Complex World: The Grand Challenge of Teaching Socio-Scientific Issues in Science Education." In *Science|Environment|Health. Towards a Renewed Pedagogy for Science Education*, edited by A. Zeyer and R. Kyburz-Graber, 7–29. Dordrecht: Springer.

Funk, Cary, Alec Tyson, Brian Kennedy, and Courtney Johnson. 2020. "Science and Scientists Held in High Esteem Across Global Publics." *Pew Research Center*, September 29, 2000. https://www.pewresearch.org/science/2020/09/29/science-and-scientists-held-in-high-esteem-across-global-publics/.

Gauchat, G. 2012. "Politicization of Science in the Public Sphere: A Study of Public Trust in the United States, 1974 to 2010." *American Sociological Review* 77: 167–87. https://doi.org/10.1177/0003122412438225.

Ghandi, L. "A History of 'Snake Oil Salesmen.'" *Code Switch*, NPR, August 26, 2013. https://www.npr.org/sections/codeswitch/2013/08/26/215761377/a-history-of-snake-oil-salesmen.

Guyatt, G. H. 1991. "Evidence-Based Medicine." *ACP Journal Club* 114, no. 2: A16. https://doi.org/10.7326/acpjc-1991-114-2-a16.

Hendriks, F., D. Kienhues, and R. Bromme. 2020. "Replication Crisis = Trust Crisis? The Effect of Successful vs Failed Replications on Laypeople's Trust in Researchers and Research." *Public Understanding of Science* 29, no. 3: 270–88. https://doi.org/10.1177/0963662520902383.

Herndon, Astead, host. "Rural Tennessee's Vaccine Hesitators." The Daily (podcast). May 10, 2021. Accessed February 10, 2022. https://www.nytimes.com/2021/05/10/podcasts/the-daily/covid-vaccine-hesitancy-white-republicans.html?showTranscript=1.

Institute of Medicine (US) Immunization Safety Review Committee. 2004. *Immunization Safety Review: Vaccines and Autism.* Washington, DC: National Academies Press.

Ioannidis, J. P. 2005. "Why Most Published Research Findings Are False." *PLOS Medicine* 2, no. 8: e124. https://doi.org/10.1371/journal.pmed.0020124.

Jenkins, E. 2000. "Science for All: Time for a Paradigm Shift?" In *Improving Science Education: The Contribution of Research*, edited by R. Millar, J. Leach, and J. Osborne, 207–26. Buckingham: Open University Press.

Johnson, B. B., and P. Slovic. 1995. "Presenting Uncertainty in Health Risk Assessment: Initial Studies of Its Effects on Risk Perception and Trust." *Risk Analysis: An Official Publication of the Society for Risk Analysis* 15, no. 4: 485–94. doi:10.1111/j.1539-6924.1995.tb00341.x.

Keselman, A., C. Arnott Smith, A. C. Murcko, and D. R. Kaufman. 2019. "Evaluating the Quality of Health Information in a Changing Digital Ecosystem." *Journal of Medical Internet Research* 21, no. 2: e11129. https://doi.org/10.2196/11129.

Keselman, A., C. Arnott Smith, G. Leroy, and D. R. Kaufman. 2021. "Factors Influencing Willingness to Share Health Misinformation Videos on the Internet: Web-Based Survey." *Journal of Medical Internet Research* 23, no. 12: e30323. https://doi.org/10.2196/30323.

Keselman, A., D. R. Kaufman, and V. L. Patel. 2004. "'You Can Exercise Your Way Out of HIV' and Other Stories: The Role of Biological Knowledge in Adolescents' Evaluation of Myths." *Journal of Science Education* 88, no. 4: 548–73.

Layton, D., E. Jenkins, S. Macgill, and A. Davey. 1993. *Inarticulate Science? Perspectives on the Public Understanding of Science and Some Implications for Science Education.* Leeds, England: University of Leeds.

Lee, S.-Y. D., A. M. Arozullah, Y. I. Cho, K. Crittenden, and D. Vicencio. 2009. "Health Literacy, Social Support, and Health Status among Older Adults." *Educational Gerontology* 35, no. 3: 191–201.

Moore, R., D. E. Willis, S. K. Shah, R. S. Purvis, X. Shields, and P. A. McElfish. 2021 "'The Risk Seems Too High': Thoughts and Feelings About COVID-19 Vaccination." *International Journal of Environmental Research and Public Health* 18, no. 16. https://doi.org/10.3390/ijerph18168690.

Murri, Nelda. 2021. "Dimethyl Fumarate (TECFIDERA): A New Small Molecule Disease-Modifying Drug for Multiple Sclerosis." *Medscape.* https://www.medscape.com/viewarticle/821109.

National Academies of Sciences, Engineering, and Medicine. 2016. *Science Literacy: Concepts, Contexts, and Consequences.* Washington, DC: The National Academies Press. https://doi.org/10.17226/23595.

Next Generation Science Standards Lead States. 2013. *Next Generation Science Standards: For States, By States.* Washington, DC: The National Academies Press.

Organisation for Economic Cooperation and Development. 2019. *PISA 2018 Assessment and Analytical Framework*. Paris: OECD Publishing. https://doi.org/10.1787/b25efab8-en.

Pinto, M., J. A. Cordón, and R. Gómez Díaz. 2010. "Thirty Years of Information Literacy (1977–2007): A Terminological, Conceptual and Statistical Analysis." *Journal of Education for Library and Information Science* 42, no. 1: 3–19. https://doi.org/10.1177/0961000609345091.

Pogue, K., J. L. Jensen, C. K. Stancil, D. G. Ferguson, S. J. Hughes, E. J. Mello, R. Burgess et al. 2020. "Influences on Attitudes Regarding Potential COVID-19 Vaccination in the United States." *Vaccines* (Basel) 8, no. 4. https://doi.org/10.3390/vaccines8040582.

Riddle, M. C., W. T. Cefalu, P. H. Evans, H. C. Gerstein, M. A. Nauck, W. K. Oh, A. E. Rothberg, et al. 2021. "Consensus Report: Definition and Interpretation of Remission in Type 2 Diabetes." *Diabetes Care*. https://doi.org/10.2337/dci21-0034.

Roberts, K. J. 1999. "Patient Empowerment in the United States: A Critical Commentary." *Health Expectations* 2, no. 2 (May): 82–92. https://doi.org/10.1046/j.1369-6513.1999.00048.x.

Sackett, D. L., W. M. Rosenberg, J. A. Gray, R. B. Haynes, and W. S. Richardson. 1996. "Evidence Based Medicine: What It Is and What It Isn't." *British Medical Journal* 312, no. 7023: 71–72. https://doi.org/10.1136/bmj.312.7023.71.

Sivaramakrishnan, M., and V. L. Patel. 1993. "Role of Traditional Knowledge in Explanation of Childhood Nutritional Deficiency by Indian Mothers." *Journal of Nutrition Education* 25: 121–29.

Snowden, D. J., and M. E. Boone. 2007. "A Leader's Framework for Decision Making. A Leader's Framework for Decision Making." *Harvard Business Review* 85, no. 11: 68–76, 149. https://www.ncbi.nlm.nih.gov/pubmed/18159787.

Solomon, M. 2021. "Trust: The Need for Public Understanding of How Science Works." *Hastings Center Report* 51, Suppl 1: S36–S39.

Tinari, Paul D. n.d. "Circumcision Permanently Alters the Brain." Circumcision Resource Center. Accessed February 10, 2022. https://circumcision.org/circumcision-permanently-alters-the-brain/.

Tomeny, T. S., C. J. Vargo, and S. El-Toukhy. 2017. "Geographic and Demographic Correlates of Autism-Related Anti-Vaccine Beliefs on Twitter, 2009-15." *Social Science Medicine* 191: 168–75. https://doi.org/10.1016/j.socscimed.2017.08.041.

US Food and Drug Administration. n.d. "Milestones of Drug Regulation in the United States." Accessed February 7, 2022. https://www.fda.gov/media/109482/download.

Vosniadou, S. 2019. "The Development of Students' Understanding of Science." *Frontiers in Education* 4, no. 32. pp. 1–6.

White, S., J. Chen, and R. Atchison. 2008. "Relationship of Preventive Health Practices and Health Literacy: A National Study." *American Journal of Health Behavior* 32, no. 3: 227–42. https://doi.org/10.5555/ajhb.2008.32.3.227.

Zahid, H. M., and M. A. Alsayb. 2021. "Assessing the Knowledge and Attitude toward COVID-19 Vaccination in Saudi Arabia." *International Journal of Environmental Research and Public Health* 18, no. 15. https://doi.org/10.3390/ijerph18158185.

Zeyer, A. 2021. "Coping with Structural Uncertainty in Complex Living Systems." In *Science|Environment|Health. Towards a Science Pedagogy of Complex Living Systems. Towards a Renewed Pedagogy for Science Education*, edited by A. Zeyer and R. Kyburz-Graber, 11–29. Dordrecht: Springer.

Zhukivska S, Lambert FB. 2021. Autism. [Essential Evidence Topics] Editors MH Ebell, MA Smith and GF Ferenchick. Accessed February 14, 2022. Available from https://www.essentialevidenceplus.com/.

8

An Examination of the Multiple Dimensions of Public Trust in Science as Health Misinformation Roadblocks

Alla Keselman and Amanda J. Wilson

Disclaimer: The opinions expressed by the authors are their own and this material should not be interpreted as representing the official viewpoint of the US Department of Health and Human Services, the National Institutes of Health, or the National Library of Medicine.

Does the Spread of Health Misinformation Imply Mistrust in Science?

THE SPREAD OF ONLINE health misinformation is a phenomenon that cannot be explained away by the lack of reliable information. It also cannot be fully accounted for by the public's lack of awareness of the views of the health establishment. There are certainly cases when people hold health beliefs without realizing that their beliefs are inconsistent with the prevailing expert opinion of the day. However, there are also many cases when people hold beliefs and take actions while knowing that these are not endorsed by the medical and public health establishment.

We are writing this chapter during the second year of the COVID-19 pandemic. At this time, three vaccines are authorized and recommended in the United States, where the authors live. These vaccines were developed by scientists working for major biotechnology companies and leading federal biomedical research organizations, tested in clinical trials, approved by the Food and Drug Administration (FDA), and recommended by the Centers for Disease Control and Prevention (CDC) as safe and effective. Yet, many Americans are hesitant to get vaccinated, despite ample encouragement from the CDC, federal and local governments, and health professionals.

Skepticism about conventional public health recommendations and medical treatments, as well as preference for nonevidence-based measures, is not unique to the COVID-19 era. In discussing this phenomenon, media commentators often talk about the decline of trust in science in American society (Jewett 2020; Parikh 2021). Are Americans mistrustful of science? What, exactly, does this mean, and how can this trust be regained? This chapter is our attempt to address these questions.

Attitudes toward Science and Scientists

Trust in science is not a simple concept; it is multidimensional (Achterberg et al. 2017). People may differ in their trust in the scientific method as a way of generating knowledge, or in their trust in specific techniques that scientists use. They may also differ in their trust in scientists and scientific institutions. Achterberg et al. (2017) show that trust in the scientific method and trust in scientific institutions are distinct concepts, and the correlation between the two is low. Trust in scientists can be further subdivided into distinctive dimensions, related to the perception of their expertise, care, honesty, and commitment (Hovland et al. 1953; Peters et al. 1997). People may view scientists as skillful and knowledgeable (i.e., having expertise) but be unsure about their commitment to the public good. People may also perceive scientists as experts, but cold rather than caring, and not committed to solving problems of interest to the communities in which people live.

Additionally, people may differ in their attitudes toward various societal and economic forces that affect scientific enterprise: funding organizations that determine research priorities, academic institutions that confer legitimacy on scientists, the government that determines science and public health policies, corporations that bring their financial interests to the table, media that communicates scientific findings, and many others. Assessing whether Americans trust science requires starting with the definition of "trust in science." Different studies define it differently, focusing on different dimensions of this trust.

Despite frequently stated concerns about declining trust in science, overall, American willingness to profess trust in scientists has been rather stable over the past decades. Since 1972, the General Social Survey has been polling Americans about their trust in different institutions and leaders (NORC, n.d.). Compared with trust in other social institutions, such as Congress, the military, and major companies, trust in science as an institution has been both relatively high and stable over the polled period, with 37–46 percent of respondents expressing "a great deal of confidence" in the people "running the institution" (Krause et al. 2019). Yet, while the relative standing of science among other societal institutions is high, the absolute numbers point out that, no matter what year we take, going back to 1970s, most people in the United States voice less than "a great deal of confidence" in the people running scientific institutions.

Trust in the scientific method appears to be higher than trust in the people who run science. In a 2019 Pew Research study involving a large sample of US adults, the majority (63 percent) believed that the scientific method "generally produces accurate conclusions." A significant minority (35 percent) felt that the scientific method "can be used to produce any conclusions the researcher wants." While confidence in science was strongly influenced by the level of science knowledge, the effect interacted with political partisanship. For example, individuals with a high level of science knowledge—only 14 percent of Democrats, but 40 percent of Republicans—believed that science "can be used to produce any conclusions the researcher wants" (Funk 2020). The methodology of the Pew survey underscores the complexity of interpreting trust in science responses as assessed by a simple questionnaire. While the question was meant to assess trust in the scientific method, someone stating that the method can be used to produce any result may be expressing mistrust in the people manipulating the method, rather than the method itself.

Americans are most optimistic about science when the question is phrased in terms of its benefits to society, with 73 percent feeling that the societal impact is "mostly positive," 3 percent believing it is "mostly negative," and 23 percent calling it mixed (Funk 2020). Attitudes toward the impact of science are also affected by science knowledge. Among respondents with a high level of science knowledge, the percentage of Americans who view the societal impact of science as mostly positive is 89 percent, while among those with a low level of science knowledge, it is 54 percent (Funk 2020).

Achterberg et al. (2017) investigated whether there was a gap between the public's trust in the scientific method and the public's confidence in scientific institutions, with stronger trust in the method, the phenomenon the authors called *science confidence gap*. They noted that, observationally, groups that the science mainstream viewed as antiscience did not actually reject the value of the scientific method. For example, anti-vaccine groups and proponents of alternative treatments frame their arguments in the language of scientific discourse and referred to "data" and "studies," albeit collected outside the corruption of the establishment. The study, indeed, found evidence of the gap, as well as a strong association between the gap and education level. For those with less education, the gap was significantly greater. Testing two explanatory models, the authors concluded that the gap was rooted in cultural discomfort induced by modernity among those with less education and income. According to the authors, people who are socially disadvantaged are more likely to experience the world as threatening, rapidly changing, and devoid of meaning, feeling disillusioned about the value of science in their lives and not trusting its institutions.

Americans' level of trust in science is comparable to that of citizens of other developed countries (Gallup 2019). An exception that distinguishes the United States from the rest of the world is the strength of the effect of ideology and political party membership on trust in science. While in many places around the world conservatives are less trusting of science, the difference is most prominent in the United States (Gallup 2019).

Public Understanding of the Nature of Science and Uncertainty

Trust in science has to be linked to a certain vision of science, the kind of questions it addresses, the perceived likelihood of errors and controversies, and ways to handle them. This vision is usually acquired through K–12 school science education. Unfortunately, the way the scientific process is taught in schools is rather different from the process as it is practiced by scientists; science taught in schools is reduced to simple models—linear and idealized (Fensham 2012; Zeyer 2021). Researchers in the growing field of science/environment/health point out that over 90 percent of school science focuses on simple problems, such as predicting an outcome from a few well-defined known variables. In contrast, the most pressing twenty-first-century problems, largely related to health and the environment, are very complex, with a high degree of uncertainty in the models (Fensham 2012; Zeyer 2021). Moreover, real-world science is an evolving process that, like all human enterprises, is open to errors, biases, and special interests. In recognition of those risks, science has developed corrective mechanisms that include experimental controls, peer review, and attempts at replication of findings. Consensus is built through dialogue and may never be quite reached on all the nuances.

When trust in science is connected to a simplistic vision of science, there is a risk of disillusionment. When people hold such simplistic visions, they expect science to provide certainty and feel disappointed by science's failure to make an accurate prediction or a lack of consensus among scientists. Scientific debate may then signify to them that science is flawed and unreliable. Vested interests exploit this unrealistic vision of science, stressing uncertainty and lack of consensus on certain issues as a way to influence public opinion about large areas of study. Interest groups (e.g., tobacco and climate) fuel suspicion about uncertainty, presenting scientific debate as abnormal and exaggerating disagreement among scientists (Solomon 2021).

The public's difficulty in understanding and accepting uncertainty poses a problem for the media and public health. Kreps and Kriner (2020) note two ways in which media can deal with uncertainty: (1) acknowledging and addressing it and (2) presenting the public with a simplification. Kreps and Kriner (2020) studied the effect of scientific uncertainty surrounding COVID-19 on the public trust. They found that "acknowledging and explaining the uncertainty embedded in models does not increase trust for science and its role in policymaking." They also found "conditional evidence that criticism of COVID-19 science emphasizing uncertainty can erode public confidence in some contexts."

Johnson and Slovic (1995) studied the impact of discussing risk magnitude uncertainties of environmental hazards on respondents' perception of an environmental agency. They found that while reporting uncertainty increased the perception of an agency's honesty, about a third of the participants viewed such reports as a sign of incompetence. Perception of honesty did not offset the perception of incompetence, as it was possible to view the agency as more honest and less competent simultaneously. Those with a better understanding of uncertainty in science were more likely to view reporting uncertainty as a sign of honesty and *not* incompetence. Yet, participants generally had little understanding of uncertainty in science.

Kreps and Kriner (2020) conclude that, in the short run, presenting the public with a simplification is a better strategy. Sadly, each approach has disadvantages when trust in science is concerned. While, given the negative impact of addressing uncertainty, the approach has an appeal in a pandemic, which was the context of the Kreps and Kriner's study, its disadvantages are also clear. When public health agencies and mainstream media do not address uncertainty, both uncertainties and the official choice to ignore them will be exploited and exaggerated by those wishing to minimize the danger of the pandemic. This will also provide fuel for conspiracy theories.

The most appropriate place for introducing people to the concept of uncertainty in science is the K–12 science classroom. Given the complexity of the topic, shortcuts are hard to build. The K–12 classroom is also the place for teaching students to be educated consumers of scientific information. In a powerful essay, Solomon (2021), a philosopher of science, writes that school science the way it is currently taught "does not include many of the epistemic tools needed to do and evaluate science." She also stresses that today's school science education does not present science as a process characterized by dissent, which hurts trust in science when people invariably encounter this dissent in socially charged science matters. Solomon distinguishes between legitimate scientific dissent and scientific denialism (Longino 1990; Solomon 2021).

When two parties disagree on matters within a scientific domain (e.g., vaccination effectiveness), members of the public often do not have the knowledge needed to evaluate the content of arguments. However, they can evaluate how the parties participate in discourse. This involves evaluating the level of expertise presented by each party, their openness to have their ideas investigated, their responsiveness to criticism, and commitment to empirical accuracy. Solomon (2021) stresses that science education should normalize scientific dissent, distinguish it from denialism, and provide people with tools for discriminating between the two.

The Role of Trust in Government

Trust in government is important when it comes to trust in science and evidence-based health information. After all, people realize that a significant amount of scientific research is funded and supported by the government and that the government is involved in many aspects of health care. A Gallup survey (2019) found that, across the world, people's level of trust in their national institutions, such as the government, the military, and the judiciary system, predicted their trust in science.

Americans have been showing declining trust in the federal government since the era of the Vietnam War and Watergate (Cooper 2018). When measured in 2010, only 22 percent of respondents said they could trust the "government in Washington . . . almost always or most of the time" (Kohut 2010). However, similar to trust in science, trust in government is not a simple concept, as the government has many functions and is represented by many organizations and institutions. Questions about trust in the CDC or the National Institutes of Health (NIH) may produce different associations and elicit different responses than questions about trust in the "government in Washington." According to the Gallup 2019 survey, 61 percent of Americans trust medical and health advice from the government.

Several studies investigated Americans' trust in the government's public health recommendations during epidemics. For example, Freimuth et al. (2014) studied the public's trust in the government's public health recommendations during the early stages of the 2009 H1N1 epidemic. These authors conceptualized trust as a multidimensional concept consisting of openness, honesty, benevolence (acting in the public's best interests), protective intent, and a sense of responsibility. They found that trust in the government was low, averaging 2.3 out of 4 on their scale. In another study, Vardavas et al. (2020) found that, of the surveyed residents of G7 countries, Americans reported the second lowest level of trust in their government's future decisions concerning COVID-19 containment measures. In Freimuth et al. (2014), trust in the government positively correlated with education, self-reported level of knowledge about H1N1, attention to news about H1N1, and presence of H1N1 cases in the respondent's community. With respect to specific government entities, participants generally trusted the CDC more than their local public health officials (Freimuth et al. 2014). Studies also show that on matters of health, people trust their doctors and nurses more than governmental agencies (92 percent vs. 61 percent of respondents in the Gallup 2019 survey) (Freimuth et al. 2014; Gallup 2019).

Unsurprisingly, trust in government recommendations translates into action. Quinn et al. (2013) and Mesch and Schwirian (2015) found that trust in the federal government during the H1N1 pandemic correlated with willingness to receive vaccines. Perception of honesty and the government officials' willingness to live their advice is very important. The immunization of President Obama's daughters significantly increased trust in government as a source of recommendation (Quinn et al. 2013).

On some topics, mistrust in the government increases sharply, especially in groups affected by discrimination and socioeconomic disparities. For example, in the Whetten et al. (2006) study of individuals living with HIV, 47 percent of minority respondents and 23 percent of nonminority respondents either believed or allowed for the possibility that the government "created AIDS to kill minorities." Those with more trust were more likely to utilize care appropriately.

Political Ideology and Trust in Science and Scientists

Political ideology, defined as a position on the conservative/liberal axis, exerts a very strong influence on trust in science among Americans, with conservatives expressing greater mistrust (Funk et al. 2020). While 67 percent of Americans who self-identify as liberal Democrats report having strong trust in scientists, only 17 percent of conservative Republicans do. While party affiliation also matters, it is less important than self-proclaimed ideology, and the two do not always align (Gauchat 2012). For example, in the above Pew Research Center survey (Funk et al. 2020), 43 percent of moderate and conservative Democrats and 26 percent of moderate and liberal Republicans have strong trust in scientists, evidencing a much smaller gap than between liberal Democrats and conservative Republicans, 17 versus 50 percentage points. While the effect of ideology on trust in science is rather universal, the magnitude of this effect in the US samples is more prominent than in other countries (Funk et al. 2020).

US conservatives' distrust of the scientific enterprise is a relatively recent phenomenon. In the analysis of the 1972–2010 General Social Survey (GSS) data on trust in science (NORC, n.d.), Gauchat (2012) compared the trajectory of trust in the "scientific community" among liberals, conservatives, and moderates. He found that conservatives started the almost forty-year-long period with the highest level of trust in the scientific community and finished it with the lowest. The change cannot be accounted for by a decline in science education among conservatives, as conservatives did not become less educated, but, rather, educated conservatives lost trust in science (Gauchat 2012).

The effect of ideology on attitudes toward science, however, differs depending on scientific issues. Not all science issues involve a partisan divide in trust. For example, a large majority of Americans of all ideologies value space exploration and see the findings of its research program as reliable. On the other end of the spectrum are questions of climate change, evolution, vaccination, and stem cell research, where respondents who identify as conservatives voice greater skepticism about relevant research findings and express less trust toward scientists (Lewandowski and Oberauer 2021). Growing prominence of these issues in the societal discourse on science co-occurs with the decline in conservative trust in science. For example, the time of the writing of this chapter is marked by a striking partisan divide among US conservatives and liberals in their attitudes toward COVID-19 vaccination. Overall, trust in science and scientists during the pandemic has been significantly lower among conservatives than among liberals (Agley et al. 2020).

Researchers interested in the impact of ideology on attitudes toward science have postulated several hypotheses as to why the phenomenon of the conservatives' mistrust of science exists. One possibility is the economic advantage of the mistrust, as many socially controversial scientific issues of the day, such as climate change, pose conclusions that have negative implications for conservative-backed corporate interests (Gauchat 2012). Additionally, the growing importance of these issues in the past several decades gave rise to regulatory science and regulatory organizations such as the EPA, which also conflict with some corporate interests and conservative viewpoints (Gauchat 2012). Some scientific questions and resulting modern biomedical developments and social views clash with conservative morality, particularly those pertaining to gender, sexuality, and reproduction (Frazzetto 2004).

In addition to potential clashes between conservative interests and viewpoints with some science agendas, there may be conservative concerns about the scientists' values. For example, there is (largely accurate) public perception that academia is a liberal institution, because liberals tend to self-select into academic careers (Gross 2013). This may lead conservatives to mistrust scientists, whom they may perceive as belonging to "the opposite camp."

Some researchers attempted to look for an explanation in the broader epistemology of conservatism. For example, Gauchat (2011) posits that, compared to liberals, conservatives are more likely to define science not as a method, but as one of many forms of knowledge, others being religion and common sense. According to this view, to be trustworthy, science needs to conform to the other forms. When there is a discrepancy, science does not automatically take precedence.

Now is a good time to recall that "trust in science" is a multidimensional concept. Mann and Schleifer (2020) note that conservatives who do not trust the scientific community still often believe that scientific research is beneficial for society. In fact, while conservatives' trust in the scientific community has declined significantly since the 1970s (Gauchat 2012; NORC, n.d.), their belief about science benefitting society does not change. Mann and Schleifer (2020) also point out that in the societal discourse about science, conservatives do not wish to cede scientific epistemology and the value of the scientific method to liberals. Rather than criticizing science as a way of gaining knowledge, they criticize the objectivity and methodologies of what they see as a biased, government-sponsored, liberal-leaning scientific establishment. To counter that, they have established conservative scientific institutions (Mann and Schleifer 2020) like think tanks and evangelical universities, thus, aiming to challenge scientific consensus using its own language and legitimization criteria.

Religion and Trust in Science

Studies that look at the impact of ideology on trust in science and scientists often also look at the impact of religion. For example, Agley et al. (2020) found a significant negative association between high religious commitment and trust in science. The relationship holds when controlled for political ideology, income, and science knowledge. Gauchat (2011, 2012) examined a correlation between frequent church attendance and distrust in science. The GSS data for the period between the late 1970s and 2018 also shows this discrepancy between Christians (the US religious majority) and the non-Christians (Krause et al. 2019). In GSS, the level of confidence in science among non-religious Americans increased, widening the trust gap between Christians and the non-religious.

When it comes to the compatibility of scientific and religious perspectives, the thorniest misalignment is between scriptural literalism and studies of the origin of the universe and the theory of evolution. When religion and science are in disagreement, the majority of religious Americans believe in the religious explanation (Gallup 2019). In this choice, religious Americans are different from religious citizens of other high-income countries (Gallup 2019). For example, Rissler et al. (2014) found that religious students are more likely to reject the theory of evolution than non-religious students, even when they understand that the theory is not contested by scientists. As literalism conflicts with some science subject matter, and, therefore, may make religious individuals doubt the methods used to derive information they perceive as conflicting with indisputable truth, this may extend to doubts about the scientific method in general (Evans 2013).

Another possible contributing factor that exacerbates the mistrust of scientists in the eyes of some religious Americans is the scientists' perceived and actual non-religiosity (Beauchamp and Rios 2020). Beauchamp and Rios (2020) point out that while 80 percent of Americans say they believe in God, only 25 percent of scientists at elite universities do. As Americans view atheists as less moral than believers (Brown-Iannuzzi et al. 2018), they may view scientists as unconcerned about the moral consequences of their work (Rutjens and Heine 2016). In support of this hypothesis, Beauchamp and Rios (2020) find that religious people perceive atheist scientists as less trustworthy than religious scientists.

Education Level and Trust in Science

When it comes to trust in science, education matters, but not as much as we would have predicted or wished. According to Gallup (2019), at the global level, "having the opportunity to learn science at school is the single most influential predictor of trust in scientists." Certainly, people with secondary education feel more at ease with science as part of the modern societal discourse than people who did not attend secondary school. Consequently, trust in science and scientists is greater in the countries where the overwhelming majority receive secondary education. However, in the developed world, the effect of education is relatively small—while having very little education is detrimental, having a great deal of education can still leave one mistrustful of science and scientists (Lewandowski et al. 2013).

Those with more education have an overall better understanding of the scientific method and more trust in it (Achterberg et al. 2017). This effect, however, does not persist across all science topics, becoming weak or non-existent as topics grow controversial. For example, Gallup (2019) finds no relationship between the level of science education and attitudes toward vaccination. While in some places, including North America, people with more education tend to believe that vaccines are safe, the opposite is true in some other regions (e.g., Eastern Europe).

Drummond and Fischhoff (2017) studied the impact of general education level on the interaction between ideology and trust in science. They found that for controversial issues, such as human evolution and climate change, education widened, rather than narrowed, the divide. Greater general education, science education, and science literacy were associated with greater polarization between political liberals and conservatives on their willingness to accept the scientific consensus. The authors note that such findings are compatible with two explanations, both in line with psychological and educational literature. The first is "motivated reasoning" (Kunda 1990), or human tendency to go to great lengths to protect their worldviews. In doing so, individuals employ many strategies like selective evidence search and selective attention to evidence, seeking information to justify a position, rather than solve a problem. Education may make people more adept at this justification construction. The existence of previously mentioned conservative scientific institutions creates a framework within which educated conservatives can mistrust science and value it at the same time (Mann and Schleifer 2020). Another hypothesis is "miscalibration," when education-induced confidence in one's knowledge grows faster than the actual knowledge (Moore and Healy 2008).

As explained in "Public Understanding of the Nature of Science and Uncertainty," we interpret the limited effect of education on trust in science as related to how science is taught in schools, rather than by the lack of connection between understanding the nature of science and trust in science and scientists.

Social Contextual Factors, Medical Mistrust, and Trust in Science

Understanding trust in science among diverse populations is a growing area of research (Jaiswal 2019). In addition to the lens of race and ethnicity, other social contextual factors—particularly those contributing to health disparities—influence trust (Petersen et al. 2020; Larson et al. 2018; Jamison et al. 2019). Although all populations experience a lack of trust in science (Whetten et al. 2006), when it comes to science as an evidence base for medicine, the constellation of trust factors for those experiencing health disparities is even more complex and includes the concept of medical mistrust (Jaiswal 2019). While biomedical researchers, health professionals, and health policymakers work with the public in related but distinct roles, communities affected by health disparities may see these roles as a hostile conglomerate representing "the other." The affected communities' attitude toward this "other" may be shaped by the quality (and their perception) of medical care they receive, history of abuse by biomedical researchers, and the overall history of social injustice and inequities (Best et al. 2021; Jaiswal et al. 2019; Jamison et al. 2019). For racial and ethnic minorities, those with low socioeconomic status, and other populations experiencing health disparities, medical mistrust influences not only trust in science but also health behaviors (Benkert et al. 2019). It is important to note that mistrust, an active distrust (Christopher et al. 2008), is not the same as the absence of trust (Webb Hooper et al. 2019; Jaiswal 2019). Rather, mistrust is distinct from interpersonal trust and a consequence of historical and ongoing racism and social exclusion (Benkert et al. 2019; Best et al. 2021; Evans and Gusmano 2021; Jamison et al. 2019; Jaiswal and Halkitis 2019). In a social context, trust in science and research and mistrust in medicine are often intertwined.

Contributing factors to health disparities and other health inequalities are social determinants of health (SDoH), the conditions affecting health, functioning, and quality of life based on where people are born, live, learn, work, play, worship, and age (Healthy People 2030, n.d.). Added to that are the beliefs and attitudes toward institutions of those experiencing health disparities building over time. Best et al. (2021), in discussing implications for ethical public health practice in COVID-19 response, document how the effects of inequities and injustices accumulate over time and are transferred intergenerationally to the Black community. Morton et al. (2013) developed a tribal institutional review board (IRB) as part of the Native American Research Center for Health (NARCH) "to create new levels of trust and a more beneficial atmosphere for research and recruitment" (2161). Several characteristics and requirements of the IRB were specifically designed to address both trust and the widely held beliefs that tribal members would be "guinea pigs" for researchers (Morton et al. 2013). Efforts to build resilience to health misinformation by addressing trust in science are compounded in the context of SDoH, requiring multilevel, multi-actor solutions (Benkert et al. 2019; Best et al. 2021; Evans and Gusmano 2021; Jaiswal 2019; Jaiswal and Halkitis 2019; Jaiswal et al. 2020).

Webb Hooper et al. (2019) categorized five different levels at which trust needed to be addressed in an urban community through a phenomenological listening study: intrapersonal, interpersonal, institutional, community, and policy. Their work revealed higher medical distrust levels in Black and deaf/hearing impaired participants than in other participant groups; they found that community distrust is a multilevel problem; and they indicated that "low trust and distrust also result from perceived inequities created and maintained by institutions, community structural factors, and policy" (sec. 4). Evans and Gusmano (2021) found that among Black mothers, a contributing factor of HPV vaccine hesitancy was fueled by mistrust of science, medicine, and the government. Participants' attitudes were shaped by their own lived experiences and perceived experiences of others in the context of racial discrimination in health care and structural racism. Their recommended intervention is racial justice actions at the interpersonal, institutional, community, and policy levels over the short- and long-term, with the caveat that "trust and reciprocity are inseparable" (last para.). Policy actions targeting SDoH and structural inequalities are part of the multilevel and multi-actor solutions needed to address mistrust and enhance trust across all social contexts.

Media and Attitudes toward Science

Much of the time, the public learns about scientific advances and their practical applications from the media. This gives media the opportunity to shape attitudes. Quality coverage of science news may promote a positive image of science and scientists and foster science literacy. These impacts may increase trust in science and science-based public health recommendations. For example, in a 2009 study by Quinn, following the news more closely was associated with a greater willingness to get vaccinated against the H1N1 virus (Quinn et al. 2013).

Conversely, partisan coverage may reduce trust in science. In the United States, liberal and conservative media outlets send different messages about issues such as climate change and vaccine efficacy. Viewers exposed to conservative channels that espouse skepticism about global warming have beliefs concordant with that skepticism (Feldman et al. 2012). Hmielowski et al. (2014) show that the media effect on public opinion about global warming is mediated by its effect on trust in scientists. Exposure to conservative media decreases trust in scientists, which, in turn, leads to climate beliefs that diverge from the scientific consensus. The same study notes that liberal media, however, increases trust in scientists. Recently, Dhanani and Franz (2020) looked at how news consumption patterns affected vulnerability to COVID-19 misinformation. They found that people who relied on Fox News and Facebook as their information sources for COVID-19 scored significantly higher on misinformation, while those who relied on CNN scored significantly lower on misinformation. Dhanani and Franz (2020) did not measure the relationship between media choices and trust in science and public health agencies. However, this relationship may be suggested by the finding that participants with lower misinformation scores had higher trust in the CDC.

As discussed in "Attitudes toward Science and Scientists," the public's simplistic vision of science may result in a situation where media coverage of complex and controversial topics arouses mistrust in science. Additionally, as media sources are in competition for viewership and readership, and sensations and controversies attract greater audiences, controversies may receive a disproportionate amount of media spotlight (Cooper et al. 2008)."Newsworthy" science topics are also more likely to include contradictory messages. Nagler (2014) found that when people are exposed to contradictory media messages about controversial health and nutrition topics, they lose trust in health advice from nutritional scientists, even about topics that are not controversial. More research is needed on public perception of the coverage of scientific complexity in the media.

Interventions

Several themes emerge when reviewing interventions to build or regain the public's trust in science that appear in the literature: the choice of spokesperson, increasing trust in scientists, and institutional actions to demonstrate trustworthiness. More often than not, engagement is central to these activities. Empirically derived instruments that define and assess trust in science include communications items, from which interventions can be developed (Dave et al. 2018; Nadelson et al. 2014; Nandyal et al. 2021; Todd et al. 2018). Example items include *We cannot trust science because it moves too slowly* (Nadelson et al. 2014), *Scientists don't care if laypersons understand their work* (Nadelson et al. 2014), and *Regarding the information about the COVID-19 pandemic, I hope to see the interpretation of authoritative scientists* (Gu and Feng 2021).

Using trusted messengers—in the form of community leaders and influencers who are equipped with evidence-informed recommendations—to address these and other trust-scale items is a common starting point (Freimuth et al. 2014; World Health Organization 2020). Abadie et al. (2018) recommend the use of community advisors and/or community-based organizations, as well as culturally competent staff, to maintain trust, while admonishing that trust is earned, nontransferable, and incrementally built over time. Messengers are a critical, not sole, component of any strategy to build or regain trust.

Other interventions aim to engender trust in scientists. Rolfe et al.'s (2014) systematic review found only three studies evaluating provider behavior interventions to increase trust, and the findings were inconclusive. Focusing on political ideology and trust in science, Mann and Schleifer (2020) recommend "humanizing the scientific community and correcting misperceptions of scientists themselves" (325) as a more effective outreach tool to enhance trust than a simple promotion of the science (Larson and Broniatowski 2021) or providing information about the science (Scherer et al. 2016). Jaiswal et al. (2019) recommend that health care professionals and providers be trained to acknowledge and address the causes of mistrust. Further, Morton et al. (2013) found that researchers creating multiple touchpoints for dialogue and learning with participants, as well as shared opportunities to shape and refine research for the tribal community, enhanced trust. Similarly, Ramos et al. (2019) recommend that researchers demonstrate trustworthiness through "authenticity, respectful interaction, clear, honest, and thorough explanations, and consistent provision of the power of choice on behalf of the participant or patient" (para. 34), and they regularly return research results to participants.

Institutionally, trust in science can be addressed with structural actions. Fleming et al. (2021) found that adopting terminology of the participants, adjusting language, making space for unintended ethical conversations, and implementing the patient-developed protocols strengthened trust. Best et al. (2021) recommend that public health institutions focus on demonstrating trustworthiness (1) by acknowledging and addressing untrustworthy actions, (2) through community engagement to situate research and recommendations in the local community context, and (3) by using sources the community trusts to deliver information. Similarly, Jamison et al. (2019) call on institutions to critically reflect not on the causes of distrust but on whether enough has been done to enable the institution to be viewed as trustworthy by its stakeholder communities, which "will require consistent attention to agency actions . . . and sensitivity to concerns of minority groups who often have different experiences with government agencies" (sec. 4).

Public engagement with science (PES) is a growing area of building trust in science (Cohen et al. 2008; National Academies of Sciences, Engineering, and Medicine 2015; Todd et al. 2018). PES is a bidirectional process that brings scientists, the public, and other groups together to exchange knowledge and perspectives, learn, and inform decision-making and social action. In PES, mutual learning by all parties is facilitated through a variety of methods, including informal science learning, forums and science cafes for conversation and deliberation, and science festivals (Todd et al. 2018). Forums for dialogue, in particular, are an intervention evaluated in multiple contexts and shown to be effective in enhancing trust because they invite others to be part of the scientific process (Teteh et al. 2019; Todd et al. 2018).

Along with engagement as a medium, interventions focusing on online communities are growing in the literature. Larson et al. (2021) advocate for new interventions using internet-mediated communication and social media to build trust. One example is Agley et al.'s (2021) large, randomized trial exposing participants to an infographic about the scientific process to increase trust. Promisingly for scalability, the clinical trial results did show a small increase in trust in science and that trust may have decreased the believability of COVID-19 misinformation. It is also important to note that, with the increasing use of technology in health care, such as digital health (Adjekum et al. 2018) and Healthcare 4.0 (Li and Carayon 2021), trust in technology adds complexity to any intervention aiming to build or regain the public's trust in science.

Conclusions

Trust in science is a complex, multidimensional concept that involves not only attitudes toward the scientific method as a way of generating knowledge but also toward beliefs, ethics, and intentions of individual scientists and the scientific establishment. When trust in science is low, it is rarely because people reject the scientific method as a whole. They are more likely to question the goodwill of science as the establishment; mistrust designs of specific studies, especially in domains where findings of studies run counter to the individuals' ideological and religious beliefs; and choose nonscience-based narratives that align with those same beliefs over scientific results. Mistrust of science is likely exacerbated by the discordance between an individual's perception of the nature of science, shaped by simplistic models imparted by how science is taught at school, and encounters with the uncertainties of real-world science, which may lead to disillusionment. For groups experiencing disparities, attitudes toward science are also affected by the history of abuse and neglect by the government, research, and health care establishment. While Americans generally hold positive views of science as a societal institution, there are many caveats that affect trust of specific groups on certain issues, and many of these issues are health-related.

In light of the above, how can we increase trust? We believe that, first and foremost, community engagement efforts should never label people as "antiscience," as this is not only offensive and divisive but inaccurate. Interventions should promote the understanding of science as powerful—but complex—and characterized by uncertainty, which is reduced through experimentation and dialogue. Internet-mediated technology, including social media, should also be a primary platform for interventions. Programs should emphasize the difference between productive dissent and denialism. It is important to understand that science literacy efforts will not build trust in science without social, relational engagement interventions. These interventions should bring together community members, researchers, representatives of the science establishment, and health care professionals for respectful, repeated, multidirectional conversations.

Acknowledgment

This work was carried out by staff of the National Library of Medicine (NLM), National Institutes of Health, with support from NLM.

References

Abadie, Roberto et al. 2018. "Establishing Trust in HIV/HCV Research among People who Inject Drugs (PWID): Insights from Empirical Research." *PLOS ONE* 13, no. 12: e0208410. doi:10.1371/journal.pone.0208410.

Achterberg, P., W. de Koster, and J. van der Waal. 2017. "A Science Confidence Gap: Education, Trust in Scientific Methods, and Trust in Scientific Institutions in the United States, 2014." *Public Understanding of Science* 26, no. 6: 704–720.

Adjekum, Afua, Alessandro Blasimme, and Effy Vayena. 2018. "Elements of Trust in Digital Health Systems: Scoping Review." *Journal of Medical Internet Research* 20, no. 12: e11254. doi:10.2196/11254.

Agley, J. 2020. "Assessing Changes in US Public Trust in Science Amid the COVID-19 Pandemic." *Public Health* 183: 122–25.

Agley, J., Y. Xiao, E. E. Thompson, X. Chen, and L. Golzarri-Arroyo. 2021. "Intervening on Trust in Science to Reduce Belief in COVID-19 Misinformation and Increase COVID-19 Preventive Behavioral Intentions: Randomized Controlled Trial." *Journal of Medical Internet Research* 23, no. 10: e32425. doi:10.2196/32425.

Beauchamp, A. L., and K. Rios. 2020. "Secularism in Science: The Role of Religious Affiliation in Assessments of Scientists' Trustworthiness." *Public Understanding of Science* 29, no. 2: 194–210.

Benkert, Ramona, Adolfo Cuevas, Hayley S. Thompson, Emily Dove-Meadows, and Donulae Knuckles. 2019. "Ubiquitous Yet Unclear: A Systematic Review of Medical Mistrust." *Behavioral Medicine* 45, no. 2: 86–101. doi:10.1080/08964289.2019.1588220.

Best, Alicia L., Faith E. Fletcher, Mika Kadono, and Rueben C. Warren. 2021. "Institutional Distrust among African Americans and Building Trustworthiness in the COVID-19 Response: Implications for Ethical Public Health Practice." *Journal of Health Care for the Poor and Underserved* 32, no. 1: 90–98. doi:10.1353/hpu.2021.0010.

Brown-Iannuzzi, J. L., S. McKee, and W. M. Gervais. 2018. "Atheist Horns and Religious Halos: Mental Representations of Atheists and Theists." *Journal of Experimental Psychology: General* 147, no. 2: 292–97.

Christopher, Suzanne, Vanessa Watts, Alma Knows His Gun McCormick, and Sara Young. 2008. "Building and Maintaining Trust in a Community-Based Participatory Research Partnership." *American Journal of Public Health* 98, no. 8: 1398–406. doi:10.2105/AJPH.2007.125757.

Cohen, Emma R. M., Hassan Masum, Kathryn Berndtson, Vicki Saunders, Tom Hadfield, Dilzayn Panjwani, Deepa L. Persad et al. 2008. "Public Engagement on Global Health Challenges." *BMC Public Health* 8, no. 168. doi:10.1186/1471-2458-8-168.

Cooper, J. 2018. *Congress and the Decline of Public Trust.* New York: Taylor and Francis.

Cooper, L. Z., H. J. Larson, and S. L. Katz. 2008. "Protecting Public Trust in Immunization." *Pediatrics* 122, no. 1: 149–53.

Dave, G., Leah Frerichs, Jennifer Jones, Mimi Kim, Jennifer Schaal, Stefanie Vassar, Deepthi Varma et al. 2018. "Conceptualizing Trust in Community-Academic Research Partnerships Using Concept Mapping Approach: A Multi-CTSA Study." *Evaluation and Program Planning* 66: 70–78.

Dhanani L. Y., and B. Franz. 2020. "The Role of News Consumption and Trust in Public Health Leadership in Shaping COVID-19 Knowledge and Prejudice." *Front Psychology* 11: 560828.

Drummond, C., and B. Fischhoff. 2017. "Individuals with Greater Science Literacy and Education Have More Polarized Beliefs on Controversial Science Topics." *Proceedings of the National Academy of Sciences of the United States of America* 114, no. 36: 9587–92.

Evans, John H. 2013. "The Growing Social and Moral Conflict between Conservative Protestantism and Science." *Journal for the Scientific Study of Religion* 52: 368–85.

Evans, Kiameesha R., and Michael K. Gusmano. 2021. "Civic Learning, Science, and Structural Racism." *The Hastings Center Report* 51, Suppl 1: S46–S50. doi:10.1002/hast.1229.

Feldman, L., E. W. Maibach, C. Roser-Renouf, and A. Leiserowitz. 2012. "Climate on Cable: The Nature and Impact of Global Warming Coverage on Fox News, CNN, and MSNBC." *International Journal of Press/Politics* 17, no. 1: 3–31.

Fensham, P. J. 2012. "Preparing Citizens for a Complex World: The Grand Challenge of Teaching Socio-Scientific Issues in Science Education." In *Science|Environment|Health. Towards a Renewed Pedagogy for Science Education*, edited by A. Zeyer and R. Kyburz-Graber, 7–29. Dordrecht: Springer.

Fleming, Perry R., Makayla M. Swygert, Coen Hasenkamp, Jessica Sterling, Ginny Cartee, Rebecca Russ-Sellers, Melanie Cozad, Renee J. Chosed, William E. Roudebush, and Ann Blair Kennedy. 2021. "Patient Engagement in Fertility Research: Bench Research, Ethics, and Social Justice." *Research Involvement and Engagement* 7: 1–29. doi:10.1186/s40900-021-00278-x.

Frazzetto, G. 2004. "Embryos, Cells and God." *EMBO Reports* 5, no. 6: 553–55.

Freimuth, Vicki S., D. Musa, K. Hilyard, S. C. Quinn, and K. Kim. 2014. "Trust During the Early Stages of the 2009 H1N1 Pandemic." *Journal of Health Communication* 19, no. 3: 321–39. doi:10.1080/10810730.2013.811323.

Funk, C. 2020. "Key Findings About Americans' Confidence in Science and Their Views on Scientists' Role in Society." *Pew Research Center*, February 12, 2020. https://pewrsr.ch/2Hgq31S.

Funk, Cary, Alec Tyson, Brian Kennedy, and Courtney Johnson. 2020. "Science and Scientists Held in High Esteem Across Global Publics." *Pew Research Center*, September 29, 2020. https://www.pewresearch.org/science/2020/09/29/science-and-scientists-held-in-high-esteem-across-global-publics.

Gallup. 2019. "Wellcome Global Monitor—First Wave Findings." Accessed February 14, 2022. https://wellcome.org/reports/wellcome-global-monitor/2018.

Gauchat, G. 2012. "Politicization of Science in the Public Sphere: A Study of Public Trust in the United States, 1974 to 2010." *American Sociological Review* 77: 167–87.

Gauchat, Gordon. 2011. "The Cultural Authority of Science: Public Trust and Acceptance of Organized Science." *Public Understanding of Science* 20: 751–70.

Gross, Neil. 2013. *Why Are Professors Liberal and Why Do Conservatives Care?* Cambridge: Harvard University Press.

Gu, Chao, and Yi Feng. 2021. "Influence of Public Engagement with Science on Scientific Information Literacy During the COVID-19 Pandemic: Empirical Evidence from College Students in China." *Science & Education*: 1–15. doi:10.1007/s11191-021-00261-8.

Healthy People 2030. n.d. "Social Determinants of Health." Accessed February 12, 2022. https://health.gov/healthypeople/objectives-and-data/social-determinants-health.

Hmielowski, J. D., L. Feldman, T. A. Myers, A. Leiserowitz, and E. Maibach. 2014. "An Attack on Science? Media Use, Trust in Scientists, and Perceptions of Global Warming." *Public Understanding of Science* 23, no. 7: 866–83. doi:10.1177/0963662513480091.

Hovland, C. I., I. L. Janis, and H. H. Kelley. 1953. *Psychological Studies of Opinion Change*. New Haven: Yale University Press.

Jaiswal, Jessica. 2019. "Whose Responsibility Is It to Dismantle Medical Mistrust? Future Directions for Researchers and Health Care Providers." *Behavioral Medicine* 45, no. 2: 188–96. doi:10.1080/08964289.2019.1630357.

Jaiswal, Jessica, and Perry N. Halkitis. 2019. "Towards a More Inclusive and Dynamic Understanding of Medical Mistrust Informed by Science." *Behavioral Medicine* 45, no. 2: 79–85. doi:10.1080/08964289.2019.1619511.

Jaiswal, Jessica, Stuart N. Singer, Karolynn Siegel, and Helen-Maria Lekas. 2019. "HIV-Related 'Conspiracy Beliefs': Lived Experiences of Racism and Socio-Economic Exclusion Among People Living with HIV in New York City." *Culture, Health & Sexuality* 21, no. 4: 373–86. doi:10.1080/13691058.2018.1470674.

Jamison, Amelia M., Sandra Crouse Quinn, and Vicki S. Freimuth. 2019. "'You Don't Trust a Government Vaccine': Narratives of Institutional Trust and Influenza Vaccination Among African American and White Adults." *Social Science & Medicine* 221: 87–94. doi:10.1016/j.socscimed.2018.12.020.

Jewett, Andrew. 2020. "How Americans Came to Distrust Science." *Boston Review*, December 8, 2020. https://bostonreview.net/articles/andrew-jewett-science-under-fire/.

Johnson, B. B., and P. Slovic. 1995. "Presenting Uncertainty in Health Risk Assessment: Initial Studies of its Effects on Risk Perception and Trust." *Risk Analysis* 15, no. 4: 485–94.

Kohut, Andrew. 2010. "Distrust Discontent, Anger and Partisan Rancor: The People and Their Government." *Pew Research Center*, April 18, 2010. https://www.pewresearch.org/politics/2010/04/18/distrust-discontent-anger-and-partisan-rancor.

Krause, N. M., D. P. Brossard, D. A. Scheufele, M. A. Xenos, and K. Franke. 2019. "Trends—Americans' Trust in Science and Scientists." *Public Opinion Quarterly* 83, no. 4: 817–36.

Kreps, S. E., and D. L. Kriner. 2020. "Model Uncertainty, Political Contestation, and Public Trust in Science: Evidence from the COVID-19 Pandemic." *Science Advances* 6, no. 43: eabd4563.

Kunda, Z. 1990. "The Case for Motivated Reasoning." *Psychology Bulletin* 108: 480–98.

Larson, Heidi J., Richard M. Clarke, Caitlin Jarrett, Elisabeth Eckersberger, Zachary Levine, Will S. Schulz, and Pauline Paterso. 2018. "Measuring trust in vaccination: A systematic review." Human Vaccines & Immunotherapeutics 14(7):1599–1609. doi: 10.1080/21645515.2018.1459252.

Larson, H. J., and D. A. Broniatowski. 2021. "Why Debunking Misinformation Is Not Enough to Change People's Minds About Vaccines." *American Journal of Public Health* 111: 1058–60. doi:10.2105/AJPH.2021.306293.

Larson, Heidi J., Isabelle Sahinovic, Madhava Ram Balakrishnan, and Clarissa Simas. 2021. "Vaccine Safety in the Next Decade: Why We Need New Modes of Trust Building." *BMJ Global Health* 6, Suppl 2: e003908. doi:10.1136/bmjgh-2020-003908.

Lewandowsky, S., and K. Oberauer. 2021. "Worldview-Motivated Rejection of Science and the Norms of Science." *Cognition* 215: 104820.

Lewandowsky, S., G. Gignac, and S. Vaughan. 2013. "The Pivotal Role of Perceived Scientific Consensus in Acceptance of Science." *Nature Climate Change* 3: 399–404.

Li, J., and P. Carayon. 2021. "Health Care 4.0: A Vision for Smart and Connected Health Care." *IISE Transactions on Healthcare Systems Engineering* 11, no. 3: 171–80. doi:10.1080/24725579.2021.1884627.

Longino, H. E. 1990. *Science as Social Knowledge: Values and Objectivity in Scientific Inquiry.* Princeton, NJ: Princeton University Press.

Mann, Marcus, and Cyrus Schleifer. 2020. "Love the Science, Hate the Scientists: Conservative Identity Protects Belief in Science and Undermines Trust in Scientists." *Social Forces* 99, no. 1: 305–32. doi:10.1093/sf/soz156.

Mesch, G. S., and K. P. Schwirian. 2015. "Confidence in Government and Vaccination Willingness in the USA." *Health Promotion International* 30, no. 2: 213–21. doi:10.1093/heapro/dau094.

Moore, D. A., and P. J. Healy. 2008. "The Trouble with Overconfidence." *Psychology Review* 115: 502–517.

Morton, Deborah J., Joely Proudfit, Daniel Calac, Martina Portillo, Geneva Lofton-Fitzsimmons, Theda Molina, Raymond Flores, Barbara Lawson-Risso, and Romelle Majel-McCauley. 2013. "Creating Research Capacity Through a Tribally Based Institutional Review Board." *American Journal of Public Health* 103, no. 12: 2160–64. doi:10.2105/AJPH.2013.301473.

Nadelson, Louis, Cheryl Jorcyk, Dazhi Yang, Mary Jarratt Smith, Sam Matson, Ken Cornell, and Virginia Husting. 2014. "I Just Don't Trust Them: The Development and Validation of an Assessment Instrument to Measure Trust in Science and Scientists." *School Science and Mathematics* 114(2): 76–86. doi:10.1111/ssm.12051.

Nagler, R. H. 2014. "Adverse Outcomes Associated with Media Exposure to Contradictory Nutrition Messages." *Journal of Health Communication* 19, no. 1: 24–40.

Nandyal, Samantha, David Strawhun, Hannah Stephen, Ashley Banks, and Daniel Skinner. 2021. "Building Trust in American Hospital-Community Development Projects: A Scoping Review." *Journal of Community Hospital Internal Medicine Perspectives* 11, no. 4: 439–45. doi:10.1080/20009666.2021.1929048.

National Academies of Sciences, Engineering, and Medicine. 2015. *Trust and Confidence at the Interfaces of the Life Sciences and Society: Does the Public Trust Science? A Workshop Summary.* Washington, DC: The National Academies Press. doi:10.17226/21798.

NORC. n.d. "The General Society Survey." Accessed February 12, 2022. https://gss.norc.org/.

Parikh, Sudip. 2021. "Why We Must Rebuild Trust in Science." *Pew Trend Magazine*, February 9, 2021. https://www.pewtrusts.org/en/trend/archive/winter-2021/why-we-must-rebuild-trust-in-science.

Peters, R. G., V. T. Covello, and D. B. McCallum. 1997. "The Determinants of Trust and Credibility in Environmental Risk Communication: An Empirical Study." *Risk Analysis* 17, no. 1: 43–54.

Peterson, Emily B., Wen-Ying Sylvia Chou, Dannielle E. Kelley, and Brad Hesse. 2020. "Trust in National Health Information Sources in the United States: Comparing Predictors and Levels of Trust

Across Three Health Domains." *Translational Behavioral Medicine* 10, no. 4: 978–88. doi:10.1093/tbm/ibz066.

Quinn, S. C., J. Parmer, V. S. Freimuth, K. M. Hilyard, D. Musa, and K. H. Kim. 2013. "Exploring Communication, Trust in Government, and Vaccination Intention Later in the 2009 H1N1 Pandemic: Results of a National Survey." *Biosecurity and Bioterrorism* 11, no. 2: 96–106.

Ramos, S. Raquel, Rueben Warren, Michele Shedlin, Gail Melkus, Trace Kershaw, and Allison Vorderstrasse. 2019. "A Framework for Using eHealth Interventions to Overcome Medical Mistrust Among Sexual Minority Men of Color Living with Chronic Conditions." *Behavioral Medicine* 45, no. 2: 166–76. doi:10.1080/08964289.2019.1570074.

Rissler, L. J., Sarah I. Duncan, and N. M. Caruso. 2014. "The Relative Importance of Religion and Education on University Students' Views of Evolution in the Deep South and State Science Standards across the United States." *Evolution: Education and Outreach 7, 24.* doi.org/10.1186/s12052-014-0024-1

Rolfe, Alix, Lucinda Cash-Gibson, Josip Car, Aziz Sheikh, and Brian McKinstry. 2014. "Interventions for improving patients' trust in doctors and groups of doctors." Cochrane Database of Systematic Reviews 2014(3): CD004134. doi:10.1002/14651858.CD004134.pub3.

Rutjens, B. T., and S. J. Heine. 2016. "The Immoral Landscape? Scientists Are Associated with Violations of Morality." *PLoS ONE* 11, no. 4: e0152798.

Scherer, Laura D., et al. 2016. "Can the Vaccine Adverse Event Reporting System Be Used to Increase Vaccine Acceptance and Trust?" *Vaccine* 34, no. 21: 2424–29. doi:10.1016/j.vaccine.2016.03.087.

Solomon, M. 2021. "Trust: The Need for Public Understanding of How Science Works." *Hastings Center Report* 51, Suppl 1: S36–S39.

Teteh, D. K., et al. 2019. "Use of Community Forums to Increase Knowledge of HPV and Cervical Cancer in African American Communities." *Journal of Community Health* 44, no. 3: 492–99.

Todd, Katie, Gretchen Haupt, Elizabeth Kunz Kollmann, and Sarah Pfeifle. 2018. "Fostering Conversation about Synthetic Biology Between Publics and Scientists: A Comparison of Approaches and Outcomes." *Journal of Microbiology & Biology Education* 19, no. 1. doi:10.1128/jmbe.v19i1.1434.

Vardavas, C., S. Odani, K. Nikitara, H. El Banhawi, C. Kyriakos, L. Taylor, and N. Becuwe. 2020. "Public Perspective on the Governmental Response, Communication and Trust in the Governmental Decisions in Mitigating COVID-19 early in the Pandemic across the G7 Countries." *Preventive Medicine Reports* 21: 101252.

Webb Hooper, Monica, Charlene Mitchell, Vanessa J. Marshall, Chesley Cheatham, Kristina Austin, Kimberly Sanders, Smitha Krishnamurthi, and Lena L. Grafton. 2019. "Understanding Multilevel Factors Related to Urban Community Trust in Healthcare and Research." *International Journal of Environmental Research and Public Health* 16, no. 18: 3280. doi:10.3390/ijerph16183280.

Whetten, K., J. Leserman, R. Whetten, J. Ostermann, N. Thielman, M. Swartz, and D. Stangl. 2006. "Exploring Lack of Trust in Care Providers and the Government as a Barrier to Health Service Use." *American Journal of Public Health* 96, no. 4: 716–21.

World Health Organization. 2020. "Managing the COVID-19 Infodemic: Promoting Healthy Behaviours and Mitigating the Harm from Misinformation and Disinformation." Accessed July 12, 2022. https://www.who.int/news/item/23-09-2020-managing-the-covid-19-infodemic-promoting-healthy-behaviours-and-mitigating-the-harm-from-misinformation-and-disinformation.

Zeyer, A. 2021. "Chapter 2. Coping with Structural Uncertainty in Complex Living Systems." In *Science|Environment|Health. Towards a Science Pedagogy of Complex Living Systems. Towards a Renewed Pedagogy for Science Education*, edited by A. Zeyer and R. Kyburz-Graber, 11–29. Dordrecht: Springer.

9

Critical Cultural Literacy Education as a Bridge to Improving Health Disparities in BIPOC Communities

Jason Alston and Nicole A. Cooke

On March 31, 2019, Airmiess Joseph Asghedom, a thirty-three-year-old Black hip-hop musician better known by his stage name "Nipsey Hussle," was fatally shot in his hometown of Los Angeles, California. Arrested for the crime was twenty-nine-year-old Eric Ronald Holder Jr. Holder, reportedly a member of the Rollin 60s Neighborhood Crips street gang, allegedly killed Asghedom after Asghedom accused Holder of being a "snitch" (Dillon 2019). Despite law enforcement officers charging and arresting Holder just three days after the fatal killing, conspiracy theories rapidly spread online and through social media that linked Asghedom's slaying to the American medical establishment and pharmaceutical companies (Bell 2019). At the time of his death, Asghedom was producing a documentary about Alfredo Bowman, better known as "Dr. Sebi" (Bell 2019). Bowman was a self-proclaimed doctor who claimed to be able to heal various diseases, such as AIDS, with herbs and other natural remedies (Farrow 2019). Other false claims from Bowman included asserting that alkaline foods could control blood acidity and that there was an "African gene" to be found within Sub-Saharan Africans and the African Diaspora (Jarry 2019).

Bowman had little known training and no formal licensure as a medical doctor and was seen as a quack by the established medical community in the United States, as well as other nations (Barrett 2016). However, after Asghedom's death and the resultant conspiracy theories, online interest in the bogus teachings of Bowman spiked. Compounding this renewed interest in Bowman—whose flawed medical information had actually been making rounds within the African American community since the 1980s—was the fact that Bowman had served as a medical advisor to several high-profile African American celebrities, such as comedian Eddie Murphy and singers Lisa "Left Eye" Lopes and Michael Jackson (Giacomazzo 2021). To this day, discussion of and adherence to Bowman's flawed teachings persist on social media, particularly among African Americans. The persistence of these falsehoods can be at least partially attributed to deficiencies in information and media literacy and racial literacy, two literacy prongs within the subject of this chapter: critical cultural literacy.

Misinformation is information that is false, vague, and/or misleading (Cooke 2018). The dietary and genetic pseudoscience advanced by Bowman and his followers is just one of many examples of misinformation easily found on the internet or through social media that may result in specific or disproportional harm to "Black, Indigenous, and People of Color" (BIPOC). For instance, there is also significant misinformation and disinformation (mis/dis) online related to COVID-19 and the resultant vaccine hesitancy, tobacco and alcohol usage, eating disorders, HIV and AIDS, mental illness, and other ailments that disproportionately impact BIPOC communities and result in inequal seeking of quality treatment. Treatment inequities are also influenced by racism and implicit biases held by medical professionals who believe foolish and inhumane stereotypes that result in deficient medical care (Hoffman et al. 2016; Sabin and Greenwald 2012). BIPOC awareness of such racism and implicit bias among medical professionals may make BIPOC justifiably reluctant to seek quality care from actual medical professionals (Fletcher 2020). Because mis/dis is intensified and exacerbated by social media, even though the health care professions are trying to account for harm done and do better in the future (University of Pittsburgh 2020), they will continue to contend with the deep, long-term, and justifiable mistrust that BIPOC communities feel toward their professions (Jaiswal, LoSchiavo, and Perlman 2020; White 2005).

With these complicated health dilemmas in mind, these questions remain: How can health misinformation immunity be built and strengthened? How can information professionals and educators of BIPOC information consumers make a dent in the imbalance between health disparities between BIPOC and their white peers? This chapter proposes critical cultural literacy education as a bridge to improving these health disparities in BIPOC communities and building health misinformation immunity. The chapter should be primarily helpful to educators—in K–12 or higher education—who are charged with teaching BIPOC information literacy skills, as well as information professionals who assist BIPOC with retrieving and accessing health information.

Critical cultural literacy challenges educators to teach strategies to resist mis/dis by using elements of cultural competence, critical information literacy, media literacy, historical literacy (systemic oppression and structural inequities in health care services and its relation to BIPOC health disparities), emotional literacy, racial literacy, and health literacy (mis/dis can actually come from health professionals and from within health organizations) (Cooke 2021). This contextual approach looks at the larger ecology of mis/dis and situates mis/dis as an ongoing and dynamic phenomenon to be dealt with instead of a transactional static problem to be solved (Cooke 2021).

Critical cultural literacy education benefits everyone, not just BIPOC communities. Educating BIPOC and white information consumers, especially youth consumers, will equip them with skills and critical thinking strategies that will enable them to identify mis/dis and to question the status quo when faced with health mis/dis. By teaching critical cultural literacy skills to all races, educators and information professionals are equipping these individuals to become personal and community health advocates within and for BIPOC communities, and they will also be building a more robust pipeline of future culturally competent health professionals.

Health and Medical Misinformation Abounds on the Internet and Social Media

The internet and social media sites provide an environment for information consumers to be saturated with a copious amount of health mis/dis that must be vetted for the truth. The health sciences community has long been aware that health mis/dis is prevalent on the internet, but the actual degree of prevalence is undetermined. Included here are some examples of relevant studies about online health mis/dis.

In 2011, a team of researchers reviewed the first 1,300 Google-returned website results for infant sleep safety and found that 28.1 percent of the websites provided inaccurate information, while 28.4 percent of the websites provided information that was irrelevant (Chung et al. 2012). Kedzior et al. (2019) extracted 135 claims about conception from websites and social media in 2017 and deemed only 81 of the 135 claims (60 percent) to be accurate. Lee et al. (2018) reviewed 243 websites for information about obstructive sleep apnea and concluded that most of the websites with information about this condition were "not reliable" and "inaccurate." Ferreira et al. (2019) reviewed 1,125 website recommendations for dealing with lower back pain and found 36.2 percent of the recommendations to be inaccurate with another 20.5 percent being unclear. Plambeck et al. (2021) reviewed 44 websites with information about penile implants and prostheses and found that at least half of the information on 20 of the 44 websites was inaccurate. The researchers concluded that most of the health information websites on this subject matter were "reasonably accurate" but that the "majority of websites are low quality and written at too high a level for the average patient to understand." On a more positive note, Towne et al. (2021) did a study on the accuracy of posts made on Facebook pages for patients with endometriosis and found that 93.93 percent of the "educational posts" were accurate.

Furthermore, social media and the excitement that surrounds sensationalist falsehoods have exacerbated the reach of mis/dis and made controlling the spread nearly impossible (Merchant and Asch 2018; Vosoughi, Roy, and Aral 2018). Social media entities have less control over the distribution and gatekeeping of information on their platforms, so access to false and fabricated information on these platforms is difficult to counter (Li and Scott 2020). False information spreads faster and reaches more people on social media than true information (Vosoughi, Roy, and Aral 2018); also, most people who encounter false information through social media are not going to be exposed to corrections or clarifications posted as updates (Southwell and Thorson 2015). Social media users are not necessarily sharing information with the goal of informing people but may instead be sharing information to court likes from other social media users. For these users, verifying that information is factual is not a priority and is often not done (Pennycock and Rand 2019).

Again, misinformation is information that is false, vague, and/or misleading; whereas disinformation is misinformation that is deliberately misleading and/or manipulated (Cooke 2018). Additionally, there is the term "malinformation," which actually appears to have at least two conflicting definitions. Wardle and Derakhshan (2017) have identified the concept of malinformation as occurring when true information is intentionally used to cause harm to a person, organization, population, or community. Cooke (2021), however, identifies this term as "false information that is shared with a distinct intent to cause harm, and in the case of racism, to maintain the status quo." This chapter will rely on Cooke's definition of malinformation.

Health mis/dis on the internet can spread quickly and has the potential to be dangerous if internet users believe it to be true. Deciding whether to believe all or some of the health information presented can be difficult for information consumers who lack multiliteracy skills (Cooke 2018). Educating information consumers on how to critically view health information is vital to building health misinformation immunity, especially for racially and ethnically marginalized communities who experience disproportionate health outcomes. Native Americans, for example, are reported to have a higher mortality rate than whites and a higher percentage of individuals with poor health than the total population (National Academies of Sciences, Engineering, and Medicine 2017).

Disproportionate health outcomes of BIPOC have been a national concern for decades (Milburn et al. 2019). Although federal and national organizations have made commitments to achieving health equity among BIPOC groups, the wide reach of false and misleading health information makes achieving health equity even more challenging (Chou et al. 2018). Moreover, a history of medical abuse and institutionalized racism has caused BIPOC to distrust health professionals and health care systems (Bajaj and Stanford 2021). For example, historical medical abuses such as the experiments on enslaved Black women performed by "father of gynecology" James Marion Sims, the unethical use of Henrietta Lacks's cells by medical researchers, and the US government-approved USPHS Syphilis Study—also known as the Tuskegee experiment—contribute to Black people's skepticism of medical practitioners and researchers (Abbasi 2021).

Researchers attempting to recruit Black and Latinx people for participation in the first Phase 3 trial for a COVID-19 vaccine reported struggling to secure participants (Duran 2020). Also, sometimes trust can unfortunately be misguided; in the Latinx community, videos purporting cures and treatments for rheumatoid arthritis have been viewed at three times the rate of factual videos about the condition, which has no cure (Bushak 2021). Latinx people often have a learned distrust for authorities and authoritative information due to government corruption in Latin America and may seek health and other online information from sources that should not be trusted (Guerrero 2021). Latinx people, like Black people in the United States, have also been historically subjected to cruel and unethical medical practices, such as forced sterilization (Novak and Lira 2018).

Online Health Mis/Dis and Its Effect on BIPOC Communities

BIPOC may actually be more susceptible to some misinformation, disinformation, and malinformation regarding online information than white populations. Low-income, older Black adults show a particular susceptibility to digital misinformation, even when compared to similar age groups of people from other ethnic backgrounds and economic statuses; this might be due to low levels of digital access (Seo et al. 2020). Black women especially have to cope with an immense amount of everyday challenges and may have been susceptible to a "Black Immunity Myth" that spread online during the beginning of the COVID-19 pandemic as a coping mechanism wherein they would have one less concern to worry about (Chandler et al. 2020). At times, data specifically about Sub-Saharan African or Caribbean Black populations may be applied to Black people residing in the United States without proper context; during the COVID-19 pandemic, data about low COVID-19 rates among Sub-Saharan Africans fueled Black immunity myths about the virus even though these low rates had little to do with genetics and were likely the result of international travel behavior among Sub-Saharan Africans (Collins-Dexter 2020). Also, social media outlets may be taking misinformation and disinformation largely affecting Black populations less seriously and therefore implementing remedies more slowly, if at all (Collins-Dexter 2020).

A Democratic strategist noted in 2020 that Latinx people were exposed to repetitive Spanish-language memes and other social media posts about COVID-19 vaccine side effects and that this repetition may have altered opinions over time (Sesin 2020). There is a paucity of reliable Spanish-language information online for American Latinx audiences, particularly when it comes to health information (Sesin 2020). Latinx communities are particularly vulnerable to misinformation and disinformation spread through the app WhatsApp; this app is extremely popular among users who have family and friends in other countries, and the Latinx community uses WhatsApp at a significantly higher rate than the American general public, but false information is harder to monitor on WhatsApp (Sabin 2020).

Asian Americans and Pacific Islanders face the unique obstacle of language diversity when dealing with online misinformation and disinformation; since online mis/dis is often presented to Asian Americans and Pacific Islanders in their native language, it is difficult to track this false information because there are so many native languages that are read and spoken among Asian Americans and Pacific Islanders (AAPI) (Nguyen 2020a). First-generation Americans of AAPI heritage are possibly susceptible to false claims generated in the United States against nations they feel hostility toward; for example, AAPI individuals—especially Taiwanese Americans—who had negative attitudes toward China may have more readily accepted false claims that former US president Donald Trump made about China and COVID-19 (Nguyen 2020a). In addition to language diversity, AAPI also have diverse preferences in social media platforms, which compounds the difficulty in tracking false information (Nguyen 2020a).

Indigenous Americans have a long-standing distrust of American health providers and also experience less satisfaction with the health care they receive than their white counterparts (Guadagnolo et al. 2009). Kashani et al. (2019) found that a prevailing obstacle in convincing Indigenous Americans to vaccinate their children for human papillomavirus (HPV) was misinformation about the HPV vaccine. Wright, VanEvery, and Miller (2021) posited that Indigenous Canadian mothers of infants utilize the internet to find health information for their babies, but that they may be challenged by rampant web misinformation and an inability to interpret complex medical information and to discern high-quality sources from low-quality sources. Liddell et al. (2018) executed a qualitative study of Indigenous women residing in South Dakota and found that some of the women involved in the study were negatively impacted by misinformation about cancer treatments; this, combined with pressure from health care providers to submit to medical treatments that they were not comfortable with, caused hesitance among the study participants to seek beneficial medical treatment (Liddell et al. 2018).

Online Political Disinformation Campaigns Target BIPOC

BIPOC may also be specifically targeted for misinformation, disinformation, and malinformation campaigns. Much of what is discussed in this section of the chapter concerns the targeting of BIPOC with online political disinformation, rather than online health disinformation. However, if bad-faith actors and malevolent figures are willing to target BIPOC with detrimental political disinformation, it is not unreasonable to consider that they may also—currently or in the future—target BIPOC with detrimental health disinformation. This section is therefore included in this chapter to encourage vigilance among BIPOC, as tactics used to disinform and therefore harm BIPOC politically could also be used against BIPOC to disinform and therefore harm them as far as their health is concerned. Information within this section may provide insight into how such online health disinformation campaigns might be carried out. Historical injustices like the aforementioned forced sterilization programs against Black and Latinx Americans reveal that BIPOC should not assume that their actual physical well-being would not be infringed upon for political reasons. Also, critical cultural literacy binds political literacy to several other literacies. Politics is inherently entangled with health care in the United States. Therefore, exploring how BIPOC are targeted for online political disinformation is relevant to the discussion of BIPOC and online health disinformation.

Freelon et al. (2020) found that some social media accounts that appeared to belong to Black activists and Black progressives were actually created by Russian troll farms to disinform

Black Americans. Black American communities have also been targeted with disinformation campaigns suggesting that young Black males are disproportionately susceptible to developing autism if they take the MMR vaccine (DiResta and Wardle 2020).

Latinx populations in the United States have recently been targeted in online disinformation campaigns aiming to spread falsehoods about the coronavirus and voting; these campaigns may or may not be related but are branded as broad and parts of a "largely undetected movement to depress turnout and spread disinformation" (Weissert 2021). After former US president Donald Trump won more Hispanic votes in 2020 than expected, political strategists deduced that Hispanic voters were targeted with online disinformation about then-candidate Joe Biden, including that he supported Castro-style socialism, was a "fake Catholic," and supported abortion up until the moment of birth (Ghaffary 2020). Immediately after the 2020 presidential election, the *New York Times* reported that there were Spanish-language posts claiming that Donald Trump had won reelection spreading online (Mazzei and Perlroth 2020). Particularly clear here when examining the entanglement of political information and health information is the false information regarding Biden's stance on abortion; abortion is not just a political issue but a women's health issue. False information regarding Biden's stance on abortion therefore should not be seen as a mere exercise in political disinformation, but health disinformation as well.

Concerning AAPI, the Epoch Times media company has been accused of using its Asian-language affiliates like New Tang Dynasty TV and China Uncensored to disseminate anti-China and other political disinformation (Nguyen 2020a). Chinese American voters were targeted in a disinformation campaign that sprang up on Chinese-owned mobile app WeChat in 2020, wherein claims that the federal government was mobilizing against riots on election day were spread to frighten Chinese American voters into staying home and not voting (Rodriguez, Lin, and Huseman 2020). WeChat has even reportedly been used to target the Chinese American community with health disinformation, specifically about COVID-19; Chinese-language media outlets in the United States have attempted to combat this targeted spread of disinformation, though the effectiveness of these countermeasures is unknown (Fuchs 2020). A commonality among first- and second-generation AAPI and Latinx populations is pronounced distrust of communist regimes; this distrust has made both populations susceptible to falsehoods linking leftist American political figures to communism, and the internet is abundant with such falsehoods (Nguyen 2020b).

Indigenous American populations are also targeted with disinformation. A "cyber reconnaissance company" called GroupSense claimed in 2020 to have identified Facebook and Twitter profiles masquerading as profiles of Indigenous Americans that were disseminating disinformation about politics using Indigenous-themed hashtags (Andrea 2020). Harb and Henne (2019) posited that both the US and Canadian governments regularly surveil Indigenous populations, specifically Indigenous protestors and activists, and target disinformation to them as part of these state surveillance efforts (Harb and Henne 2019). There is a precedent for health disinformation to be targeted at Indigenous Americans, though not specifically online health disinformation. Specifically, there are long-enduring "firewater myths" targeted at Indigenous communities that suggest that Indigenous people are genetically more susceptible to alcohol abuse; firewater myths may lead to a lack of self-efficacy among Indigenous populations to drink moderately, which in turn may lead to negative physical health outcomes (Gonzalez and Skewes 2016). Though the motivations for the original targeting of firewater myths to Indigenous populations do not appear to be documented, such disinformation could theoretically be advanced online for nefarious purposes.

Educating BIPOC to consume online political information through a critical cultural lens is one approach that can help build misinformation immunity within these communities. Again, due to the entanglement of politics and health care in the United States, educating BIPOC to consume online political information through a critical cultural lens could be a gateway to conditioning BIPOC to view online health information through a critical cultural lens as well. As we see in some of the previous examples, such as the disinformation about COVID-19 on WeChat and the disinformation regarding President Joe Biden's stance on abortion, the entanglement of political and health care issues is such that using critical cultural literacy to enhance recognition of mis/dis in one of these areas could facilitate abilities to recognize mis/dis in the other.

The What and the Why of Critical Cultural Literacy

Critical cultural literacy is a competence that threads together seven distinct literacies with an intent to situate mis/dis as an "ongoing and dynamic phenomenon" (Cooke 2021) that must be systemically combated by using the component literacies in cooperation to challenge and dismantle existent power structures. The seven literacies are: racial, cultural, emotional, historical, political, design, and information/media. Critical cultural literacy builds upon foundations established within critical information literacy and media literacy. Critical information literacy, "as expressed by its literature, examines the social construction and political dimensions of information, and problematizes information's development, use, and purposes with the intent of prompting students to think critically about such forces and act upon this knowledge" (Tewell 2015). Meanwhile, media literacy "is how information consumers can address messages portrayed by the media and challenge them, looking at the messages with healthy skepticism and a critical eye" (Cooke 2021). When information and media literacy are enjoined with the remaining literacies that compose critical cultural literacy, it equips information consumers who have cultural competence and cultural humility with the aptitudes needed to confront and interrogate the information they encounter, vetting it for accuracy, usefulness, and intent.

Critical cultural literacy does not provide a one-size-fits-all solution to racialized mis/dis or malinformation (Cooke 2021). Context varies from situation to situation and critical cultural literacy emphasizes context. But racialized mis/dis and malinformation are so engrained in the information consumed by the American people—BIPOC included—that at least some of the components of this threaded competency will often be applicable when vetting potential mis/dis and malinformation.

Cooke offers, as an example, using critical cultural literacy to engage hatred-laden information about AAPI during the COVID-19 pandemic. Through traditional information literacy, Cooke asserts that information consumers can come to the conclusion that Chinese people and other AAPI are not responsible for the COVID-19 pandemic, even if elected officials explicitly blame them for it (Cooke 2021). Critical information literacy, per Cooke, would take it a step further, with information consumers recognizing that "catchy phrases" and other rhetoric that scapegoats AAPI for the COVID-19 pandemic are racist stereotypes and caricatures. With critical cultural literacy, information consumers will understand that increased racism toward and harassment of AAPI during specific global phenomena is not new; AAPI were also subjected to increased harm in the United States following the attack on Pearl Harbor and in the immediate aftermath of the Vietnam War (Mineo 2021), among other examples. Cooke (2021) writes:

> (T)here is a progression from traditional information and media literacy where the goal is essentially to know how to fact-check claims with vetted and credible sources. There is absolutely a place and need for this kind of literacy, but it has to be acknowledged for what it is: addressing mis/dis in the moment and in isolation. If the real goal is to effectively push back and repudiate mis/dis and racist malinformation, then contextual and consistent education—critical cultural literacy education—is what is needed.

Critical Cultural Literacy in Action

To see how the component literacies of critical cultural literacy work together, we can work through a previous example of common early misconceptions of Black/African American susceptibility to COVID-19 infections. In her publication *Canaries in the Coal Mine: COVID-19 Misinformation and Black Communities*, Brandi Collins-Dexter noted that toward the beginning of the COVID-19 global pandemic, many Black Americans were believing misinformation suggesting that Black people could not or did not die from COVID-19. Belief in this misinformation was supported by myriad variables, but among these variables were reports that COVID-19 was having a less devastating effect in Sub-Saharan Africa than in many other parts of the world (Soy 2020). Health misinformation online, however, led some to believe that since COVID-19 was not claiming as many lives among Black people in Sub-Saharan Africa, Black people had lower susceptibility to the SARS-CoV-2 virus. Contrarily, COVID-19 was actually hitting Black communities in the United States especially hard.

Black Americans may phenotypically resemble Black Sub-Saharan Africans, but assumptions that these populations are especially genetically similar because of their physical appearances reflect issues around racial literacy. Black Americans in reality might not have the perceived genetic adjacency to Black Sub-Saharan Africans because (a) Sub-Saharan Africans are more genetically diverse and dissimilar to one another than human populations are within any other continent (Campbell and Tishkoff 2008), and (b) most Black Americans who descend from enslaved Africans have European ancestry and genetic admixture versus being "purely Black." Understanding that Black Americans who descend from enslaved Africans tend to have European ancestry as well also involves historical literacy.

Additional contrasts between the effects of COVID-19 on Black American communities versus Sub-Saharan African communities are grounded in other literacies that comprise the critical cultural literacy model. International travel patterns and other behaviors affected the speed of COVID-19's spread in Africa versus other areas of the world; these behaviors are rooted in African culture and politics (cultural and political literacy). Unlike the United States, many African nations quickly introduced public health measures once COVID-19 cases were recorded in the continent—including avoiding handshakes, frequent hand-washing, social distancing, and wearing of face masks—which citizens obeyed without emotional resistance (Soy 2020) (emotional and political literacy). Several West African nations had good community health systems in place to deal with viral pandemics in response to an Ebola virus pandemic that had occurred a few years earlier (Soy 2020) (design literacy). Finally, Sub-Saharan Africans tend to trust their governments' information regarding COVID-19 and governmental responses to the pandemic, though trust in COVID-19 vaccinations is lacking in Sub-Saharan Africa (Sanny 2021) (information and media literacy). The example used here does lend itself rather neatly to the established critical cultural literacy model, so it is worth repeating that critical cultural literacy does not provide a one-size-fits-all solution to racialized mis/dis or malinformation and that context will vary by situation.

The objective of critical cultural literacy in building health misinformation immunity within BIPOC communities is to equip community members with tools to read the world through a critical consciousness that acknowledges and understands the existence and impact of multi-systemic oppression. If BIPOC can interrogate the online health information they encounter through the critical cultural literacy lens, they will be able to refute the health mis/dis they encounter and prevent it from becoming engrained and readily accepted malinformation and the unchallenged status quo. Critical cultural literacy cannot be achieved in an environment where the learner is simply given information and expected to receive it without questioning or thinking critically about the information given, the lived experiences of the person delivering the information, or the conscious and unconscious racial bias that may be rooted within the information. Critical cultural literacy education empowers the learner to be curious about why the world, and the people in it, are the way they are.

Conclusion: What Information Professionals Can Do

While this chapter focuses on the need of BIPOC at large to use critical cultural literacy and its component literacies to interrogate online health information, someone needs to make BIPOC communities aware of critical cultural literacy and teach these communities how to confront health information with the seven component literacies in mind. Information professionals, namely librarians, will be key in filling this role.

For librarians and library personnel who deliver instruction sessions to students in K–12 or higher education, critical cultural literacy can be applied by weaving the component competencies into lesson plans. Librarians can determine whether or not the actual concept of critical cultural literacy needs to be explained to their audience. For college students, explaining critical cultural literacy itself may be appropriate. Academic librarians can develop modules and instruction plans that teach critical cultural literacy and its component frameworks, and give students exercises that test their knowledge and understanding of the component literacies. Librarians can also have college students retrieve health information and then determine if what they have found is sound per critical cultural literacy; the process can be similar to what is demonstrated in the "Critical Cultural Literacy in Action" section of this chapter.

For K–12 students, however, librarians can deliver instruction related to the component literacies without explicitly tasking the students with learning what critical cultural literacy is. Even at the elementary level, for instance, students can learn to use their budding understandings of history, race, culture, politics, and the remaining literacies to be critical of the health information they encounter. Elementary school students can build confidence in their information-vetting behaviors by recognizing, for example, that information with noticeable historical inconsistencies or inaccuracies may be untrustworthy. Elementary school may even be the best time to teach students to avoid believing things just because they have an emotional desire to believe them to be true; by high school, and certainly by college, it may be too late for this. The competencies within critical cultural literacy can be taught at the elementary school level without burdening the students with understanding the threaded competency of critical cultural literacy itself.

Librarians, especially public librarians, who help adult users retrieve health information can discuss the elements of critical cultural literacy when explaining why retrieved information is or is not reliable. Usually, adult users will not be captive audiences for lesson-planned instruction in critical cultural literacy, but librarians can still explain to these users how encountered information is or is not reliable per the critical cultural literacy components. When opportunities arise, however, public librarians, too, can explain what critical cultural literacy is and point library users to resources to learn more.

The internet and social media will continue—for the foreseeable future—to be the first stops for information seekers seeking health and other types of information. Bad-faith actors know this and will use the internet and social media to misinform, disinform, and malinform. Knowing this is the case, the public must be armed with tools such as critical cultural literacy to combat and reject unreliable information.

References

Abbasi, Isha. 2021. "From Tuskegee to Today: The Fraught History of Black Americans with the Medical Field, and the Contemporary Issues Faced Under the Coronavirus." *Michigan Journal of Race and Law* 26. https://mjrl.org/2021/03/21/from-tuskegee-to-today-the-fraught-history-of-black-americans-with-the-medical-field-and-the-contemporary-issues-faced-under-the-coronavirus/.

Andrea, Lawrence. 2020. "Foreign Actors Seeking to Sow Divisions by Targeting Native American Populations, Cyber Intelligence Firm Says." *Milwaukee Journal Sentinel*, August 27, 2020. https://www.jsonline.com/story/news/politics/elections/2020/08/27/election-trolls-targeting-native-populations-cyber-group-says/5481408002/.

Bajaj, Simir Singe, and Fatima Cody Stanford. 2021. "Beyond Tuskegee: Vaccine Distrust and Everyday Racism." *The New England Journal of Medicine* 384, no. 5: e12. https://10.1056/NEJMpv2035827.

Barrett, Stephen. 2016. "A Skeptical Look at the Late 'Dr. Sebi.'" *Quackwatch*, August 16, 2016. https://quackwatch.org/11Ind/sebi/.

Bell, Chris. 2019. "Conspiracy Theories Spread After Nipsey Hussle Shooting." *BBC News*, April 2, 2019. https://www.bbc.com/news/blogs-trending-47785688.

Burnette, Catherine E., Soonhee Roh, Jessica Liddell, and Yeon-Shim Lee. 2018. "American Indian Women Cancer Survivor's Needs and Preferences: Community Support for Cancer Experiences." *Journal of Cancer Education* 34: 592–99. https://doi-org.proxy.mul.missouri.edu/10.1007/s13187-018-1346-4.

Bushak, Lecia. 2021. "Study: Health Misinformation Rampant in Hispanic Communities." *PR Week*, August 17, 2021. https://www.prweek.com/article/1725019/study-health-misinformation-rampant-hispanic-communities.

Campbell, Michael C., and Sarah A. Tishkoff. 2008. "African Genetic Diversity: Implications for Human Demographic History, Modern Human Origins, and Complex Disease Mapping." *Annual Review of Genomics and Human Genetics* 9: 403–33. https://dx.doi.org/10.1146%2Fannurev.genom.9.081307.164258.

Chandler, Rasheeta, Dominique Guillaume, Andrea G. Parker, Amber Mack, Jill Hamilton, Jemea Dorsey, and Natalie D. Hernandez. 2020. "The Impact of COVID-19 Among Black Women: Evaluating Perspectives and Sources of Information." *Ethnicity & Health* 26, no. 1: 80–93. https://doi-org.proxy.mul.missouri.edu/10.1080/13557858.2020.1841120.

Chou, Wen-Ying S., April Oh, and William M. P. Klein. 2018. "Addressing Health-Related Misinformation on Social Media." *JAMA* 320, no. 23. https://doi:10.1001/jama.2018.16865.

Chung, Matthew, Rosalind P. Oden, Brandi L. Joyner, Alexandra Sims, and Rachel Y. Moon. 2012. "Safe Infant Sleep Recommendations on the Internet: Let's Google It." *The Journal of Pediatrics* 161, no. 6: 1080–84. https://doi-org.proxy.mul.missouri.edu/10.1016/j.jpeds.2012.06.004.

Collins-Dexter, Brandi. 2020. *Canaries in the Cold Mine: COVID-19 Misinformation and Black Communities.* Cambridge, MA: Harvard Kennedy School. https://shorensteincenter.org/wp-content/uploads/2020/06/Canaries-in-the-Coal-Mine-Shorenstein-Center-June-2020.pdf.

Cooke, Nicole. 2018. *Fake News and Alternative Facts: Information Literacy in a Post-Truth Era.* Chicago: ALA Editions.

Cooke, Nicole. 2021. "Tell Me Sweet Little Lies: Racism as a Form of Persistent Malinformation." *Project Information Literacy*, August 11, 2021. https://projectinfolit.org/pubs/provocation-series/essays/tell-me-sweet-little-lies.html.

Dillon, Nancy. 2019. "Alleged Killer Eric Holder Shot Nipsey Hussle with Two Guns After 'Snitch' Accusation, Grand Jury Transcripts Say." *New York Daily News*, June 27, 2019. https://www.nydailynews.com/news/national/ny-nipsey-hussle-grand-jury-transcripts-snitch-comments-alleged-20190627-z5as2lo4fra7ziygeiml3kvfce-story.html.

DiResta, Renee, and Claire Wardle. 2020. *Online Misinformation About Vaccines.* The Sabin-Aspen Vaccine Science & Policy Group. https://www.sabin.org/sites/sabin.org/files/sabin-aspen-report-2020_meeting_the_challenge_of_vaccine_hesitancy.pdf.

Duran, Gil. 2020. "Unmasked in the Plandemic: Misinformation During the Novel Coronavirus (SARS-CoV-2) Pandemic." Master's thesis, University of San Francisco.

Farrow, Kenyon. 2019. "No, Dr. Sebi Did Not Have the Cure for HIV–Despite Nipsey Hussle's Planned Documentary." *The Body*, April 2, 2019. https://www.thebody.com/article/dr-sebi-did-not-cure-hiv-nipsey-hussle-documentary.

Ferreira, Giovanni, Adrian C. Traeger, Gustavo Machado, Mary O'Keefe, and Christopher G. Maher. 2019. "Credibility, Accuracy, and Comprehensiveness of Internet-Based Information About Lower Back Pain: A Systematic Review." *Journal of Medical Internet Research* 21, no. 5. https://doi.org/10.2196/13357.

Fletcher, Michael A. 2020. "Black Americans See a Health-Care System Infected by Racism, New Poll Shows." *National Geographic*, October 16, 2020. https://www.nationalgeographic.com/history/article/black-americans-see-health-care-system-infected-racism-new-poll-shows.

Freelon, Deen, Michael Bossetta, Chris Wells, Josephine Lukito, Yiping Xia, and Kirsten Adams. 2020. "Black Trolls Matter: Racial and Ideological Asymmetries in Social Media Disinformation." *Social Science Computer Review* 39, no. 2. https://doi-org.proxy.library.umkc.edu/10.1177%2F0894439320914853.

Fuchs, Chris. 2020. "How Chinese-Language Media in the U.S. are Debunking WeChat Coronavirus Misinformation." NBC News, March 13, 2020. https://www.nbcnews.com/news/asian-america/how-chinese-language-media-u-s-are-debunking-wechat-coronavirus-n1156621.

Ghaffary, Shirin. 2020. "How Fake News Aimed at Latinos Thrives on Social Media." *Vox*, November 19, 2020. https://www.vox.com/recode/21574293/social-media-latino-voters-2020-election.

Giacomazzo, Bernadette. 2021. "Meet Dr. Sebi, the Controversial 'Herbalist' Who Claimed He Could Cure Any Disease." *All That's Interesting*, October 4, 2021. https://allthatsinteresting.com/dr-sebi.

Gonzalez, Vivian M., and Monica C. Skewes. 2016. "Association of the Firewater Myth with Drinking Behavior Among American-Indian and Alaska Native College Students." *Psychology of Addictive Behaviors* 30, no. 8: 838–49. https://dx.doi.org/10.1037%2Fadb0000226.

Guadagnolo, B. Ashleigh, Kristin Cina, Petra Helbig, Kevin Molloy, Mary Reiner, E. Francis Cook, and Daniel G. Petereit. 2009. "Medical Distrust and Less Satisfaction with Healthcare Among Native Americans Presenting for Cancer Treatment." *Journal of Healthcare for the Poor and Underserved* 20, no. 1: 210–26. https://doi.org/10.1353/hpu.0.0108.

Guerrero, Jean. 2021. "Op-Ed: How Conspiracy Theories About COVID-19 Prey on Latinos." *Los Angeles Times*, May 2, 2021. https://www.latimes.com/opinion/story/2021-05-02/latinos-covid-vaccines-resistance-skepticism.

Harb, Jenna, and Kathryn Henne. 2019. "Disinformation and Resistance in the Surveillance of Indigenous Protesters." In *Information, Technology and Control in a Changing World.* Springer International Publishing. Editors: Blayne Haggart, Kathryn Henne, and Natasha Tusikov. Publisher: Cham, Switzerland. pp. 187–212.

Hoffman, Kelly M., Sophie Trawalter, Jordan R. Axt, and M. Norman Oliver. 2016. "Racial Bias in Pain Assessment and Treatment, Recommendations, and False Beliefs About Biological Differences Between Blacks and Whites." *Proceedings of the National Academy of Sciences of the United States of America* 113, no. 16: 4296–4301. https://www.pnas.org/content/113/16/4296.

Jaiswall, J., C. LoSchiavo, and D. C. Perlman. 2020. "Disinformation, Misinformation and Inequality-Driven Mistrust in the Time of COVID-19: Lessons Unlearned from AIDS Denialism." *AIDS and Behavior* 24, no. 10: 2776–80. https://www.ncbi.nlm.nih.gov/pmc/articles/PMC7241063/.

Jarry, Jonathan. 2019. "Dr. Sebi: What do We Make of this Non-Doctor?" McGill. Last modified April 12, 2019. https://www.mcgill.ca/oss/article/quackery/dr-sebi-what-do-we-make-him.

Kashani, Beeta M., Melissa Tibbits, Rachel C. Potter, Rosa Gofin, Li Westman, and Shinobu Watanabe-Galloway. 2019. "Human Papillomavirus Vaccination Trends, Barriers, and Promotion Methods Among American Indian/Alaska Native and Non-Hispanic White Adolescents in Michigan 2006-2015." *Journal of Community Health* 44: 436–43. https://doi-org.proxy.mul.missouri.edu/10.1007/s10900-018-00615-4.

Kedzior, Sophie G. E., Tina Bianco-Miotto, James Breen, Kerrilyn R. Diener, Martin Donnelley, Kylie R. Dunning et al. 2019. "It Takes a Community to Conceive: An Analysis of the Scope, Nature, and Accuracy of Online Sources of Health Information for Couples Trying to Conceive." *Reproductive Biomedicine & Society Online* 9: 48–63. https://doi-org.proxy.mul.missouri.edu/10.1016/j.rbms.2019.08.004.

Lee, Jongmin, Woo Ho Ban, Hyun Kyung Park, Eunbyeol Na, Sug Kyung Kim, Hyeon Hui Kang, and Sang Haak Lee. 2018. "Accuracy and Reliability of Internet Resources Providing Information on Obstructive Sleep Apnea." *Journal of Clinical Sleep Medicine* 14, no. 10: 1717–23. https://dx.doi.org/10.5664%2Fjcsm.7380.

Li, Bo, and Olan Scott. 2020. "Fake News Travels Fast: Exploring Misinformation Circulated Around Wu Lei's Coronavirus Case." *International Journal of Sport Communication* 13, no. 3: 505–13. https://doi.org/10.1123/ijsc.2020-0056.

Liddell, Jessica L., Catherine E. Burnette, Soonhee Roh, and Yeon-Shim Lee. 2018. "Healthcare Barriers and Supports for American Indian Women with Cancer." *Social Work in Health Care* 57 (8): 656–673. https://doi.org/10.1080/00981389.2018.1474837.

Mazzei, Patricia, and Nicole Perlroth. 2020. "False News Targeting Latinos Trails the Election." *New York Times*, November 4, 2020. https://www.nytimes.com/2020/11/04/us/spanish-language-misinformation-latinos.html.

Merchant, Raina M., and David A. Asch. 2018. "Protecting the Value of Medical Science in the Age of Social Media and 'Fake News.'" *JAMA* 320, no. 23: 2415–16. https://doi:10.1001/jama.2018.18416.

Milburn, Norweeta G., Alison B. Hamilton, Susana Lopez, and Gail E. Wyatt. 2019. "Mentoring the Next Generation of Behavioral Scientists to Promote Health Equity." *American Journal of Orthopsychiatry* 89, no. 3: 369–77. https://content.apa.org/doi/10.1037/ort0000415.

Mineo, Liz. 2021. "Rise of Violence, Harassment Amid Pandemic Part of Continuing Tale of Racism in the U.S." *The Harvard Gazette*, March 24, 2021. https://news.harvard.edu/gazette/story/2021/03/a-long-history-of-bigotry-against-asian-americans/.

National Academies of Sciences, Engineering, and Medicine. 2017. "Appendix A: Native American Health: Historical and Legal Context." In *Communities in Acton: Pathways to Health Equity*. Washington, DC: National Academies Press. https://nap.nationalacademies.org/catalog/24624/communities-in-action-pathways-to-health-equity. pp. 507–518.

Nguyen, Terry. 2020a. "The Challenge of Combating Fake News in Asian-American Communities." *Vox*, November 27, 2020. https://www.vox.com/identities/21579752/asian-american-misinformation-after-2020.

Nguyen, Terry. 2020b. "Asian-American Voters Face Misinformation Campaigns." Interview by Debbie Elliot. *NPR*, December 6, 2020.

Novak, Nicole L., and Natalie Lira. 2018. "California Once Targeted Latinas for Forced Sterilization." *Smithsonian Magazine*, March 22, 2018. https://www.smithsonianmag.com/history/california-targeted-latinas-forced-sterilization-180968567/.

Pennycook, Gordon, and David G. Rand. 2019. "Fighting Misinformation on Social Media Using Crowdsourced Judgments of News Source Quality." *Proceedings of the National Academy of Sciences* 116, no. 7: 2521–26. https://doi.org/10.1073/pnas.1806781116.

Plambeck, Benjamin, Jinfeng Jiang, David Fu, Alexandra Colvin, and Deibert Christopher. 2021. "MP27-07 Exploring the Readability, Quality and Accuracy of Online Health Information for Penile Implants/Protheses." *Journal of Urology* 206, no. 3 supplemental: e474–e474. https://doi.org/10.1097/JU.0000000000002024.07.

Rodriguez, Joe F., Shannon Lin, and Jessica Huseman. 2020. "Misinformation Image on WeChat Attempts to Frighten Chinese Americans Out of Voting." *ProPublica*, November 2, 2020. https://www.propublica.org/article/misinformation-image-on-wechat-attempts-to-frighten-chinese-americans-out-of-voting.

Sabin, Janice A., and Anthony G. Greenwald. 2012. "The Influence of Implicit Bias on Treatment Recommendations for 4 Common Pediatric Conditions: Pain, Urinary Tract Infection, Attention Deficit Hyperactivity Disorder and Asthma." *American Journal of Public Health* 102, no. 5: 988–95. https://pubmed.ncbi.nlm.nih.gov/22420817/.

Sabin, Sam. 2020. "Hispanic Adults Use WhatsApp More than the General Public. Disinformation Campaigns are Targeting that Vulnerability." *Morning Consult*, October 30, 2020. https://morningconsult.com/2020/10/30/hispanic-adults-use-whatsapp-more-than-the-general-public-disinformation-campaigns-are-targeting-that-vulnerability/.

Sanny, Josephine A. 2021. "African Citizens Support Their Governments' Pandemic Responses, Mostly: They're Not Sure About Vaccines." *Washington Post*, August 27, 2021. https://www.washingtonpost.com/politics/2021/08/27/african-citizens-support-their-governments-pandemic-responses-mostly-theyre-not-sure-about-vaccines/.

Sesin, Carmen. 2020. "Mistrust, Disinformation Among Latinos on COVID Vaccine Worries Hispanic Doctors." NBC News, December 20, 2020. https://www.nbcnews.com/news/latino/mistrust-disinformation-among-latinos-covid-vaccine-worries-hispanic-doctors-n1251636.

Seo, Hyunjin, Matthew Blomberg, Darcey Altschwager, and Hong Tien Vu. 2020. "Vulnerable Populations and Misinformation: A Mixed-Methods Approach to Underserved Older Adults' Online Information Assessment." *New Media & Society* 23, no. 7: 2012–33. https://doi-org.proxy.library.umkc.edu/10.1177%2F1461444820925041.

Southwell, Brian G., and Emily A. Thorson. 2015. "The Prevalence, Consequence, and Remedy of Misinformation in Mass Media Systems." *Journal of Communication* 65, no. 4: 589–95. https://doi-org.proxy.mul.missouri.edu/10.1111/jcom.12168.

Soy, Anne. 2020. "Coronavirus in Africa: Five Reasons Why COVID-19 Has Been Less Deadly than Elsewhere." BBC News, October 8, 2020. https://www.bbc.com/news/world-africa-54418613.

Tewell, Eamon. 2015. "A Decade of Critical Information Literacy: A Review of the Literature." *Communications and Information Literacy* 9, no. 1: 24–43. https://doi.org/10.15760/comminfolit.2015.9.1.174.

Towne, Jordan, Yasmine Suliman, Kaleigh A. Russel, Mallory A. Stuparich, Samar Nahas, and Sadikah Behbehani. 2021. "Health Information in the Era of Social Media: An Analysis of the Nature and Accuracy of Posts Made by Public Facebook Pages for Patients with Endometriosis." *Journal of Minimally Invasive Gynecology* 28, no. 9: 1637–42. https://doi-org.proxy.mul.missouri.edu/10.1016/j.jmig.2021.02.005.

University of Pittsburgh. 2020. "Modern-Day Hippocrates: Incoming School of Medicine Students Write Their Own Oath." *PittWire*, September 11, 2020. https://www.pitt.edu/pittwire/features-articles/modern-day-hippocrates-incoming-school-medicine-students-write-their-own-oath.

Vosoughi, Soroush, Deb Roy, and Sinan Aral. 2018. "The Spread of True and False News Online." *Science* 359, no. 6380: 1146–51. https://doi.org/10.1126/science.aap9559.

Wardle, Claire, and Hossein Derakhshan. 2017. *Information Disorder: Toward an Interdisciplinary Framework for Research and Policy Making*. Council of Europe.

Weissert, Will. 2021. "From Vote to Virus, Misinformation Campaigns Target Latinos." AP News, March 7, 2021. https://apnews.com/article/joe-biden-donald-trump-race-and-ethnicity-media-misinformation-9696392bf389ba8ca3441d2314abcefa.

White, Robert M. 2005. "Misinformation and Misbeliefs in the Tuskegee Study of Untreated Syphilis Fuel Mistrust in the Healthcare System." *Journal of the National Medical Association* 97, no. 11: 1566–73. https://pubmed.ncbi.nlm.nih.gov/16334509/.

Wright, Amy L., Rachel VanEvery, and Vicky Miller. 2021. "Indigenous Mothers' Use of Web- and App-Based Information Sources to Support Healthy Parenting and Infant Health in Canada: Interpretive Description." *JMIR Pediatrics and Parenting* 4, no. 2: e16145. https://doi.org/10.2196/16145.

III

PRACTICE

10

When Medical Practice Meets Medical Myth

Confronting Misinformation in the Clinical Encounter

Jamie L. Wood, Erin Eckert, Megan von Isenburg, Joseph Jackson, and Brian G. Southwell

In the summer of 2021, the surgeon general issued an advisory regarding health misinformation as a threat to public health and societal well-being (Murthy 2021, 4–7). While this advisory generated news headlines, the phenomenon of misinformation has been a dilemma for health care professionals (HCPs) for many years (Granter and Papke 2018; Murthy 2021, 4). HCPs globally face challenges during interactions with patients and their families when dealing with inaccurate, misleading, and problematic information. These problematic sources have seen a sharp increase concurrent with the increase in users of multiple social media platforms (Suarez-Lledo and Alvarez-Galvez 2021).

Consider the experiences of one of us. Dr. Joseph Jackson is a practicing pediatrician in Durham, North Carolina, who regularly encounters patients referring to misinformation in their exchanges with him. Below are two examples of his experiences in the clinical setting written as fictionalized composites to represent both the types of misinformation patients espouse and their motivations for doing so. We note that these vignettes do not represent any individual patient and are not taken directly from medical records.

> Encounter 1—S.K. is a twelve-month-old African American male who presents to the clinic with his mom for a scheduled well-child visit. In addition to reviewing growth and development, S.K. is scheduled to receive his routine twelve-month vaccinations, which include the measles, mumps, and rubella (MMR) vaccine as per CDC guidelines ("Birth-18 Years Immunization Schedule | CDC" 2021). When asked to consent for vaccinations, his mom reports hearing from a close friend who recently read an article about the increased potential for African American boys to develop autism following the administration of the MMR vaccine. His mother also has a cousin who was diagnosed with autism, so she remains highly resistant to continuing with any of the remaining childhood immunizations given this perceived concern. Although his mom remains open to discussing vaccines, she has decided to refuse all childhood immunizations given her mounting mistrust of the medical establishment.

> Encounter 2—B.J. is a seventeen-year-old male who presents to the clinic for a routine annual visit prior to leaving for his first year of college. He is interested in receiving a COVID-19 vaccine which his university has recommended. However, his parents are reluctant for him to move forward with COVID-19 vaccination because they read an article claiming the vaccine was never properly studied

and may have received emergency approval without credible evidence from the former president of the United States. B.J.'s parents are concerned he might contract COVID-19 when he is away at college, but they are equally concerned that the testing to determine the safety and efficacy of the vaccine for use in young people is insufficient. Therefore, they believe B.J. should not receive the shot.

The preceding examples illustrate just two of the many types of misinformation Dr. Jackson has encountered in over fifteen years of practice. What can we learn from such situations? Clearly, misinformation is a pervasive threat. However, not all misinformation is the same, and it can sometimes be weaved together with legitimate concerns that patients want to discuss with their HCP.

Dr. Jackson is not alone in encountering medical misinformation from his patients. In 2020, we surveyed physicians and physician assistants in North Carolina about their experiences with medical misinformation. When asked if patients had referred to medical misinformation in a clinical encounter within the past year, 94 percent of our respondents said yes (Wood et al. 2021).

The COVID-19 pandemic has heightened public awareness of misinformation related to health, medicine, and wellness (Bellware 2020; Mian and Khan 2020; Tasnim, Hossain, and Mazumder 2020; Wang et al. 2019). With increased patient access to both information and misinformation via the internet and social media platforms (Jacobs, Amuta, and Jeon 2017), the medical community has responded with calls for HCPs to engage with their patients on the topic of misinformation (O'Connor and Murphy 2020; Sturgill 2021; Wu and Mccormick 2018). This poses a challenge for HCPs to figure out the best methods and tools to do so.

Here, we discuss the patient's challenge of medical misinformation, how it impacts the clinical encounter, and the lack of preparation and training HCPs receive to discuss such misinformation with patients. We will also discuss the Duke Program on Medical Misinformation, which we developed with others in 2020–2021. We offer a process that other academic medical institutions can use as a model or supplement to potentially mitigate the spread of medical misinformation.

Scope of the Problem

HCPs in the United States face tremendous challenges in executing their work. Time to talk with patients is often limited, patients often have access to a wide array of both accurate and inaccurate information that can influence their decision-making, and clinician training often emphasizes medical care over the nuances of interacting with patients who refer to inaccurate information.

Time Constraints

Data from Medscape's 2018 Physician Compensation Report (which excluded psychiatrists) show that 62 percent of respondents spend an average of thirteen to twenty-four minutes with their patients (Kane 2018). Since contact time is a scarce and valuable resource, both the HCP and patient must choose what is most important for discussion in the clinical setting. If patients opt to refer to inaccurate information found online (which they do not know to be inaccurate), part of the challenge lies in the time available to explore and discuss that (mis) information. Considering this perspective, some HCPs may tend to either simply dismiss a patient's reference to misinformation without engaging with it or attempt to quickly contradict them by referring to peer-reviewed studies. This tendency is understandable, but such choices threaten the patient-HCP relationship.

Time constraints in office (or telehealth) visits are also relevant to our discussion because of their suppressive effect. If patients perceive time is lacking during a clinic visit, they may choose to withhold information about supplements they are taking or prescribed medication they have chosen not to take. This withholding might be detrimental to patient health and could even prove fatal. For HCPs to uncover any relevant and potentially dangerous patient-held misinformation, they may need to specifically ask and probe in a type of conversation that requires trust between the patient and HCP.

The Prevalence of Misinformation

Currently, little data in the peer-reviewed literature describes how HCPs specifically encounter medical misinformation espoused by patients in a clinical setting, but anecdotal evidence highlights concern among researchers and HCPs alike (Bellware 2020; Tasnim, Hossain, and Mazumder 2020). Wood et al. (2021) recently published pilot survey data from 2,183 licensed practitioners in North Carolina that suggests that the problem HCPs face is dramatic. In addition to the near-ubiquity of encounters with medical misinformation reported by respondents, they also reported the frequency of encounters with misinformation related to five specific topics: COVID-19, vaccines, statins, essential oils, and alternative therapies to cancer. Respondents most often noted patient references to misinformation about vaccines, with 65.5 percent (1375/2100) reporting "often" or "sometimes" encountering what they deemed to be vaccine misinformation. Respondents also frequently encountered misinformation ("often" or "sometimes") on the topics of COVID-19 origin (54.1 percent), treatment (56.2 percent), and essential oils (52.4 percent) (Wood et al. 2021).

Importantly, medical misinformation is not all the same. Despite news headlines decrying the prevalence of misinformation, we should keep in mind that misinformation varies in reach and consequence. If a piece of misinformation is seen and shared by only a small group of people, the impact of that misinformation is limited in terms of public health. Medical misinformation becomes problematic for public health when many people not only see and share the misinformation but then engage in a behavior based on that misinformation. Southwell and colleagues (2019) point to the example of questionable information that urges consumers to consume lemon and cayenne pepper to "detox" and reduce the risk of cancer, despite a lack of evidence supporting this as prevention or treatment for cancer. If only a small network of people sees such misinformation, it is likely limited both in terms of audience reach and in terms of whether consequentially unhealthy behavior is being promoted. After all, consuming these two ingredients is unlikely to have serious health-related consequences. However, misinformation surrounding the COVID-19 vaccine includes the mistaken belief that taking the vaccine will change the recipient's DNA. This misinformation has a large reach across social media and other platforms and has likely resulted in some people refusing the COVID-19 vaccine. This does have serious consequences for public health, as the pandemic will persist with fewer people being vaccinated.

An Imbalance in Training and Perspective

HCPs receive extensive training in the basic science of the body, interpretation of clinical data (vital signs, lab analysis, scan results, etc.), and skills related to the patient encounter before they practice professionally. Those who hold degrees in their field (e.g., MDs, DOs, PAs, BSNs, DPTs, etc.) generally complete significant coursework in the sciences and research methodologies, which is less likely to be the case with their patients. Data from the 2020 US Census show that 53.4 percent of the population has completed high school or some college, while only 37.5 percent attained a bachelor's degree or higher (https://www.census.gov/content/dam/Census/library/visualizations/time-series/demo/fig_2.png). As such, HCPs and patients are likely to approach health-related questions and potential answers, both accurate and misinformed, from different starting points. HCPs and patients may not tap into the same well of resources to access information regarding health and disease. HCPs are generally familiar with, and have easier access to, costly subscription-based academic databases and medical literature because of their education and professional affiliations. Patients likely will not have access to nor familiarity with these resources unless they have similar institutional affiliations and educations. One consequence is that clinician and patient might both earnestly look for information on a particular topic, but differences in resources mean the patient is more likely to encounter misinformation during their search. Websites and social media content that support misinformation are often easier for patients to access and understand (Murthy 2021, 5). Therefore, when patients bring health-related information into the clinical encounter with the HCP, both may be operating in good faith without fully understanding the perspective, motivation, resources, and rationale of the other.

One curricular content area required in most academic health care professions programs and relevant to discussing information and evidence with patients is evidence-based practice (EBP). EBP curricula can vary based on school and profession but are generally defined as "the conscientious, explicit and judicious use of current best evidence in making decisions about the care of individual patients" (Sackett et al. 1996, 71). A 2018 Delphi study and survey identified sixty-eight consensus-based core EBP competencies that are organized into the five primary EBP domains: asking clinical questions, acquiring the evidence, appraising and interpreting studies, applying the evidence in the care of individual patients, and evaluating the process (Albarqouni et al. 2018). Applying the evidence includes taking the individual patient's preferences and values into consideration as well as engaging the patient in shared decision-making. However, specifically engaging in discussions of misinformation with patients is not typically included in EBP curricula. Although EBP approaches clearly offer useful information to structure and guide informed decision-making by clinicians and patients working together, it is unclear how many EBP trainings explicitly address how to overcome biases that can stem from the inaccurate information base on which patients sometimes rely. After all, the typical EBP focus is on avoiding reliance on such inaccurate and invalid information in the first place.

HCPs also typically receive training in shared decision-making, in which patients and clinicians work together to make informed decisions about patient care options (Oshima Lee and Emanuel 2013), and motivational interviewing, a technique designed to help patients make a change using a guiding, rather than directing, style (Rollnick et al. 2010). Recent reviews of shared decision-making and motivational interviewing curricula in medical schools show that while these courses are heterogeneous and lack standardization, they do frequently include content on communicating with patients (Durand et al. 2018; Kaltman and Tankersley 2020). It is unknown how much, if any, training in these areas specifically addresses patient interactions directly involving health misinformation. When licensed practitioners in North Carolina were surveyed and asked about formal training relating to engaging patients in conversation on medical misinformation, only 18 percent of respondents said they could recall receiving such formal training (Wood et al. 2021). Simply stated, many clinicians do not have formal training for a situation that almost all clinicians report facing regularly.

We want our HCPs to be well-trained in reviewing clinical trial data and well-versed in guiding patients to the best treatment options. However, this likely leaves less time to teach HCPs how to understand the motivations of why a patient may seek an alternate or unproven treatment that is based on misinformation or clinically untested hypotheses. We can speculate as to what may be primary drivers for patients to believe medical misinformation: fervent hope for a cure to a disease, a cheaper alternative treatment, or beliefs based on religion/cultural/political identity (Scherer and Pennycook 2020). Additionally, patients in these circumstances may lean more into the tendency of accepting information as true with less stringent critical analysis of that information.

We see an example of imbalance in information analysis between HCPs and patients in recent study results. Boudewyns et al. (2021) studied primary care providers (PCPs) and patients enrolled in an experiment to determine if these groups would detect deceptive and misleading information as the amount of that information increased. Each group of participants viewed a mock website advertising a hypothetically realistic but nonexistent drug to treat chronic pain. Participants were randomly assigned to see one of three versions of the website: one with no deceptive or misleading claims, one with a few deceptive or misleading claims, and one with many. The authors found that exposure to more deceptive claims or tactics did not increase suspicion about the accuracy of the website among patients. In contrast, PCPs demonstrated a different pattern; exposure to more deceptive claims and tactics led to a greater perception that the website in question was deceptive and also predicted lower acceptance of deceptive claims. Although everyone is vulnerable to misinformation under some circumstances, patients appear to be more vulnerable to nuanced medical misinformation than PCPs, and similar patterns are likely for other types of practitioners. Despite some potential advantages in deception detection, HCPs are not necessarily trained to translate that knowledge clearly for their patients. With training in EBP, but little to none in psychology, social science, or misinformation specifically, HCPs may lack the skills to discuss patient-held misinformation thoughtfully and with empathy.

Ideally, we want to strive for HCP-patient interactions that not only maintain strength and trust in the relationship but also remove potential "blinders" HCPs might have given their extensive training. For example, suppose a patient presents to her PCP with a severe cough and chest pain. The PCP diagnoses the patient with pneumonia and recommends a standard antibiotic. The patient refuses the medication, stating that she eats only organic food and will use a specific combination of essential oils to cure the infection. From the perspective of the PCP, this response may seem foolish and potentially life threatening. The PCP knows the pathophysiology of pneumonia and the pharmacology of antibiotics, having learned the basic science of the body, and is likely aware of the lack of credible peer-reviewed evidence to support alternative treatment. But if the PCP simply "throws the facts" at this patient without accounting for the values that led the patient to her stance or without accounting for patient psychology, it is unlikely to change her mind and may even undermine the relationship. If this is the tactic used, the PCP might never learn that the patient had a previous allergic reaction to an antibiotic and has vowed to never take another one. Or, perhaps, that she read an article from a health blog that espoused the "harm" antibiotics will do to the natural microbial community in her body. In this age of misinformation, HCPs should expect and be prepared to discuss patient ideas or preferences that are misaligned with the latest peer-reviewed evidence.

Social science suggests that general misinformation poses a challenging problem for society (Southwell, Thorson, and Sheble 2018, 1–11), but medical misinformation specifically can invite potentially life-threatening consequences. However, all hope is not lost. We know the majority of Americans have a positive view of both medical doctors and medical research scientists ("Trust in Medical Scientists Has Grown in U.S., but Mainly Among Democrats" 2020, 19). Nonetheless, the challenge of widely available medical misinformation threatens the trusted relationships that typically exist between patients and practitioners. The threat in this instance lies not only in problematic decisions that patients might make but also in the interactions between clinicians and patients that can occur when medical misinformation is a factor. Support for clinicians in addressing the conversational opportunities that lie ahead seems to be a vital but perhaps overlooked part of the equation for the future of health care.

HCP Training as a Mitigation Strategy

In December 2020, we launched the Duke Program on Medical Misinformation at Duke University. The program has two codirectors—Jamie L. Wood, PhD, and Brian G. Southwell, PhD; Erin Eckert, MPA, CPPS of the Duke Center for Healthcare Safety and Quality, has overseen program logistics in the initial phase of the initiative. We also invited an advisory board of medical professionals representing a broad spectrum of health care fields and medical education, including medicine, nursing, pharmacy, and library sciences. Megan von Isenburg, MSLS, and Joseph Jackson, MD, serve on the board.

From January to June of 2021, we offered monthly, online workshops with the following goals:

1. To help HCPs understand the patient psychology of misinformation and the information environment.
2. To provide practice conversations using case-based scenarios of patient reference to misinformation in a clinical encounter.

We opened our workshops to anyone working in a health-related profession who wanted to learn more about medical misinformation and how to discuss it with patients. We believe this initial offering directly meets the need for training identified in the Wood et al. (2021) study, which suggested that most providers in North Carolina have not received training to discuss medical misinformation meaningfully with patients during clinical encounters. Due to COVID-19 restrictions, we used Zoom as our online platform to host the workshops. This did complicate interpersonal interaction but also underscored the need for such a training program, as misinformation related to COVID-19 and prevention measures spread widely in the United States and around the world during this period (Southwell, Wood, and Navar 2020). The virtual setting also opened the door to global participation; we welcomed participants from four countries and various states (including North Carolina). The geographic diversity of participants appears to have been a strength of the approach; as participants shared anecdotal examples of their experiences with medical misinformation, the details varied, but underlying themes of patient access to misinformation and challenging discussions were nearly universal.

In a typical session, we ask participants for their professional identities and experiences with medical misinformation both as icebreaker questions and to gather additional background information. The first thirty-five minutes of the workshop is a didactic session exploring the context of medical misinformation, how patients experience it, and why they may be persuaded to believe it. Some of the theoretical approach—which emphasizes human vulnerability to misinformation and the need for compassion for patients—draws on essays such as those by Southwell, Thorson, and Sheble (2017) and Southwell, Wood, and Navar (2020, 2021). We place particular emphasis on the human need for social connection and hope for the future, noting the absence of either is a fertile breeding ground for misinformation and a challenge for science communication. One example we use comes from an analysis of the rapid dissemination of a news article touting a cure for cancer (Vincent 2019). The original article, published in the *Jerusalem Post* on January 28, 2019, was picked up by multiple other news outlets, which then led to over four million shares of the articles in three weeks on social media (predominately Facebook). Vincent (2019) also writes that there was little fact-checking for the claim, noting that news outlets carried the original article as a "repeat" story.

The next thirty-five minutes of a typical session are devoted to participant practice with case-based scenarios. We assign participants randomly to Zoom breakout rooms with an assigned case we have created, often tailored to the anticipated composition of a particular workshop when possible. Each case focuses on a patient either refusing or questioning a conventional treatment, such as a vaccine, due to misleading information accessed via a website or other media. One example scenario we use is based on the article "The Medications That Change Who We Are," published online with the BBC Future on January 8, 2020. The article cites anecdotes of patients who developed aggressive behavior after they began taking statins, so our scenario asks participants to imagine a sixty-six-year-old female with high cholesterol now refusing to take her statin after reading the article. We ask participants to discuss how this conversation might go and provide tips for developing a productive conversation, which include being empathetic and open, acknowledging the patient's concerns, asking what they have learned outside of the clinic visit, and referring them to accurate sources of information.

After participants have time to discuss scenarios in the breakout rooms, we bring everyone back to the main Zoom room for discussion. Part of the discussion includes the question of what resources could assist in addressing identified challenges. One overarching goal of our program, in addition to individual training, is to identify the institutional or structural changes or implementations that could mitigate the spread of medical misinformation if put in place. These discussions have been helpful in that regard, suggesting, for example, the potential utility of developing learning networks of organizational partners.

Between January and June 2021, we hosted six online workshops with a total of eighty-one participants; attendance ranged from eight to twenty-four people per workshop. Individual workshop registration costs were $125 per registrant, and we were approved to offer Continuing Medical Education credit after completion. We recruited participants via internal advertising at Duke University, promotion via the Duke Center for Healthcare Safety and Quality Twitter account, and personal outreach efforts via the codirectors. Participants attended from across the United States and from around the globe, including Israel, the United Kingdom, and Canada. Of those who indicated their profession in our background questions, approximately 40 percent were nurses or nurse practitioners, and roughly a quarter were physicians, which might point to some differences in time pressures faced by various groups for even a ninety-minute session. Other attendees included nonclinical professionals, allied health professionals, a physician assistant, and others such as medical students.

In post-workshop surveys, feedback has been overwhelmingly positive, which may indicate both an interest in the subject matter and a need for this type of training. Almost all of our participants (96 percent through mid-2021) either agree or strongly agree with the following statement: This workshop will help me initiate conversations about medical misinformation and talk with patients about inaccurate information they encounter. When asked "I would recommend this workshop to others," 93 percent of respondents said yes. Overall, our participants reported that they gained new knowledge and insight into the complexity of medical misinformation and that they could immediately *apply* this knowledge to patients in the clinic. Survey respondents highlighted these ideas (see examples below) when responding to this question: "I would recommend this workshop to others. Why or why not?"

"This workshop highlights a gap in providing ways to address misinformation as presented by patients. The experience provides for practical ways to address this gap and triggers thought on the issue of misinformation in health and what an individual can do in certain circumstances."

"You provided me with a gift of words that I can use. Thank you."

An additional theme that emerged from our feedback survey was the commonality of medical misinformation across borders and fields of health care, as this example highlights:

"This is a topic that all members of the healthcare team need to be facile in. Our patients bring us information from all corners of the earth, and it is our responsibility to help them translate it to improve their health."

Noting the interprofessional nature of mitigating medical misinformation was not a specific goal we had in mind when starting these workshops. In retrospect, however, this theme makes sense, especially when one reflects on the challenges and opportunities related to trust that all HCPs face in their professional work. For example, patients may be more comfortable discussing topics with a nurse rather than a physician based on many factors, including gender, ethnicity, or language barriers.

Following the initial development of our program, we have identified many potential directions for growth, expansion, and collaboration. One model is a "train the trainer" approach, which could expand the reach of our key ideas. Pending necessary support, we also could do follow-up "check-ins" with previous participants to see how what they learned is serving them, and what else, if anything, is needed. Some of our advisory board also continue to be interested in research related to medical misinformation, which could dovetail with the implementation and practice of our pragmatic workshops. Finally, as mentioned earlier, we are interested in how increasing knowledge of medical misinformation can lead to institutional changes within medical practice. For example, do we need new "quick access" databases for HCPs containing the most common pieces of misinformation and how to discuss it? What role can our medical librarians play in helping patients understand and critically analyze available information? What should departments do if HCPs are serving as *sources* of medical misinformation? These are large questions about a complex topic, and it is likely that one simple strategy will not be the answer.

Finally, our effort is part of a growing chorus of educational efforts. At the time of this writing, Duke is not alone in offering courses on misinformation. For example, the Mayo Clinic now offers a course titled "COVID-19: Countering an 'Infodemic' of Misinformation," and the Stanford Center for Continuing Medical Education has created a three-part webinar series (CME credit available) titled "Medicine, Media & Misinformation." The University of Minnesota has developed an elective course for medical students titled "COVID-19: Outbreaks and the Media," which teaches students how to share accurate public health information while correcting misinformation. These courses are relevant and timely and the continued expansion of courses about health-related misinformation will be vital even after the COVID-19 pandemic is over.

Conclusion

With each new scientific discovery, the potential for propagation of misinformation exists. Consider for a moment the human gut microbiome. A flourishing microbial community resides within the human gastrointestinal (GI) tract that serves many physiological functions, including roles in digestion and immunity (Thursby and Juge 2017). Researchers have studied this community for decades, but advances in genetic sequencing developed in the mid-2000s made groundbreaking discoveries possible. Scientists have identified the specific species present in the GI tract (Tang 2019) and have learned that an individual's microbiome is unique (Dickson 2019). Replacing a patient's gut microbiome via fecal transplants has been tested in randomized controlled trials for *C. difficile* infections (Moayyedi et al. 2017) and ulcerative colitis (Costello et al. 2019; Kelly and Ananthakrishnan 2019) with demonstrated effectiveness. However, as scientific discovery of the microbiome grows, so does the potential for and documentation of misinformation about it. Recent studies document the rise in articles classified as "microbiome hype" (Marcon, Turvey, and Caulfield 2021, 5) that deal with research methods linking the gut microbiome and brain (Hooks, Konsman, and O'Malley 2020), and the dubious connection between gut health and "immune boosting" as related to the COVID-19 pandemic (Rachul et al. 2020). In reviewing multiple narratives in the popular press regarding the microbiome and its potential effects on overall health, Bik (2016) reminds readers that correlation does not equal causation and notes along with Marcon (2020) that many products marketed to improve or "boost" gut health have little credible evidence to support them.

Misinformation surrounding the gut microbiome is only one drop in a large ocean of health-related misinformation. For those working as HCPs, medical educators, patient educators, or librarians and information scientists, mitigating the spread of misinformation can seem like bailing out this ocean with a teaspoon. This complex problem will require many approaches; we focused on the relationships between HCPs and patients, noting that HCPs will likely need specific training to discuss misinformation with patients. Other strategies, some of which are addressed by other authors in this text, include increasing science/health literacy within the lay public, investing in high-quality science journalism by the popular press, and creating resources with accurate information that are easily accessible and understood by general audiences. We also acknowledge the many structural barriers in place that deter mitigation efforts, one of which is equal access to high-quality, easily understandable health information.

If the COVID-19 pandemic has taught us anything, it is that navigating patient-held beliefs based on misinformation requires time, patience, and empathy, particularly when that misinformation affects public health and involves politics and group identity. HCPs have long-standing relationships with patients in which they can use their empathy and be patient. By providing HCPs with the proper training to discuss medical misinformation with patients, we can further strengthen trust in these relationships and add one more tool in the toolbox of misinformation mitigation.

References

Albarqouni, Loai, Tammy Hoffmann, Sharon Straus, Nina Rydland Olsen, Taryn Young, Dragan Ilic, Terrence Shaneyfelt, R. Brian Haynes, Gordon Guyatt, and Paul Glasziou. 2018. "Core Competencies in Evidence-Based Practice for Health Professionals." *JAMA Network Open* 1 (2). https://doi.org/10.1001/jamanetworkopen.2018.0281.

BBC Future. 2020. "The Medications that Change Who We Are." https://www.bbc.com/future/article/20200108-the-medications-that-change-who-we-are.

Bellware, K. 2020. "The Coronavirus Is Spreading Rapidly. So Is Misinformation about It." *The Washington Post*, February 10, 2020. https://www.washingtonpost.com/health/2020/02/10/coronavirus-is-spreading-rapidly-so-is-misinformation-about-it/.

Bik, Elisabeth M. 2016. "The Hoops, Hopes, and Hypes of Human Microbiome Research." *Yale Journal of Biology & Medicine* 89(3): 363–373.

"Birth-18 Years Immunization Schedule | CDC." 2021. Centers for Disease Control and Prevention. February 12, 2021. https://www.cdc.gov/vaccines/schedules/hcp/imz/child-adolescent.html#note-rotavirus.

Boudewyns, Vanessa, Kevin R. Betts, Mihaela Johnson, Ryan S. Paquin, Amie C. O'Donoghue, and Brian G. Southwell. 2021. "Experimental Evidence of Consumer and Physician Detection and Rejection of Misleading Prescription Drug Website Content." *Research in Social and Administrative Pharmacy* 17 (4): 733–43. https://doi.org/10.1016/j.sapharm.2020.06.019.

Costello, Samuel P., Patrick A. Hughes, Oliver Waters, Robert v. Bryant, Andrew D. Vincent, Paul Blatchford, Rosa Katsikeros et al. 2019. "Effect of Fecal Microbiota Transplantation on 8-Week Remission in Patients With Ulcerative Colitis." *JAMA* 321 (2). https://doi.org/10.1001/jama.2018.20046.

Dickson, Iain. 2019. "Stability and Individuality of Adult Microbiota." *Nature*, June 17, 2019. https://www.nature.com/articles/d42859-019-00012-4.

Durand, Marie-Anne, Peter R. DiMilia, Julia Song, Renata W. Yen, and Paul J. Barr. 2018. "Shared Decision Making Embedded in the Undergraduate Medical Curriculum: A Scoping Review." *PLoS ONE* 13 (11). https://doi.org/10.1371/journal.pone.0207012.

Granter, Scott R., and David J. Papke. 2018. "Opinion: Medical Misinformation in the Era of Google: Computational Approaches to a Pervasive Problem." *Proceedings of the National Academy of Sciences* 115 (25). https://doi.org/10.1073/pnas.1808264115.

Hooks, Katarzyna B., Jan Pieter Konsman, and Maureen A. O'Malley. 2020. "Microbiota-Gut-Brain Research: A Critical Analysis." *Behavioral and Brain Sciences* 42. https://doi.org/10.1017/S0140525X18002133.

Jacobs, Wura, Ann O. Amuta, and Kwon Chan Jeon. 2017. "Health Information Seeking in the Digital Age: An Analysis of Health Information Seeking Behavior among US Adults." *Cogent Social Sciences* 3 (1). https://doi.org/10.1080/23311886.2017.1302785.

Kaltman, Stacey, and Amelia Tankersley. 2020. "Teaching Motivational Interviewing to Medical Students." *Academic Medicine* 95 (3). https://doi.org/10.1097/ACM.0000000000003011.

Kane, Leslie. 2018. "Medscape Physician Compensation Report 2018." Published April 11, 2018. https://www.medscape.com/slideshow/2018-compensation-overview-6009667#32.

Kelly, Colleen R., and Ashwin N. Ananthakrishnan. 2019. "Manipulating the Microbiome With Fecal Transplantation to Treat Ulcerative Colitis." *JAMA* 321 (2). https://doi.org/10.1001/jama.2018.20397.

Marcon, A. 2020. "Microbiome Research, Nutrition, and Social Media: A Messaging Muddle." https://www.unscn.org/en/Unscn-news?idnews=2082.

Marcon, Alessandro R., Stuart Turvey, and Timothy Caulfield. 2021. "'Gut Health' and the Microbiome in the Popular Press: A Content Analysis." *BMJ Open* 11 (7). https://doi.org/10.1136/bmjopen-2021-052446.

Mian, Areeb, and Shujhat Khan. 2020. "Coronavirus: The Spread of Misinformation." *BMC Medicine*. BioMed Central Ltd. https://doi.org/10.1186/s12916-020-01556-3.

Moayyedi, Paul, Yuhong Yuan, Harith Baharith, and Alexander C. Ford. 2017. "Faecal Microbiota Transplantation for Clostridium Difficile-Associated Diarrhoea: A Systematic Review of Randomised Controlled Trials." *Medical Journal of Australia*. Australasian Medical Publishing Co. Ltd. https://doi.org/10.5694/mja17.00295.

Murthy, Vivek H. 2021. "Confronting Health Misinformation: The U.S. Surgeon General's Advisory on Building a Healthy Information Environment." Washington, D.C. Publisher: U.S. Department of Health and Human Services. https://pubmed.ncbi.nlm.nih.gov/34283416/.

O'Connor, Cathal, and Michelle Murphy. 2020. "Going Viral: Doctors Must Tackle Fake News in the Covid-19 Pandemic." *BMJ* 368 (m1090). https://doi.org/10.1136/bmj.m1587.

Oshima Lee, Emily, and Ezekiel J. Emanuel. 2013. "Shared Decision Making to Improve Care and Reduce Costs." *New England Journal of Medicine* 368 (1). https://doi.org/10.1056/NEJMp1209500.

Rachul, Christen, Alessandro R. Marcon, Benjamin Collins, and Timothy Caulfield. 2020. "COVID-19 and Immune Boosting' on the Internet: A Content Analysis of Google Search Results." *BMJ Open* 10 (10). https://doi.org/10.1136/bmjopen-2020-040989.

Rollnick, S., C. C. Butler, P. Kinnersley, J. Gregory, and B. Mash. 2010. "Motivational Interviewing." *BMJ* 340 (April 27). https://doi.org/10.1136/bmj.c1900.

Sackett, D. L., W. M. C. Rosenberg, J. A. M. Gray, R. B. Haynes, and W. S. Richardson. 1996. "Evidence Based Medicine: What It Is and What It Isn't." *BMJ* 312 (7023). https://doi.org/10.1136/bmj.312.7023.71.

Scherer, Laura D., and Gordon Pennycook. 2020. "Who Is Susceptible to Online Health Misinformation?" *American Journal of Public Health* 110 (Suppl 3): S276–S277. https://doi.org/10.2105/AJPH.2020.305908.

Southwell, Brian G., Jeff Niederdeppe, Joseph N. Cappella, Anna Gaysynsky, Dannielle E. Kelley, April Oh, Emily B. Peterson, and Wen-Ying Sylvia Chou. 2019. "Misinformation as a Misunderstood Challenge to Public Health." *American Journal of Preventive Medicine* 57 (2). https://doi.org/10.1016/j.amepre.2019.03.009.

Southwell, Brian G., Emily A. Thorson, and Laura Sheble. 2017. "The Persistence and Peril of Misinformation." *American Scientist* 105 (6). https://doi.org/10.1511/2017.105.6.372.

Southwell, Brian G., Emily A. Thorson, and Laura Sheble. 2018. "Misinformation among Mass Audiences as a Focus for Inquiry." In *Misinformation and Mass Audiences*, edited by Brian G. Southwell, Emily A. Thorson, and Laura Sheble, 1–11. Austin: University of Texas Press.

Southwell, Brian G., Jamie L. Wood, and Ann Marie Navar. 2020. "Roles for Health Care Professionals in Addressing Patient-Held Misinformation beyond Fact Correction." *American Journal of Public Health*. American Public Health Association Inc. https://doi.org/10.2105/AJPH.2020.305729.

———. 2021. "Función de Los Profesionales de La Salud de Rectificar La Información Errónea Que Tienen Los Pacientes Más Allá de Corregir Los Hechos." *Revista Panamericana de Salud Pública* 45 (May). https://doi.org/10.26633/RPSP.2021.60.

Sturgill, Amanda. 2021. "Health Care Providers Can Help Combat Harmful Misinformation About the Pandemic." *North Carolina Medical Journal* 82 (1): 68–70. https://doi.org/10.18043/ncm.82.1.68.

Suarez-Lledo, Victor, and Javier Alvarez-Galvez. 2021. "Prevalence of Health Misinformation on Social Media: Systematic Review." *Journal of Medical Internet Research* 23 (1): e17187. https://doi.org/10.2196/17187.

Tang, Lei. 2019. "Sequence-Based Identification of Human-Associated Microbiota." *Nature*, June 17, 2019. https://www.nature.com/articles/d42859-019-00011-5.

Tasnim, Samia, Mahbub Hossain, and Hoimonty Mazumder. 2020. "Impact of Rumors and Misinformation on COVID-19 in Social Media." *Journal of Preventive Medicine and Public Health*. Korean Society for Preventive Medicine. https://doi.org/10.3961/JPMPH.20.094.

Thursby, Elizabeth, and Nathalie Juge. 2017. "Introduction to the Human Gut Microbiota." *Biochemical Journal*. Portland Press Ltd. https://doi.org/10.1042/BCJ20160510.

"Trust in Medical Scientists Has Grown in U.S., but Mainly Among Democrats." 2020. www.pewresearch.org.

Vincent, Emmanuel. 2019. "Here is Who Repeated an Unsupported Claim about 'A Complete Cure for Cancer in a Year,' Misleading Millions on Social Media." https://healthfeedback.org/who-repeated-unsupported-claim-complete-cure-for-cancer-misleading-millions-on-social-media-jerusalem-post/.

Wang, Yuxi, Martin McKee, Aleksandra Torbica, and David Stuckler. 2019. "Systematic Literature Review on the Spread of Health-Related Misinformation on Social Media." *Social Science and Medicine* 240: 1–12. https://doi.org/10.1016/j.socscimed.2019.112552.

Wood, Jamie L., Grace Y. Lee, Sandra S. Stinnett, and Brian G. Southwell. 2021. "A Pilot Study of Medical Misinformation Perceptions and Training Among Practitioners in North Carolina (USA)." *INQUIRY: The Journal of Health Care Organization, Provision, and Financing* 58 (January). https://doi.org/10.1177/00469580211035742.

Wu, Joel T., and Jennifer B. Mccormick. 2018. "AMA Journal of Ethics ® POLICY FORUM Why Health Professionals Should Speak Out Against False Beliefs on the Internet." Vol. 20. www.amajournalofethics.org.

11

Teaching Young People to Think Critically about Health Claims and Choices

Sarah Rosenbaum, Allen Nsangi, and Daniel Semakula

Why Teach Critical Thinking about Health Choices?

PEOPLE EVERYWHERE ARE bombarded by family, friends, health personnel, marketers, governments, and others with many unreliable claims about what to do to protect or improve their health (Haber et al. 2018; Walsh-Childers et al. 2018). During the COVID-19 pandemic, a tsunami of health information about "what works" or "doesn't work" has resulted in what the World Health Organization calls an "infodemic" (Zarocostas 2020): an overabundance of information, including both reliable and unreliable claims about the effects of treatments or preventive interventions (such as vaccines), that makes it hard for people to find trustworthy guidance. This flood of contradictory and uncertain information in the wake of the COVID-19 pandemic has brought public attention to the importance of an already existing problem: many people lack the ability to apply basic principles for distinguishing between reliable and unreliable claims and evidence and using this information to make informed decisions (Boutron et al. 2019; Dahlgren et al. 2021).

We define a health intervention, broadly, as an action that can improve (or potentially harm) our health—such as taking medication, using dietary supplements, administering traditional remedies, getting an operation, using equipment or devices, exercising, changing diet, or undergoing physical or psychological therapies. Health interventions may also include actions aiming to improve public health, such as closing schools or issuing face mask mandates to stop the spread of infectious diseases. Believing in and acting on unreliable claims about the effects of health interventions can lead to harm, waste of personal or public resources due to overuse of services (Brownlee et al. 2017), or resistance to health actions that might be helpful (Glasziou et al. 2017).

People in low-income settings are disproportionately affected by unreliable claims about health interventions because they can least afford to waste resources. However, people everywhere need skills to distinguish between reliable and unreliable claims when making decisions about what to believe and what to do. Without these skills, we are more vulnerable to being misled by misinformation, both online and elsewhere.

How Do People Make Judgments about the Reliability of Health Information?

Believing a health claim to be "reliable" means perceiving that it can be trusted. While researchers are trained to appraise the strength of evidence in their respective fields through established, systematic approaches, non-researchers will likely use less rigorous strategies. A systematic review of the criteria and indicators that consumers use to evaluate the quality of online health information defined low-quality information as "information that is inaccurate, incomplete, or biased" (Sun et al. 2019). Researchers found twenty-five criteria across three aspects of the information itself: design, source, and content. For instance, people may base a quality judgment on whether the appearance of a website is visually appealing; whether the source is familiar, popular, or easy to access; or whether the message is written in plain language, error-free, and found across multiple sources (giving the impression of consensus). The ways people evaluate quality vary broadly and are highly subjective and context-dependent. For example, laypersons are more likely to base judgments about information quality on superficial features, such as professional-looking design, than experts in that field (Stanford et al. 2002).

Brashier and Marsh present an overview from a cognitive processing perspective of how people construct a judgment of truth (Brashier and Marsh 2020). They found three categories of information that people use: base rates, feelings, and consistency with information retrieved from memory. This means, among other things, that the way people feel about a message (e.g., if it is easy to understand), and if they have seen it before, impacts their judgment about whether to believe it or not.

Shortcomings of Intuitive Strategies

Many conscious or unconscious strategies people employ to evaluate quality or make inferences about the trustworthiness of information are ill-suited for making accurate assessments about the reliability of claims about health interventions. Unreliable claims can be found on visually appealing platforms, promoting messages that "feel right" and are easy to read; a misleading claim may spread quickly across a wide network of platforms, so people see it "everywhere." Relying solely on the advice of experts can also be tricky, as experts may openly disagree (Nagler et al. 2020).

Solutions are not straightforward. Labeling information as coming from "research" is not sufficient: a survey commissioned by the UK Academy of Medical Sciences reported only 37 percent of the public said they trusted evidence from medical research, compared with 65 percent who trusted the experiences of their friends and families (Academy of Medical Sciences 2017). Merely pointing to government sources may not be effective. Government institutions, such as health authorities, may be juggling conflicting roles of providing the public with balanced information as well as issuing public health recommendations or mandates that they want people to comply with. This could lead them to (intentionally or unintentionally) present information in ways that distort the effects of interventions, exaggerate the benefits, or downplay potential harms (Oxman et al. 2022).

Additionally, not all people value the same sources. While many people consider government institutions to be reliable sources of health information, others are highly skeptical of information coming from authorities. A study from 2020 estimating the prevalence of conspiracy thinking among adults in the United Kingdom found that a surprisingly high number of participants exhibited mistrust in government institutions and experts, well beyond the fringe population that authors expected to find. People who perceive themselves to be socially marginalized are particularly skeptical (Freeman et al. 2020). Although important, merely teaching people to think critically about the *source* of information is not sufficient to equip them with the skills they need to differentiate between reliable and unreliable health claims.

Our Approach to This Problem

Rather than promoting skills to think critically about information sources, the Informed Health Choices (IHC) team has taken a different approach. We aim to build people's capacity to identify and think critically about the *basis* for a claim (e.g., the supporting evidence) and about the effect of health interventions, and to apply this knowledge when deciding what to believe and do. These skills can be applied to personal choices about health interventions or to debates or decisions about public policies (Informed Health Choices, n.d.).

The IHC team is a multidisciplinary, international collaboration established in 2012. We are a core group of partners in Norway, Uganda, Kenya, Rwanda, United Kingdom, and Chile, with a secretariat at the Norwegian Institute of Public Health, and additional teams participating in various related projects on five continents (Informed Healthcare Choices Group 2020). We develop, evaluate, and contextualize open access learning resources using mixed research methods and human-centered design. This chapter is about our collective efforts; therefore, "we" in this text means teams of the core IHC partners as well as some teams in the network.

Below we describe how we developed and evaluated primary school learning resources (for children ages ten to twelve) in collaboration with teachers, students, and other relevant stakeholders in East Africa, with funding from the Norwegian Research Council, and how others are contextualizing them for use in many other countries around the globe.

Why Start with Young People?

Children and teenagers make choices that impact their health, both in the presence or absence of parents or guardians. Teaching them critical thinking skills early in life can help equip them to make better choices now and later as adults. It might improve academic achievement more broadly (Pellegrino and Hilton 2012) and can help to foster desirable dispositions (Abrami et al. 2015), such as questioning the basis of claims more generally. Moreover, because misconceptions, attitudes, and behaviors developed during childhood may be resistant to change later as children grow older (National Research Council 1999, 2007), it is important to encourage critical thinking early.

Teaching people at an early age also means reaching a large segment of the population who do not have the same learning opportunities later (Unesco 2019). In several parts of the world, particularly in Sub-Saharan Africa, a high proportion of the total population is made up of young people. In Uganda, for instance, where the piloting and evaluation of the primary school resources took place, 48 percent of the population was fourteen years old or younger in 2017 (National Population Council 2017), and a third of Ugandan children who complete primary school do not advance to the next level of education (Tamusuza 2011; Deininger 2003). This is not unique to Sub-Saharan Africa; on a global scale, one-sixth of adolescents and youth are out of school.

Children have the developmental capacity to learn to think critically about claims and the strength of supporting evidence (Sandoval et al. 2014; Duschl, Schweingruber, and Shouse

2007). Learning about fair comparisons (controlled research) is already a part of the curriculum in several countries (Oxman and García 2020; Biesty et al. 2020).

A systematic review of educational interventions that aimed to improve people's ability to appraise health claims showed that educational approaches have the potential to improve knowledge and skills, both in adults and children. However, studies were of varying quality and many only measured effects in the short term (Cusack et al. 2018).

What Do People Need to Learn?

Our first step in developing an educational intervention was to establish what people needed to learn. Authors of *Testing Treatments* (Evans et al. 2011) sought to explain to a lay audience how we know if a treatment works, how we know if it has harms, and how we weigh benefits against harms to determine the risk. Building on these basic learning goals and drawing on a broader body of related literature (Oxman, Chalmers, and Austvoll-Dahlgren 2018), we developed a set of building blocks for educational interventions: IHC Key Concepts (Informed Health Choices Group 2019b). These forty-four concepts are categorized into groups of concepts about "claims," "comparisons," and "choices." See table 11.1 for examples of some of the concepts.

The IHC Key Concepts serve as standards for judgment, or principles for evaluating the trustworthiness of treatment claims (figure 11.1), comparisons, and choices. The list of concepts forms a framework from which educators or researchers can develop learning resources

TABLE 11.1
Key Concepts Included in the IHC Primary School Resources

Category	*Key Concepts in IHC Primary School Resources**
Claims: *Recognizing claims about the effects of treatments that have an unreliable basis*	• Treatments may be harmful • Personal experiences or anecdotes (stories) are an unreliable basis for assessing the effects of most treatments • Widely used treatments or treatments that have been used for a long time are not necessarily beneficial or safe • New, brand-named, or more expensive treatments may not be better than available alternatives • Opinions of experts or authorities do not alone provide a reliable basis for deciding on the benefits and harms of treatments • Conflicting interests may result in misleading claims about the effects of treatments
Comparisons: *Understanding whether comparisons of treatments are fair and reliable*	• Identifying the effects of treatments depends on making comparisons • Apart from the treatments being compared, the comparison groups need to be similar at the beginning of comparison (i.e., "like needs to be compared with like") • If possible, people should not know which of the treatments being compared they are receiving • Small studies in which few outcome events occur are usually not informative and the results may be misleading • The results of single comparisons of treatments can be misleading
Choices: *Making informed choices about treatments*	• Decisions about treatments should not be based on considering only their benefits

*These are taken from an early version of the full Key Concepts, which is updated annually. For the most recent version of all Key Concepts, see www.informedhealthchoices.org/key-concepts.

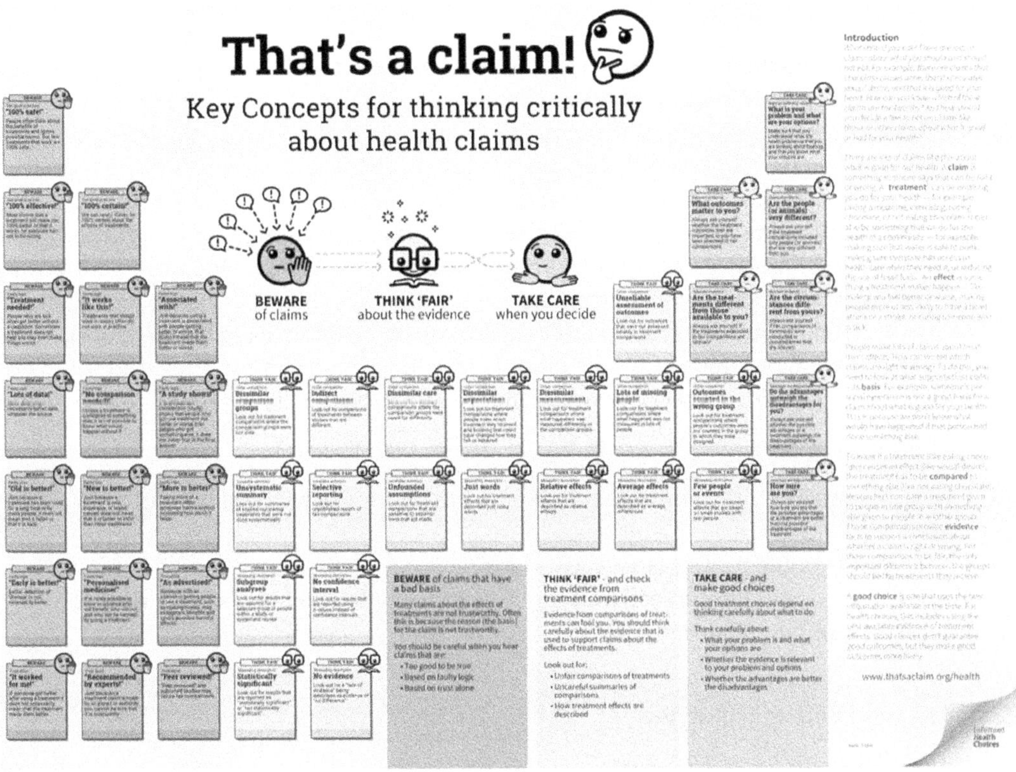

FIGURE 11.1
Poster of IHC Key Concepts for Health Claims, Accessible at Thatsaclaim.org.

tailored to different audiences or media and create questions to evaluate learning impact (see CLAIM Evaluation Tool described in more detail below). The list also functions as a taxonomy for tagging related learning resources (James Lind Initiative, n.d.).

Not all IHC Key Concepts can be taught at the same time or to the same age groups but should ideally be introduced and repeated over several school years in a spiral curriculum. The IHC primary school resources are based on twelve of the forty-four concepts (table 11.1), prioritized together with educators early in the development phase of that work, according to what students at that age could be expected to learn and how much time there was to teach concepts in one semester (Nsangi et al. 2015).

Additionally, researchers in other fields have adapted Key Concepts to thinking critically about the effect of agricultural, educational, environmental, management, and speech and therapy interventions (Aronson et al. 2019) (Informed Health Choices Group, n.d.-d).

Developing IHC Primary School Learning Resources

To develop the learning resources, we used a human-centered design approach (Giacomin 2014) characterized by the participatory involvement of multiple key stakeholders and rapid cycles of creating and testing prototypes. We worked closely with key stakeholders, international and national advisory groups, and networks of teachers and students in partner countries throughout the two-year developmental phase (Nsangi, Semakula, Rosenbaum et al. 2020).

Context Constraints and User Needs

To understand the school context and teacher/student needs, we organized workshops with teachers in Uganda, visits to some of their schools, and piloted early prototypes with students (some of which we also tried out in Norway). We discovered many constraints: basic materials were scarce, electricity was unstable, internet was not available in classrooms and equipment was mostly limited to blackboards, classes were often very large (i.e., during our trial, the teacher–student ratio was on average 1:69), resources for teacher training or printing were lacking, and school timetables were full. Although teachers felt the content was important to teach, it fell outside of their current curriculum and was new to them, making them prone to adding incorrect interpretations or examples. Additionally, although English was the official language at school, many students spoke other languages at home and struggled to some degree with English. We aimed therefore to develop resources that:

- Appealed to both teachers and students
- Could be taught over one semester (ten weeks) by a teacher without prior in-depth knowledge
- Were feasible to use in very large classrooms
- Were designed for children with varying levels of English literacy or who were learning English as a second language

Designing and Piloting Prototypes

After prioritizing a set of IHC Key Concepts that were teachable and relevant to primary school students (Nsangi et al. 2015), we carried out cycles of development over a two-year period: generating ideas, prototyping, and user and pilot testing with students and teachers in Uganda, Kenya, Rwanda, and Norway.

Several of our early ideas that worked in smaller Norwegian piloting environments, such as learning games, failed miserably in larger classrooms that were common in many places in Uganda. The initial pilots in Uganda highlighted two major problems. First, it was challenging to organize games and activities in classes with seventy to one hundred children. Second, the Key Concepts were new to the teachers, and they expressed a need for support or training. Implementing an extensive training program was not only unfeasible for our project, but it was unsustainable more broadly, as we sought to develop resources that could work on their own without our support. However, we did observe that the teachers were learning the Key Concepts together with the children.

The idea for our ultimate approach—an illustrated story in comic book format, with an accompanying teacher's guide—grew out of our efforts to find an approach that was feasible to implement despite many contextual constraints (see figure 11.2). We created and piloted several full drafts of this concept, before producing the final set of resources we used in the trial: comic book, exercise booklet, teachers' guide, activity cards for one lesson, and poster (Informed Health Choices Group, n.d.-b).

Since the comic book represented a tightly scripted, narrative solution, teachers were able to conduct a lesson with very little or no prior experience teaching the content. Illustrations provided both visual appeal and support for low-literacy learners (Nicholas 2007). Translations of key vocabulary words to Luganda and Swahili, common local languages, helped facilitate teaching to students with lower English language competence. Classes read the comic book in

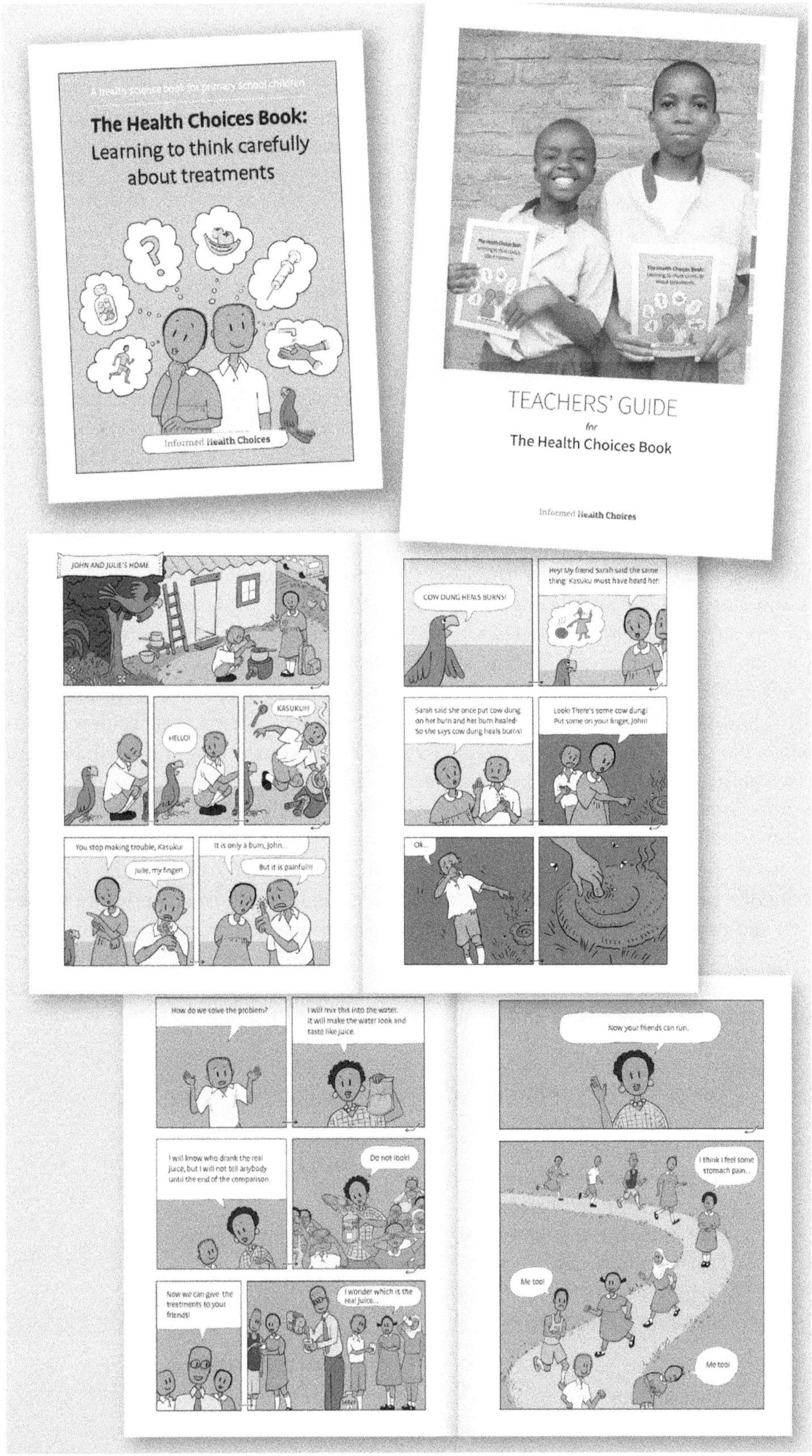

The Health Choices Book:
Learning to think carefully about treatments
Informed Health Choices
TEACHERS' GUIDE
for
The Health Choices Book
Informed Health Choices
JOHN AND JULIE'S HOME
HELLO!
KASUKU!!!
You stop making trouble, Kasuku!
Julie, my finger!
It is only a burn, John...
But it is painful!!!
COW DUNG HEALS BURNS!
Hey! My friend Sarah said the same thing. Kasuku must have heard her!
Sarah said she once put cow dung on her burn and her burn healed. So she says cow dung heals burns!
Look! There's some cow dung! Put some on your finger, John!
Ok...
How do we solve the problem?
I will mix this into the water. It will make the water look and taste like juice.
I will know who drank the real juice, but I will not tell anybody until the end of the comparison.
Do not look!
Now we can give the treatments to your friends!
I wonder which is the real juice...
Now your friends can run.
I think I feel some stomach pain...
Me too!
Me too!

FIGURE 11.2
Informed Health Choices Primary School Learning Resources.
Source: For downloadable files in several languages: www.informedhealthchoices.org/primary-school-resources.

different ways than we had planned for. Some large classes read aloud in unison, some teachers assigned students to read the different characters' roles like a play, and others read aloud for the class or instructed students to read on their own. Students also brought books home and shared them with family members. To cover printing costs for resources needed in the randomized trial, we reallocated project funds.

What Did Evaluations Show?

What We Measured

To assess a person's understanding of and ability to apply the IHC Key Concepts (including children as young as ten), we developed the CLAIM Evaluation Tool multiple-choice questions (Austvoll-Dahlgren, Semakula et al. 2017). Instead of a fixed questionnaire, CLAIM is a flexible battery of questions that can be combined according to the purpose (Informed Health Choices Group, n.d.-a). CLAIM questions can be used as tests in educational settings, in randomized trials evaluating outcomes of educational interventions, or in cross-sectional studies to gauge ability in a population. Prior to the trial, we validated the questions in a Rasch analysis in Uganda and Norway (Austvoll-Dahlgren, Guttersrud et al. 2017). Researchers in other countries have since translated and validated CLAIM in several languages and settings.

For the school trial in Uganda, we used twenty-four multiple-choice questions that covered the twelve Key Concepts that were the starting point for the primary school resources (Nsangi et al. 2017) and nine Key Concepts covered in a podcast for parents that we developed and evaluated in parallel (Semakula et al. 2017). To measure understanding rather than memorization, the questions did not reuse any of the examples or scenarios in the learning resources. The test also included questions that assessed intended behaviors, self-efficacy, attitudes, and literacy (see figure 11.3).

In the trial, our primary outcome measurement was a mean score on the CLAIM test (comparing the mean score of the group who received the learning intervention to those who didn't). In addition, we wanted to look at what percentage of each group of students "passed" and what percentage achieved a mastery of the concepts. To determine these cut-off scores, we invited experts, teachers, and methodologists to make judgments in a structured approach for establishing standards for passing and mastery (Davies et al. 2017).

Habibah has pain in her ear, and she asks her brother Hassan what to do about it. He says that once, when he had a pain like that, he rinsed his ear with hot water. The next day, his ear pain was gone. Based on his experience, he says rinsing with hot water is helpful for ear pain.

Do you agree with Hassan?

A. Yes, because this is Hassan's experience, it is likely to be true.

B. No, Hassan's experience is not enough to be sure.

C. Yes, Hassan rinsed his ear with hot water, and the next day his ear pain was gone.

FIGURE 11.3
Example of CLAIM Multiple-Choice Question.
Source: To access, see: www.informedhealthchoices.org/claim-evaluation-tools.

End-of-Term Trial

We evaluated the primary school learning resources in 2016, in a cluster-randomized trial in Uganda, including 120 primary schools and over 10,000 ten- to twelve-year-olds (Nsangi et al. 2017). Intervention schools received the IHC primary school resources and an introductory workshop to explain the process of the trial. Teachers taught the content in nine, eighty-minute lessons during one school term. We did not intervene in the control schools.

Trial results showed that these learning resources led to a large improvement in the ability of students to assess claims about the effects of health interventions (see table 11.2). Children's mean score in schools receiving the intervention was 20 percent higher than for the control schools (62.4 percent vs. 43.1 percent). Of the children in the intervention schools, 69 percent achieved a passing score compared to 27 percent in control schools, and 19 percent of children in intervention schools had a score indicating mastery of the twelve Key Concepts compared to 1 percent in the control schools. Teachers in intervention schools also performed considerably better than in control schools: 72 percent achieved a score indicating mastery compared to 15 percent in control schools.

TABLE 11.2
Results of End-of-Term Trial

End-of-Term Trial	*Control Schools* N = 4,430 children 67 teachers	*Intervention Schools* N = 5,753 children 85 teachers	*Adjusted Difference*
Mean score	43.1% (SD 15.2%)	62.4% (SD 18.8%)	**20.0%** (95% CI 17.3–22.7%)
Passing score, children (≥13 out of 24 correct answers)	27% (1,186 children)	69% (3,967 children)	**50%** (95% CI 44–55%)
Mastery score, children (≥20 out of 24 correct answers)	1% (38 children)	18.6% (1,070 children)	**18%** (95% CI 18–18%)
Mastery score, teachers (≥20 out of 24 correct answers)	15% (10 teachers)	72% (61 teachers)	**57%** (95% CI 37–70%)

One-Year Follow-Up Study

The one-year follow-up study (see table 11.3) indicated that learning is retained for at least a year (Nsangi, Semakula, Oxman et al. 2020). For the intervention schools, the mean score and the proportion of children with passing scores increased from the intervention term to the one-year follow-up term (mean score: from 62.4 percent to 68.7 percent, passing score: from 69 percent to 80 percent, and mastery score: from 18.6 percent to 28.9 percent). The mean scores in the control schools also improved from the previous year (from 43.1 percent to 53.0 percent), resulting in a somewhat smaller—albeit still large—difference between the intervention and control schools for the mean score. This means that all children improved their knowledge after one year, but the intervention school children maintained their lead over the children who hadn't received the IHC learning resources. Control schools received sets of learning resources after the study was completed.

TABLE 11.3
Results of One-Year Follow-Up

One-Year Follow-Up	*Control Schools* N = 2,844 children 64 teachers	*Intervention Schools* N = 3,943 children 78 teachers	*Adjusted Difference*
Mean score	53.0% (SD 16.8%)	68.7% (SD 18.2%)	**16.7%** (95% CI 13.9–19.5%)
Passing score, children (≥13 out of 24 correct answers)	51.5 % (1,464 children)	80.1% (3,160 children)	**39.5%** (95% CI 29.9–47.5%)
Mastery score, children (≥20 out of 24 correct answers)	4.9% (139 children)	28.9% (1,138 children)	**25.0%** (95% CI 23.2–26.5%)
Mastery score, teachers (≥20 out of 24 correct answers)	21.9% (14 teachers)	67.9% (53 teachers)	**46.3%** (95% CI 31.5–56.6%)

Process Evaluation

Our process evaluation study findings were consistent with the findings of the trial (Nsangi et al. 2019). The findings suggested that children, teachers, and parents valued the IHC school intervention and found the characters, story, and illustrations appealing. Teachers found the IHC lessons compatible with the curriculum and with their teaching styles. In addition, they appreciated the flexibility that enabled them to apply differentiated instruction. Effect modifiers included teachers' skills and competencies and positive learning environments. Our analysis concluded that these likely contributed to intermediate effects, including teachers' motivation, self-efficacy, positive attitudes, and a positive overall experience, which in turn contributed to the IHC resources having a large effect on the ability of the children to assess claims about treatment effects.

The process evaluation uncovered two major barriers to implementing the resources on a larger scale in Uganda. First, the cost of printing resources (4.00 USD per student) was prohibitive in this context. Second, despite the highly positive reception by participating schools, the content fell outside the current curriculum and was impossible to add to existing class timetables. In a new project to develop learning resources for secondary schools (2019–2024), we aim to mitigate these barriers by producing digital resources, by exploring how the IHC Key Concepts map onto existing curricula in participating countries, and by engaging earlier and more closely with curriculum developers (Informed Health Choices Group, n.d.-c).

Translation and Contextualization

Planning for and Facilitating Use in Other Settings

To ensure we didn't develop too narrowly targeted materials that were only suitable for use in Uganda, we translated the resources, carried out pilots in Rwanda, Kenya, and Norway, and incorporated findings from that work during development (Mugisha 2016; Ikirezi 2018). However, we did expect that there would be a need for additional adjustments to the content to make it suitable for use in other languages, cultural settings, and educational environments. Therefore, we developed detailed, pragmatic, open access guidance for translating and contextualizing the resources, with an emphasis on how to engage students, teachers, and other key stakeholders in this work (Informed Health Choices Group 2019a, 2017, 2019c). Our annual newsletter provides an overview of all recent or ongoing activities in each IHC network country to adapt the IHC resources to their settings (Informed Healthcare Choices Group 2020).

Translation

The original resources are in English, with key words also provided in Luganda and Kiswahili. To date (autumn 2021) they have been translated to Spanish, Norwegian, Kinyarwanda, Kiswahili, French, Italian, Greek, Croatian, Basque, Persian, Brazilian Portuguese, and Catalan, with other languages in the pipeline.

Some languages may lack good translations for central vocabulary terms. When the Ugandan team translated the glossary to Luganda, they noted difficulties with words like *anecdote*, *chance*, and *unfair* (Semakula and Nsangi 2018). Additionally, many countries have more than one official language, and some have several local languages. We provided space in the textbook for the translation of key words for multi-language settings (see figure 11.4).

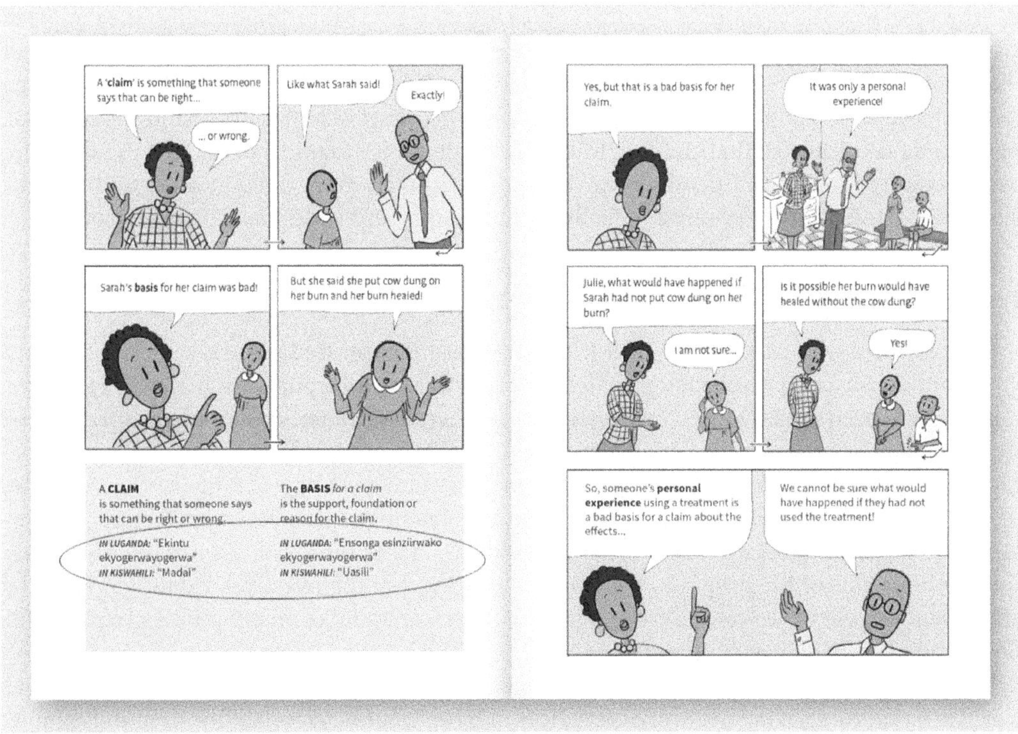

FIGURE 11.4
Space in the Layout for Translations of Key Terms to Other Locally Relevant Languages.

Other Contextualization

After language translation, other contextualization activities can include carrying out pilots in schools, changing or adapting content (texts or images), conducting context analyses, or validating the CLAIM Evaluation Tool. As of September 2021, two teams have written up contextualization results involving school pilots in settings other than East Africa: Ireland (Glynn 2020) and Italy (Alderighi, Rasoini, and Rosenbaum). Although we cannot draw firm conclusions about contextualization concerns from the two studies, several patterns resonate with what we already know.

The Irish study was led by a school principal. The Italian study was carried out by two medical doctors who translated the resources and taught lessons to two classes at a local school. Both teams recruited school classes with children aged ten to twelve. For details, see the respective publications. These teams came to many similar conclusions about students' and teachers' personal experiences of the learning resources. The Irish study, however, also included stakeholder feedback from the wider educational environment, enabling the author to identify some of the most likely barriers to the uptake of the IHC learning resources in the Irish educational system.

Children's Experiences

Children in both countries responded enthusiastically to the learning resources, like the children in East Africa and Norway. They enjoyed the comic book characters and dialog, and felt the format made it more enjoyable and easier to learn. More importantly, they enjoyed learning the Key Concepts. The Italians reported that children especially liked learning about "bad basis for claims." The Irish and Italian children did not react negatively to the story being set in Africa; on the contrary, it appeared to add to their curiosity and interest in the material. Both teams also reported that children found the content easy to understand, that the structure helped children move confidently from simpler concepts to more difficult ones, and that the illustrated comic format appeared to facilitate motivation and widespread engagement.

Teachers' Experiences

Irish teachers who participated in teaching the lessons expressed positive experiences, with their confidence and enthusiasm growing as they progressed through the material. However, some experienced negative first impressions. Teachers and other stakeholders worried that students wouldn't relate to the African setting, which stood in contrast to the students' actual experiences; there was also initial concern about the number of pages in the book and guide, the prescriptive instructions, unfamiliar names and examples, and a seemingly simplistic vocabulary. Without adaptation to improve these first impressions and champions who could speak to the value of the program, the study concluded that the resources would not likely be implemented on a wide scale in Ireland, where there are many competing new programs for slots in an already full curriculum.

In the Italian study, teachers did not participate in teaching the lessons but had an observer role. They reported having positive experiences in terms of understandability, desirability, suitability, and usefulness.

Recommended Changes to the Learning Resources

Both the Irish and Italian teams left the drawings and storyline intact but made changes to the names of some of the characters in the comic. While the Irish changed many of the extra examples in the text to treatments and diseases that were more locally relevant, the Italian team left these mostly unaltered. However, they did provide more locally relevant examples orally while delivering the lessons (e.g., the local custom of taking onion as an antiflu treatment). The Irish study recommended several physical changes to the children's book to counteract some of the negative or misleading first impressions. This included altering the layout to fit the A4 format and eliminating the exercise and activity pages in the comic book to achieve a much thinner, less overwhelming publication and slimming the teachers' guide by deleting unnecessary content (such as the embedded comic book images). They also suggested the development of flashcards and other learning resources to form a toolbox for teachers that could facilitate more diversified, less prescriptive, teaching activities. Additionally, they proposed including more explicit home-school links that would tie in with the emphasis on parent involvement in the Irish curriculum.

Teacher Training Considerations

When developing these resources for use in Uganda, we understood that although the content would likely be new to most teachers, a comprehensive teacher training program would likely be unfeasible in most countries. Therefore, we deliberately created highly scripted content that teachers could use successfully without prior training. Although this prescriptive approach did effectively enable teachers in the Ugandan trial to conduct the lessons without extensive prior training, it wasn't obvious to those teachers that they would be able to do this until they had experience teaching the lessons. Additionally, the prescriptive approach was not appreciated by the Irish teachers and stakeholders, who were used to having more freedom to employ teaching strategies of their own choosing. The Irish study highlighted the necessity of teacher training, both to build teachers' confidence that the foreign-looking resources were actually very relevant to their students and to provide them with a better knowledge basis from which to bring their own ideas and teaching strategies into play.

The Italian team used a different approach: the two doctors taught the lessons, in the presence of the class teacher who both observed and provided classroom support. As medical professionals, the doctor team already had in-depth knowledge of the Key Concepts and understood the relevance of the content for the children. They were able to present relevant examples from the medical literature not included in the materials and improvise confidently during the lessons. It is also possible that the novelty of having doctors visit the class (mirroring the comic book narrative, where two doctors engage with two school children throughout the story) had an additional positive impact on students' curiosity and attention to the content. Although not likely as sustainable as national policy, this approach, with health professionals as guest teachers, could be adopted by individual regions or schools, or in more informal learning environments, such as library or community programs.

Relevance to Curricula

Interestingly, the Irish students did not recognize the IHC lessons as connected to curricular work, and they viewed this as an advantage. The Irish stakeholders identified Social Personal and Health Education (SPHE) as the subject most likely relevant for primary school learners and mentioned Social Environmental and Scientific Education (SESE) and English reading as other possibilities.

The Italian study did not include a formalized curriculum mapping, but the authors described subjects that teachers identified as relevant and how teachers applied the learning and approaches from these lessons in other classes. For example, teachers initiated a project involving a critical approach to advertisements and another where students created figurative representations of the Key Concepts.

In more recent projects, we have conducted context analyses that include mapping the IHC Key Concepts to national curricula to make these ties explicit for teachers and facilitate teaching the content in existing subjects (Lund 2018; Mugisha et al. 2021; Senyonga et al. 2021). However, the Key Concepts represent a new type of knowledge and skills that, while relevant to many different subjects taught today, will not likely map onto most existing subjects directly. Health may not be given much space in schools' timetables (e.g., thirty minutes a week in the Irish curriculum), and critical thinking is more likely to be an overarching goal in a curriculum rather than a separate subject.

However, educational systems are moving toward competence-based curricula (Voogt and Roblin 2012), with added emphasis on thematic and cross-cutting teaching. These resources are well-suited for that purpose. In the context analyses we have performed more recently in secondary schools, we found that newer curricula may include lofty ideals for teaching across subjects, but there is little information available about how teachers are supposed to do this, and few learning resources that are designed specifically for this purpose. These resources can fill some of that gap.

Conclusions

Health literacy, according to an integrated model, includes four types of competencies: the ability to access, understand, appraise, and apply health information (Sørensen et al. 2012). A systematic review of the causes, impacts, and potential strategies of the COVID-19 infodemic points to improving health literacy as an important countermeasure (Pian, Chi, and Ma 2021). Although the ability to appraise health information could be an important defense against misinformation, few studies have investigated the effects of interventions to teach critical appraisal skills to children, patients, or the public in any country. We have developed and evaluated learning resources for primary school children and their teachers that were shown in a large, randomized trial to have a substantial impact on children's ability to think critically about claims about the effects of health interventions and to use this knowledge in decision-making scenarios. Partnering teams are translating and contextualizing these resources for use in many countries. Building on this initial work, we are currently developing a new set of flexible, digital resources for use in secondary schools that we will evaluate in randomized trials and process evaluations in East Africa and subsequently make them available for translation and contextualization (see www.informedhealthchoices.org/secondary-school-resources).

Although these studies were carried out prior to the onset of pandemic, both teachers and children acknowledged the importance of learning to think critically about the effects of health interventions. Since then, the relevance of these learning resources has become much more apparent. Halpern and Dunn present critical thinking as a model for intelligence for solving real-world problems. They make a compelling argument for how improving people's critical thinking skills, such as the ability to think critically about the basis for a claim, could have had an important impact on attitudes and behaviors related to public health interventions during the pandemic (Halpern and Dunn 2021). It is our hope that curriculum developers, principles, teachers, parents, engaged health professionals, librarians, and others will use, adopt, and adapt the materials that we have created, so young people and adults are better positioned to protect themselves from misinformation about health interventions and make informed choices for themselves, their families, and their communities.

Free to Use and Adapt

The IHC primary school resources, other related resources, guides, and publications are accessible at www.informedhealthchoices.org. Learning resources are free to download, use, reproduce, or adapt. They are protected with a Creative Commons license 4.0 international license, meaning anyone can share as well as adapt the material, provided you credit us, indicate what changes you made, and do not use it for commercial purposes. Please contact us for access to files for translating, contextualizing, or high-resolution printing.

Acknowledgments

Many thanks to Astrid Dahlgren, Dara Glynn, Camilla Alderighi, and Raaffaele Rasoini for commenting on parts of this book.

References

Abrami, Philip C., Robert M. Bernard, Eugene Borokhovski, David I. Waddington, C. Anne Wade, and Tonje Persson. 2015. "Strategies for Teaching Students to Think Critically: A Meta-Analysis." *Review of Educational Research* 85 (2): 275–314.

Academy of Medical Sciences. 2017. "Enhancing the Use of Scientific Evidence to Judge the Potential Benefits and Harms of Medicines." Accessed February 13, 2022. https://acmedsci.ac.uk/file-download/44970096.

Alderighi, Camilla, Raffaele Rasoini, and Sarah Rosenbaum. 2022. "Feasibility of Contextualizing the Informed Health Choices learning resources in Italy: A Pilot Study in a Primary School in Florence." https://zenodo.org/record/6581224.

Aronson, Jeffrey K., Eric Barends, Robert Boruch, Marnie Brennan, Iain Chalmers, Joe Chislett, Peter Cunliffe-Jones, Astrid Dahlgren, Marie Gaarder, and Andy Haines. 2019. "Key Concepts for Making Informed Choices." *Nature Publishing Group* 572(7769): 303–306.

Austvoll-Dahlgren, Astrid, Øystein Guttersrud, Allen Nsangi, Daniel Semakula, and Andrew D. Oxman. 2017. "Measuring Ability to Assess Claims about Treatment Effects: A Latent Trait Analysis of Items from the 'Claim Evaluation Tools' Database Using Rasch Modelling." *BMJ Open* 7 (5): e013185. https://doi.org/10.1136/bmjopen-2016-013185.

Austvoll-Dahlgren, Astrid, Daniel Semakula, Allen Nsangi, Andrew D. Oxman, Iain Chalmers, Sarah Rosenbaum, and Øystein Guttersrud. 2017. "Measuring Ability to Assess Claims About Treatment Effects: The Development of the 'Claim Evaluation Tools.'" *BMJ Open* 7 (5): e013184. https://doi.org/10.1136/bmjopen-2016-013184.

Biesty, Linda, Sandra Galvin, Elaine Finucane, Patricia Healy, Declan Devane, and Tom Conway. 2020. "Can Learning about Trials be Child's Play? A Qualitative Exploration of the 'Schools Teaching Awareness of Randomised Trials' (START) Initiative." *Trials* 21 (1): 1–12.

Boutron, Isabelle, Romana Haneef, Amélie Yavchitz, Gabriel Baron, John Novack, Ivan Oransky, Gary Schwitzer, and Philippe Ravaud. 2019. "Three Randomized Controlled Trials Evaluating the Impact of 'Spin' in Health News Stories Reporting Studies of Pharmacologic Treatments on Patients'/Caregivers' Interpretation of Treatment Benefit." *BMC Medicine* 17 (1): 1–10.

Brashier, Nadia M., and Elizabeth J. Marsh. 2020. "Judging Truth." *Annual Review of Psychology* 71: 499–515.

Brownlee, Shannon, Kalipso Chalkidou, Jenny Doust, Adam G. Elshaug, Paul Glasziou, Iona Heath, Somil Nagpal, Vikas Saini, Divya Srivastava, and Kelsey Chalmers. 2017. "Evidence for Overuse of Medical Services Around the World." *The Lancet* 390 (10090): 156–68.

Cusack, Leila, Chris B. Del Mar, Iain Chalmers, Elizabeth Gibson, and Tammy C. Hoffmann. 2018. "Educational Interventions to Improve People's Understanding of Key Concepts in Assessing the Effects of Health Interventions: A Systematic Review." *Systematic Reviews* 7 (1): 68.

Dahlgren, Astrid, Kjetil Furuseth-Olsen, Christopher J. Rose, and Andrew D. Oxman. 2021. "The Norwegian Public's Ability To Assess Treatment Claims: Results of a Cross-Sectional Study of Critical Health Literacy" [version 2; peer review: 1 approved, 1 approved with reservations]. *F1000Research* 9 (179). https://doi.org/10.12688/f1000research.21902.2.

Davies, Alun, Martha Gerrity, Lena Nordheim, Okebukola Peter, Newton Opiyo, Jonathan Sharples, Helen Wilson, Charles Wysonge, Astrid Austvoll-Dahlgren, and Andrew David Oxman. 2017. *Measuring Ability to Assess Claims About Treatment.* IHC Working Paper.

Deininger, Klaus. 2003. "Does Cost of Schooling Affect Enrollment by the Poor? Universal Primary Education in Uganda." *Economics of Education Review* 22 (3): 291–305.

Duschl, Richard A., Heidi A Schweingruber, and Andrew W. Shouse. 2007. "Taking Science to School: Learning and Teaching Science in Grades K-8." *Eurasia Journal of Mathematics, Science & Technology Education* 3 (2): 163–66.

Evans, Imogen, Hazel Thornton, Iain Chalmers, and Paul Glasziou. 2011. *Testing Treatments: Better Research for Better Healthcare.* Pinter & Martin Publishers.

Freeman, Daniel, Felicity Waite, Laina Rosebrock, Ariane Petit, Chiara Causier, Anna East, Lucy Jenner, Ashley-Louise Teale, Lydia Carr, and Sophie Mulhall. 2020. "Coronavirus Conspiracy Beliefs, Mistrust, and Compliance with Government Guidelines in England." Psychological Medicine 52: 251–263.

Giacomin, Joseph. 2014. "What is Human Centred Design?" *The Design Journal* 17 (4): 606–623.

Glasziou, Paul, Sharon Straus, Shannon Brownlee, Lyndal Trevena, Leonila Dans, Gordon Guyatt, Adam G. Elshaug, Robert Janett, and Vikas Saini. 2017. "Evidence for Underuse Of Effective Medical Services Around The World." *The Lancet* 390 (10090): 169–77.

Glynn, Dara. 2020. "Contextualising the Informed Health Choices (IHC) Programme and Resources for Delivery in the Irish Primary School System." Research Masters, National University of Ireland, Galway. https://www.informedhealthchoices.org/wp-content/uploads/2021/08/DaraGlynn_Thesis_2020.pdf.

Haber, Noah, Emily R. Smith, Ellen Moscoe, Kathryn Andrews, Robin Audy, Winnie Bell, Alana T. Brennan, Alexander Breskin, Jeremy C. Kane, and Mahesh Karra. 2018. "Causal Language and Strength of Inference in Academic and Media Articles Shared in Social Media (CLAIMS): A Systematic Review." *PLoS ONE* 13 (5): e0196346.

Halpern, Diane F., and Dana S. Dunn. 2021. "Critical Thinking: A Model of Intelligence for Solving Real-World Problems." *Journal of Intelligence* 9 (2): 22.

Ikirezi, Aline. 2018. "Qualitative Study Exploring the Suitability of Informed Health Choices Resources Translated into Kinyarwanda for Use in Primary Schools: Case of Remera Protestant Primary School in Kigali City." Master's thesis, University of Rwanda.

Informed Health Choices. n.d. "Informed Health Choices." Accessed February 13, 2022. www.informedhealthchoices.org.

Informed Health Choices Group. 2017. *Guide for Piloting the Informed Health Choices School Resources.* Norwegian Institute of Public Health. https://www.informedhealthchoices.org/wp-content/uploads/2016/08/GUIDE-for-piloting-IHC-primary-school-resources.pdf.

Informed Health Choices Group. 2019a. *Guide for Translating the Informed Health Choices School Resources.* Norwegian Institute of Public Heallth. https://www.informedhealthchoices.org/wp-content/uploads/2019/12/GUIDE-for-translating-IHC-school-resources_20190218.pdf.

Informed Health Choices Group. 2019b. *Key Concepts for Informed Health Choices: A Framework for Enabling People to Think Critically About Health Claims.* Norwegian Institute of Public Health. https://www.informedhealthchoices.org/wp-content/uploads/2019/12/IHC-Key-Concepts_Health_2019.pdf.

Informed Health Choices Group. 2019c. *Resource Production Guide for Translating and Adapting Informed Health Choices Learning Resources.* Norwegian Institute of Public Health. https://www.informedhealthchoices.org/wp-content/uploads/2019/12/GUIDE_ResourceProduction_20190313.pdf.

Informed Healthcare Choices Group. 2020. "Informed Health Choices Newsletter 2020." Norwegian Institute of Publich Health. Accessed February 13, 2022. https://www.informedhealthchoices.org/wp-content/uploads/2020/02/2020-Informed-Health-Choices-newsletter-1.pdf.

Informed Health Choices Group. n.d.-a. "IHC Claim Evaluation Tools." Norwegian Institute of Public Health. Accessed February 13, 2022. https://www.informedhealthchoices.org/claim-evaluation-tools/.

Informed Health Choices Group. n.d.-b. "IHC Primary School Resources." Norwegian Institute of Public Health. Accessed February 13, 2022. https://www.informedhealthchoices.org/primary-school-resources/.

Informed Health Choices Group. n.d.-c. "IHC Secondary School Resources." Norwegian Institute of Public Health. Accessed February 13, 2022. https://www.informedhealthchoices.org/secondary-school-resources/.

Informed Health Choices Group. n.d.-d. "That's a Claim. Guides for Thinking Critically About Claims." Accessed February 13, 2022. https://thatsaclaim.org/.

James Lind Initiative. n.d. "Teaching Evidence-Based Health Care." Accessed February 13, 2022. https://teachingebhc.org/about/.

Lund, Hanna Marie, Per Erlend Mathisen, Marte Evensen Rekkavik, and Enok Voll. 2018. *Teaching Critical Thinking About Health Claims: Market Analysis for Norwegian Primary and Lower Secondary School.* Norwegian Institute of Public Health. https://www.informedhealthchoices.org/wp-content/uploads/2019/04/Norwegian-market-analysis-2018-11-22.pdf.

Mugisha, Michael. 2016. "Piloting Primary School Teaching Resources for Informed Health Care Choices in an Urban School Setting in Kigali." Master's thesis, University of Rwanda.

Mugisha, Michael, Anne Marie Uwitonze, Faith Chesire, Ronald Senyonga, Matt Oxman, Allen Nsangi, Daniel Semakula, Margaret Kaseje, Simon Lewin, and Nelson Sewankambo. 2021. "Teaching Critical Thinking About Health Using Digital Technology in Lower Secondary Schools in Rwanda: A Qualitative Context Analysis." *PLoS ONE* 16 (3): e0248773.

Nagler, Rebekah H., Rachel I. Vogel, Sarah E. Gollust, Alexander J. Rothman, Erika Franklin Fowler, and Marco C. Yzer. 2020. "Public Perceptions of Conflicting Information Surrounding COVID-19: Results From a Nationally Representative Survey of U.S. Adults." *PLoS ONE* 15 (10): e0240776. https://doi.org/10.1371/journal.pone.0240776.

National Population Council. 2017. "State of Uganda Population Report." Kampala, Uganda. Accessed Febraury 13, 2022. http://npcsec.go.ug/wp-content/uploads/2013/06/SUPRE-REPORT-2017.pdf.

National Research Council. 1999. *How People Learn: Bridging Research and Practice.* National Academies Press.

National Research Council. 2007. *Taking Science to School: Learning and Teaching Science In Grades K-8.* National Academies Press.

Nicholas, Judy Lavender. 2007. "An Exploration of The Impact of Picture Book Illustrations on the Comprehension Skills and Vocabulary Development of Emergent Readers." PhD dissertation, Louisiana State University and Agricultural and Mechanical Collegess.

Nsangi, Allen, Daniel Semakula, Andrew D. Oxman, Astrid Austvoll-Dahlgren, Matt Oxman, Sarah Rosenbaum, Angela Morelli et al. 2020. "Effects of the Informed Health Choices Primary School Intervention on The Ability of Children in Uganda to Assess the Reliability of Claims about Treatment Effects, 1-Year Follow-Up: A Cluster-Randomised Trial." *Trials* 21 (1): 27. https://doi.org/10.1186/s13063-019-3960-9. https://www.ncbi.nlm.nih.gov/pubmed/31907013.

Nsangi, Allen, Daniel Semakula, Claire Glenton, Simon Lewin, Andrew D. Oxman, Matt Oxman, Sarah Rosenbaum et al. 2019. "Informed Health Choices Intervention to Teach Primary School Children in Low-Income Countries to Assess Claims About Treatment Effects: Process Evaluation." *BMJ Open* 9 (9): e030787. https://doi.org/10.1136/bmjopen-2019-030787. https://bmjopen.bmj.com/content/bmjopen/9/9/e030787.full.pdf.

Nsangi, Allen, Daniel Semakula, Andrew D. Oxman, and Nelson K. Sewankambo. 2015. "Teaching Children in Low-Income Countries to Assess Claims About Treatment Effects: Prioritization of Key Concepts." *Journal of Evidence-Based Medicine* 8 (4): 173–80.

Nsangi, Allen, Daniel Semakula, Andrew D. Oxman, Astrid Austvoll-Dahlgren, Matt Oxman, Sarah Rosenbaum, et al. 2017. "Effects of the Informed Health Choices Primary School Intervention on the Ability of Children in Uganda to Assess the Reliability of Claims about Treatment Effects: A Cluster-Randomised Controlled Trial." *The Lancet* 390 (10092): 374–88. https://doi.org/10.1016/S0140-6736(17)31226-6.

Nsangi, Allen, Daniel Semakula, Sarah Rosenbaum, Andrew D. Oxman, Matt Oxman, Angela Morelli, Astrid Austvoll-Dahlgren, et al. 2020. "Development of the Informed Health Choices Resources in Four Countries to Teach Primary School Children to Assess Claims about Treatment Effects: A Qualitative Study Employing a User-Centred Approach." *Pilot Feasibility Stud* 6 (18). https://doi.org/https://doi.org/10.1186/s40814-020-00565-6.

Oxman, Andrew D., Atle Fretheim, Simon Lewin, Signe Flottorp, and Sarah Rosenbaum. 2022. "Health Communication In and Out of Public Health Emergencies: To Persuade Or to Inform?" Preprint, submitted *Health Research and Policy Systems*.

Oxman, Andrew D., and Laura Martínez García. 2020. "Comparison of the Informed Health Choices Key Concepts Framework to Other Frameworks Relevant to Teaching and Learning How to Think Critically About Health Claims and Choices: A Systematic Review." *F1000Research* 9: 164.

Oxman, Andrew D., Iain Chalmers, and Astrid Austvoll-Dahlgren. 2018. "Key Concepts for Assessing Claims about Treatment Effects and Making Well-Informed Treatment Choices." *F1000Research* 7: 1784.

Pellegrino, James W., and Margaret L. Hilton. 2012. *Education for Life and Work: Developing Transferable Knowledge and Skills in the 21st Century*. National Academies Press.

Pian, Wenjing, Jianxing Chi, and Feicheng Ma. 2021. "The Causes, Impacts and Countermeasures of COVID-19 'Infodemic': A Systematic Review Using Narrative Synthesis." *Information Processing & Management* 58 (6): 102713.

Sandoval, William A., Beate Sodian, Susanne Koerber, and Jacqueline Wong. 2014. "Developing Children's Early Competencies to Engage with Science." *Educational Psychologist* 49 (2): 139–152.

Semakula, Daniel, and Allen Nsangi. 2018. "Using Multiple Languages In Education: Experiences from the Informed Health Choices Research Project." *EAL Journal* (blog), February 5, 2018. https://ealjournal.org/2018/02/05/experiences-from-the-informed-health-choices-project-in-using-multiple-languages/.

Semakula, Daniel, Allen Nsangi, Andrew D. Oxman, Matt Oxman, Astrid Austvoll-Dahlgren, Sarah Rosenbaum et al. 2017. "Effects of the Informed Health Choices Podcast on the Ability of Parents of Primary School Children in Uganda to Assess Claims About Treatment Effects: A Randomised Controlled Trial." *Lancet* 390 (10092): 389–98. https://doi.org/10.1016/s0140-6736(17)31225-4.

Senyonga, Ronald, Nelson K. Sewankambo, Solomon Kevin Mugagga, Esther Nakyejwe, Faith Chesire, Michael Mugisha, Allen Nsangi, et al. Forthcoming. 2022. "Learning to Think Critically About Health Using Digital Technology in Ugandan Lower Secondary Schools: A Contextual Analysis." PLoS ONE 17(2): e0260367 doi: 10.1371/journal.pone.0260367.

Sørensen, Kristine, Stephan Van den Broucke, James Fullam, Gerardine Doyle, Jürgen Pelikan, Zofia Slonska, and Helmut Brand. 2012. "Health Literacy and Public Health: A Systematic Review and Integration of Definitions and Models." *BMC Public Health* 12 (1): 1–13.

Stanford, Julianne, Ellen R. Tauber, B. J. Fogg, and Leslie Marable. 2002. *Experts Vs. Online Consumers: A Comparative Credibility Study of Health and Finance Web Sites*. Consumer Web Watch.

Sun, Yalin, Yan Zhang, Jacek Gwizdka, and Ciaran B. Trace. 2019. "Consumer Evaluation of the Quality of Online Health Information: Systematic Literature Review of Relevant Criteria and Indicators." *Journal of Medical Internet Research* 21 (5): e12522.

Tamusuza, Anthony. 2011. "Leaving School Early: The Quest for Universal Primary Education in Uganda." *Journal of Statistique Africain* 11: 110–51.

Unesco. 2019. *New Methodology Shows that 258 Million Children, Adolescents and Youth Are Out of School*. Accessed February 13, 2022. http://uis.unesco.org/sites/default/files/documents/new-methodology-shows-258-million-children-adolescents-and-youth-are-out-school.pdf.

Voogt, Joke, and Natalie Pareja Roblin. 2012. "A Comparative Analysis of International Frameworks for 21st Century Competences: Implications for National Curriculum Policies." *Journal of Curriculum Studies* 44 (3): 299–321.

Walsh-Childers, Kim, Jennifer Braddock, Cristina Rabaza, and Gary Schwitzer. 2018. "One Step Forward, One Step Back: Changes in News Coverage of Medical Interventions." *Health Communication* 33 (2): 174–87.

Zarocostas, John. 2020. "How to Fight an Infodemic." *Lancet* 395 (10225): 676.

12

Medical Professionals Using Social Media to Combat Misinformation

Lisa Mordell, Eve Bloomgarden, Shikha Jain, and Vineet Arora

The Need for Medical Professionals to Combat Misinformation

IN 2021, THE SURGEON GENERAL declared misinformation a public health crisis and called on health professionals and health care organizations to "proactively engage with patients and the public on health misinformation" and to "use technology and media platforms to share accurate health information with the public" (Murthy 2021). While a critical goal, it is important to note that most medical professionals are not trained in the nuances of fighting medical misinformation or using social media or technology platforms to address medical misinformation with their patients and communities. Moreover, there are additional risks that medical professionals who engage in advocacy around medical misinformation face on social media. As a result, it is important to consider how to best engage medical professionals in using social media to combat medical misinformation. In this chapter, the authors aim to describe a model for how medical professionals can use social media to combat misinformation with a particular focus on the COVID-19 vaccine.

Defining Types of Medical Misinformation and Reasons for Its Rise

In order to understand how to address medical misinformation, it is important to understand how false information is shared and the distinction between misinformation and disinformation. *Misinformation* is information that is misleading, inaccurate, or untrue based on currently available evidence, and the decision to share this information may not be done with malicious intent (Pan American Health Organization 2020). *Disinformation* is a category of misinformation that is deliberately created and shared with the intent to deceive, typically for some type of personal, financial, or political gain (Centers for Disease Control and Prevention 2021). The purpose of disseminating this inaccurate information is to achieve some secondary gain that often does not benefit the targeted audience. Disinformation is often then shared as misinformation.

An *infodemic* occurs when there is an overabundance of information, including mis- and disinformation, during an acute health crisis such as an epidemic. The term "infodemic" was first used during the SARS outbreak (Rothkopf 2003) and was reintroduced by World Health Organization director-general Dr. Tedros Adhanom Ghebreyesus during the Munich Security Conference in February 2020. In an infodemic, credible, authoritative, and trusted voices are diluted by mis- and disinformation, both of which are designed to elicit emotional responses, including anxiety and fear. This dilution and mixed messaging leads to confusion, mistrust in science and public health messaging, bad decision-making, as well as polarization along political lines. Misinformation causes direct and tangible harm to both individuals and the public at large. For example, prior to COVID-19 vaccine availability, misinformation about masks, social distancing, and other public health measures led to premature relaxation of mitigation measures in many states, and a subsequent rise in COVID-19 cases, hospitalizations, and deaths. Even before the COVID-19 vaccines were granted Emergency Use Authorization, disinformation was disseminated to the public by an organized anti-vaccine movement that has been active for decades. Once vaccines became available to the public, the amount of misinformation shared increased rapidly, exploiting very real fears and taking advantage of vulnerable populations. For example, one of the most popular reasons for women of reproductive age not to get vaccinated was the myth that COVID-19 vaccines caused infertility. This misinformation led to an increase in morbidity and mortality for unvaccinated pregnant women (Berry et al. 2021). Additionally, mis- and disinformation surrounding unsubstantiated treatments for COVID-19, such as hydroxychloroquine, ivermectin, and bleach, led to unnecessary illness and death due to medication toxicity, and avoidance of evidence-based interventions as well as vaccination. Furthermore, this created real harm for many people who rely on hydroxychloroquine for treatment of chronic medical conditions, as these individuals experienced relapse of chronic medical conditions, pain, and disability due to supply shortages of their essential medications (Romo 2021).

It is also worth considering the reasons for the rise of medical misinformation. According to the law of rumor, rumors arise when the ambiguity of the information is high, and the importance of the information is also high (Allport and Postman 1946). The natural information asymmetry in the doctor-patient relationship and in health care leads to high ambiguity of medical information, which is extremely important information to all because it relates to one's health and longevity. A recent paper in the *Journal of the American Medical Association* (Arora, Madison, and Simpson 2020) articulated several reasons why medical misinformation arises (see table 12.1). While this chapter was written before the pandemic, many of the types of misinformation outlined in the figure are easily recognized types of misinformation seen during the COVID-19 pandemic. For example, the COVID-19 pandemic witnessed an explosion of pseudoscience (unscientific claims) and junk science (fraudulent data) requiring retractions of multiple peer-reviewed articles that were published in well-respected journals.

Another reason for the rise of medical misinformation is due to the rapid and evolving science during a pandemic. Therefore, much of the world is not only wrestling with blatant misinformation but also outdated science, inappropriately applied science, and conflicting interpretations of science. For example, public health officials did not universally recommend masking early in the pandemic. Experts then pivoted to recommend universal masking due to the clear role that masks played in the mitigation of spread. Now, misinformation about masking continues to proliferate due to the initial message of masks not providing a benefit (outdated science). A similar phenomenon occurs when experts have conflicting interpretations of science, such as the US and UK approaches to mitigation and vaccine uptake. This has led to differences in policies around masking and other mitigation in schools. It is easy for misinformation to spread in the context of conflicting interpretations of science.

TABLE 12.1
Types, Examples, and Strategies to Address Misinformation Affecting the Patient-Clinician Relationship

Type of Misinformation	*Definition*	*Example*	*Example Strategy to Address Misinformation*
Pseudoscience	Misinformation due to unscientific claims	Goop website recommendation for "jade eggs"	Dr. Jennifer Gunter debunks jade eggs using social media
Junk science	Claims made based on fraudulent or disproven data	Fear of vaccines causing autism	Pediatricians use TikTok to spread provaccine messages
Outdated science	Due to the incremental nature of science, information is now outdated or has been reversed	Use of percutaneous coronary intervention for patients with stable angina	Cardiology professional society shares training materials for cardiologists on how to discuss this change with patients
Inappropriately applied science	Misinformation due to clinical heterogeneity that renders science not relevant to clinical context	Maintaining tight glycemic control in older patients	Patient group highlights the harm of tight glycemic control for older patients with diabetes
Conflicting interpretations of science	Misinformation perpetuated due to conflicts in two or more established guidelines, sometimes due to vested interests	US Preventive Services Task Force and American Cancer Society recommendations for breast cancer screening	Health system hosts community grand rounds with local leaders to dispel myths about mammography

Source: V. M. Arora, Madison, and Simpson 2020.

Social Media and Medical Misinformation

Medical misinformation only holds power when it reaches an audience to influence. As of October 2021, the audience of social media users is approximately 4.5 billion globally (DataReportal 2021). The online social media network also provides the perfect medium for the amplification of information and misinformation (Wang et al. 2019). According to a 2018 study, false information on social media is significantly more likely to be shared by users, spreading faster and reaching more users as compared to evidence-based or true information (Vosoughi, Roy, and Aral 2018). Misinformation and disinformation elicit stronger emotional responses, especially negative ones, which drive user engagement and the number of shares. The way that information is presented to users varies by platform and is constantly changing, but it is clear that algorithms curate information to maximize engagement by sharing information deemed relevant to that individual (Agrawal 2016). Misinformation thrives when social media algorithms promote information based on engagement, reactions, and likelihood to share a post or article, without giving weight to whether the information is true or false. Additionally, people tend to support and follow other people with similar values and opinions, and this creates an echo chamber where differing opinions are absent, and untruths become the reality (Cinelli et al. 2021).

Although social media has given rise to the spread of misinformation, it can also be harnessed to combat the COVID-19 infodemic in real-time through rapid identification of misconceptions and spreading and sharing of valid scientific information. A recent review in

Lancet of over eighty studies identified that social media during the COVID-19 pandemic can help to not only rapidly identify infodemics/misinformation but also survey public attitudes and governmental responses to the pandemic (Tsao et al. 2021). Therefore, it is not surprising that major public health organizations recognize the potential to harness individuals and groups to fight medical misinformation on social media, particularly related to the COVID-19 vaccine. The Centers for Disease Control and Prevention (CDC) maintains social media toolkits for health communicators to use and has also released sample social media messages to promote the COVID-19 vaccine (2020). Local health departments have also engaged individuals as social media ambassadors during the pandemic. For example, the Illinois Department of Public Health (2020) began offering an ambassador program for members of the general public to have access to social tools and posts to amplify information about the pandemic, and more specifically about the COVID-19 vaccine.

Health Professionals, Social Media, and Medical Misinformation

Health professionals are uniquely positioned to describe on-the-ground accounts of how mis- and disinformation influence and guide the understanding and behavior of the patients and their communities. During the pandemic, messages from health care professionals on social media not only reach more people but can also be influential in shaping people's attitudes. This is especially important since many hospitals, due to privacy and risk-aversion, are not willing or able to work with traditional media to provide on-the-ground accounts of what may be happening inside the walls of an emergency room, hospital ward, or intensive care unit. Social media use by health professionals can also be effective. For example, a randomized study showed that tweets containing personal pleas by emergency medicine physicians were perceived to be more effective in shaping attitudes toward the pandemic and more likely to be shared when compared to formal tweets by policy officials (Solnick et al. 2021).

Unfortunately, health care professionals might be reluctant to engage in social media publicly for a variety of reasons. One reason is fear of retribution from their employer. Early accounts in the pandemic highlighted these penalties, faced by those who spoke out about work conditions and lack of personal protective equipment (Way 2020), which included being terminated. In fact, the National Health Service (Johnson 2020) in the United Kingdom went so far as to counsel their workforce to avoid "commenting on political issues, such as PPE" and is said to have used intimidation tactics, such as threatening email and monitoring personal accounts, to prevent their employees from speaking out (Letsas and Mantouvalou 2020).

Another reason health care professionals are reluctant to engage is the fear of harassment. One study conducted just prior to the COVID-19 pandemic showed that roughly one in four physicians reported being personally attacked on social media (Pendergrast et al. 2021), and the most common reason for this was advocacy, particularly around vaccines. This same study showed that one in six female physicians report being sexually harassed online. Women who are subject to online harassment often reduce their online presence (Staude-Müller, Hansen, and Voss 2012), effectively limiting the likelihood of re-engaging on social media to counter misinformation. Other challenges to health professionals engaging on social media include the amount of time required to do so effectively and the fact that this work is undervalued and uncompensated.

While there are concerns that trust in health professionals is eroding, surveys of the public demonstrate that health professionals are perceived as trusted messengers by the public. According to a 2020 Gallup poll, health professionals rate highly in Americans' assessment of honesty and ethics (Saad 2020). At least six in ten US adults say that nurses, medical doctors, pharmacists, and dentists have high levels of these virtues. It is notable that nurses have ranked first in Americans' assessment of honesty and ethics for the past nineteen years (Reinhart 2020). Furthermore, trust in doctors has actually risen during the pandemic, highlighting the importance of harnessing these voices in promoting public health messaging and addressing medical misinformation.

How Health Care Professionals Can Engage in Combating Medical Misinformation: The IMPACT Model

Given the trusted status of health professionals, it is critical to empower health professionals to speak up against medical misinformation despite the challenges, reluctance, and risks outlined thus far. With this in mind, the Illinois Medical Professionals Action Collaborative Team (IMPACT) was formed in March 2020 with the explicit purpose to amplify health care worker voices and disseminate evidence-based information to combat misinformation and medical mistrust, with an initial focus on the state of Illinois.

The group formed organically after a core sector of physicians with existing social media identities and influence connected to warn about COVID-19. Following its inception, IMPACT strategically recruited members with expertise the organization needed, such as diversity and equity, lab medicine and testing, health communications scientists, pediatric advisors, immunology advisors, data analysts, pharmacists, nurses, public health specialists, and outreach specialists. This expansion has allowed IMPACT to utilize interdisciplinary approaches and deepen their credibility as a trusted health care messenger.

How IMPACT Established a Presence on Social Media: Platform Considerations for Misinformation

Before any misinformation can be combated on social media, it is first crucial to establish an individual or group's social media presence. However, a social media presence is not only the existence of a social media account; the content shared from this account needs to reach the intended audiences. Therefore, it is crucial for individuals and groups to understand how to establish and cultivate an intentional social media presence. Each social media platform is different, and for personal accounts it may be best to start initially with one social media platform. However, groups or organizations benefit from streamlined accounts across multiple platforms portraying consistent messaging and recognized branding to maximize reach and visibility. Regardless of individual or group identity, to be seen as a trusted messenger and credible expert, all platforms should be presented in a professional manner. In any platform, the goal is to catch the individual's eye with design and content that is understandable and lends itself to engagement. Across all social media platforms, images and videos tend to garner more views and shares than text-only posts, but both are effective communication techniques. Each social media platform has its own personality, appeal, and nuances that can be tailored to effectively combat misinformation.

Twitter

Twitter was a central platform for IMPACT, in part because many of the founders already had active Twitter accounts and were viewed as credible sources of information prior to the pandemic. Twitter is one of the most active social media platforms, with nearly 500 million tweets sent per day (Sayce 2019) and with one in five US adults using Twitter (Hughes and Wojcik 2019). It allows for the rapid sharing of information and real-time news updates. Additionally, the platform designates some accounts and users as "verified," adding a layer of confidence that the account is credible. Unfortunately, disinformation campaigns, fake news, and resharing of misinformation also thrive on Twitter, as the verified status is not easily obtained and does not have a category for health professionals. Furthermore, the status is primarily offered to celebrities, politicians, and influencers, and being verified does not mean that the information shared is true. An excellent way to utilize Twitter to counter misinformation is to amplify evidence-based information by posting peer-reviewed articles, or information from the news media from trusted reputable sources. When posting a photo, Twitter enables "tagging" up to ten accounts. This provides those individuals with a notification that the post exists with the goal of having that individual or group engage and amplify the information.

Twitter also has the option of creating a group direct messaging thread, allowing up to fifty individuals to be included in one group. IMPACT utilized this feature by creating an "IMPACT amplifier." IMPACT team members, partners, and other important stakeholders used this amplifier to share IMPACT posts and infographics for amplification on social media, to communicate quickly about pertinent pandemic-related questions and concerns, as well as to stay on top of rapidly changing information across the state. The amplifier also became a way to protect one another as members of the group were alerted when another member was attacked or targeted by those attempting to spread disinformation. When an individual found themselves a target, other members of the amplifier would respond with data and evidence in hopes of drowning out bad information with good information.

Facebook

There are thousands of physicians and health professional private groups on Facebook. Each group has one or more moderators who have to approve members; for many physician groups, membership requires verification that the individual is a physician. These groups are an excellent modality to crowdsource and disseminate information and tag appropriate stakeholders as necessary. When IMPACT was formed, one of the cofounders was also the Facebook moderator for Physician Mommies Chicago, a Facebook group of over 2,000 physicians. The team also recruited the moderator of a newly formed health professional group of almost 3,000 members called the Illinois COVID-19 Collective to join the team. These groups allowed IMPACT to crowdsource information from the community and other health care professionals to quickly identify concerns, address questions, and guide the narrative on truthful messages and science-based recommendations. For example, Facebook groups alerted IMPACT to PPE shortages that allowed the team to direct resources to health care professionals through IMPACT partnerships. Facebook also alerted the team to local misinformation/disinformation campaigns including anti-mask and anti-vaccine rallies.

Additionally, when the first COVID-19 vaccine doses were offered to health care professionals, IMPACT was alerted to significant challenges that many health care professionals were facing in trying to get vaccinated through these Facebook groups. The IMPACT team was then able to open vaccine events for unaffiliated health care professionals, and the information about these events was shared with these health care professional Facebook groups. Thousands of health care professionals were able to be successfully vaccinated this way (Wallia et al. 2021). IMPACT continued to then create a vaccine clearinghouse website for the public to find vaccine appointments and shared this vaccine-related information with many Facebook groups, including the Chicago Vaccine Hunters, a group of 81,000 members. Facebook allowed IMPACT to easily reach diverse communities of health professionals, as well as the general public, in order to provide resources and to counter misinformation in a novel way.

Instagram, YouTube, and TikTok

After initially establishing on Twitter and Facebook, IMPACT expanded to Instagram, YouTube, and TikTok to begin reaching a younger demographic. Instagram is a photo and video-sharing social media platform that focuses on aesthetics and is flooded with content creators and influencers (Conduct Science 2019). Similar to Twitter, Instagram also enables "tagging" individuals or accounts to facilitate amplification. The IMPACT Instagram account was managed by a group of volunteer student interns who are well-versed with strategies to target this younger demographic. IMPACT's Instagram account utilized a streamlined and consistent aesthetic to share infographics and statements combating misinformation.

YouTube is a video-sharing platform with over 2 billion users, making it the second most used social media platform (Statista 2021). It allows users to upload longer-duration videos for subscribers to like, view, comment, and share (Lua 2019). IMPACT shared video interviews called "IMPACTful Chats" on this platform, where two physician team members interviewed a wide variety of experts to answer questions about the pandemic. Video sharing provided a human face and voice to updated evidence-based information.

TikTok is also a video-sharing platform; however, TikTok videos vary in length from three to sixty seconds and are typically set to audio clips, songs, or prerecorded video footage, with creative tools and effects. Additionally, each TikTok user has a "For You" page of videos, which are videos tailored to the users' interest and watch history based on an algorithm with artificial intelligence, allowing for videos to have the potential to reach millions of users even if the original creator of a video has a small following (Sehl 2020). IMPACT did not create a TikTok account but rather recruited a team member with a large non-health care professional audience to begin repurposing IMPACT's infographics and messaging on this platform in video form.

Overall IMPACT Philosophy to Dealing with Misinformation

When engaging on social media, it is first important to remember that many people have already made up their minds and their decisions will not be able to be swayed. Therefore, the goal is to reach those individuals who are unsure which information they should believe (Clayman, Jain, and Arora 2020).

When discussing information, it is important to ensure that statements and claims are grounded in evidence and informed by respected experts in the field. The most important part of addressing misinformation, whether in person or on social media, is to identify what the misinformation is, where it is coming from, and provide evidence to the contrary. When providing evidence to the contrary, to leave an impression, the most effective public health messaging strategy is to lead with the facts (Goldstein et al. 2020). This was the method that IMPACT adopted to create debunking infographics, described in further detail below.

There are generally two approaches to addressing misinformation: a reactive approach or a proactive approach. In the reactive approach, one sees incorrect information circulating and addresses it in real-time, with articles and facts. However, in order to change the hearts and minds of those on social media, only posting links to articles and evidence will not make a difference in others' thinking. Individuals on social media often do not take the time to read an entire article. So, it is essential to summarize the key points and screenshot the important parts of the article that should be read.

When engaging in the reactive approach to misinformation on social media, IMPACT team members have found it helpful to engage with facts and to avoid emotional or negative responses that lead to the poster feeling defensive. For example, if someone posts inaccurate information, respond with an article or facts, and summarize important points in a simple way. Do not waste time arguing with those who are trying to troll or raise the temperature of the conversation. There is an important "bystander" effect that has been observed when fighting misinformation, such that the information posted is actually more influential for the other individuals who may come across this online conversation, versus changing the minds of those set in their ways and maliciously posting misinformation.

The proactive approach to addressing misinformation can be extremely successful when taken on by a team. The first step is understanding the myths and inaccurate information circulating on social media and in the community. It is important to note that this information may differ based on who is affected by the rumor, as well as cultural differences in the types of rumors or myths circulating. Once the prevalent myths are identified, a proactive, targeted, coordinated strategy can be undertaken with easy-to-understand social media posts, infographics, and messaging to quickly and rapidly stop the myths from spreading further. By partnering with other organizations and trusted community messengers, the counter-messaging can be amplified and circulated beyond one's reach.

Lastly, regardless of the proactive or reactive approach, to help persuade people, it is often very helpful to "lead from where you stand" and consider a personal anecdote or perspective. For example, as many of the IMPACT founders are physician mothers, leading with credible stories of how they were handling COVID-19 at home or with their children was often an easy place to start. Likewise, as the team has expertise in different areas, a hospitalist may take the lead to discuss bed capacity whereas a primary care physician would take the lead to discuss immunization.

Combating Misinformation in Practice: Case Studies

Development of a Rapid Response Team to React: Promoting Distancing

IMPACT's initial focus after inception at the beginning of the pandemic was on social distancing and masking using a predominantly reactive approach. The group initially came together when noting the large groups gathering for St. Patrick's Day celebrations and at O'Hare airport in Chicago (Jain 2020), and the lack of a messaging campaign to educate on the evolution and severity of the ongoing situation. Due to the observation of the already rapid dissemination of misinformation on social media, the team created a "Rapid Response Team" to identify issues and respond quickly with letters to policymakers, op-eds, statements or petitions to be published and disseminated via social media. The initial Rapid Response Team consisted of IMPACT cofounders and student interns.

Using closed Facebook groups, IMPACT identified that many health professionals felt similarly and were concerned about the lack of action around social distancing. As a result, initial efforts focused on letters and petitions sent to local policymakers and government officials requesting urgent and immediate action for social distancing practices to be initiated and a "shelter in place" order to be enacted, which was ultimately put into place (Arora 2020). These templates of letters and petitions were also shared with health care workers in other states to modify appropriately for their own use.

Strategic Growth Through Partnerships to Disseminate Information and Combat Misinformation

IMPACT established novel collaborations and partnerships with other organizations and grassroots coalitions with aligned missions to facilitate rapid communication and consistent messaging, and to build a large network of trusted and credible resources. Organizations included groups such as MasksNowIL, a group of volunteers who sewed masks to address medical supply shortages; GetMePPEChi, a coalition of Chicago medical students assessing PPE needs and coordinating donations to health care and community organizations in Chicago; Dear Pandemic, an interdisciplinary all-woman team of researchers and clinicians with expertise including nursing, mental health, health policy, and epidemiology; and This Is Our Shot, a national campaign to elevate health heroes, build trust around vaccines, and fight misinformation.

One novel partnership to note was with Bump Club & Beyond, a national network of over 150,000 new and expectant mothers. Through this partnership, team members worked collaboratively with Lindsay Pinchuk, the founder of the group, to identify key misconceptions and misinformation that expectant mothers were hearing. Through biweekly Facebook live Q&A sessions, IMPACT team members were able to speak directly to this high-risk population and answer their questions and concerns. The live sessions were recorded so that the video sessions could be watched later and shared across both groups' networks and platforms (IMPACT4HC 2021). This partnership is an excellent example of how to reach a broader audience to identify important topics that need to be addressed and then take the information to where the interested parties get their information.

Another strategy to address misinformation that was particularly successful was coordinating traditional media with social media. By creating coordinated messaging campaigns and cross-promoting initiatives across social media platforms, IMPACT established itself as a trusted source of science-based messaging, and traditional news media outlets began reaching out regularly for expert opinion or commentary. This enabled the group to establish relationships with multiple news organizations and journalists in Illinois and to share specific initiatives and content with multiple contacts. IMPACT cofounders and other members were asked to contribute both locally and nationally to the *Chicago Tribune* (Thayer 2020), *Fox32Chicago* (Fox32Chicago 2020), *TIME* (Dockterman 2021), *New York Times* (Wu 2021), *Good Morning America* (Kindelan and Lang 2020), *Wall Street Journal* (Hopkins and Campo-Flores 2020), *Chicago Sun-Times* (Walker 2020), and more. Media spotlights further increased the team's credibility, reach, and ability to disseminate information. Consistency in messaging is key when taking a social media campaign and translating it for news media. A useful strategy can be sharing relevant infographics, letters, or other resources with the news outlet prior to a scheduled interview. If published in print, ensure hyperlinks to all relevant publications, initiatives, letters, or petitions to maximize reach and also to stay consistent and on message.

Masking and Messaging: A Persistent Challenge

Guidance and policy around mask wearing exemplify how one simple public health recommendation can be mired by misinformation in every way possible. To counter misinformation and disinformation about masks and to expand evidence-based messaging outside of Illinois, IMPACT launched a campaign calling for a national mask mandate (IMPACT4HC 2020a). This campaign utilized partnerships, collaborations, and tools such as letters, and a national Change.org petition. To date, this petition has over 113,000 signatures. IMPACT team members also authored several pieces to articulate that masking is a public health issue, not a partisan one (Arora, Jain, Zimmerman et al. 2020); the importance of getting the messaging right (Arora and Jain 2020); and the need for a national approach to universal masking policy that was posted and reshared from popular health care blogs (Arora, Jain, Ranney et al. 2020). These op-eds also included direct links to the petition to increase visibility and reach. By widening the range of outlets of reach, the group's strategy was to effectively reach many different individuals from different parts of the country with consistent messaging.

Masking in schools became an issue of particular passion when IMPACT team members were alerted to the fact that groups on Facebook were organizing against masks in schools using many of the same techniques that anti-vaccine groups were using. The group wrote an op-ed (Zimmermann et al. 2020), a letter to the editor in the *Chicago Tribune* (Zimmermann et al. 2020), and a letter to the Illinois Superintendent (IMPACT4HC 2020b), specifically highlighting the need for maintaining masking in schools and alerting the public to be wary of misinformation surrounding masks.

Later in the pandemic, when *JAMA Pediatrics* published a research letter claiming that masking harmed children, IMPACT team members were alerted through social media that the letter was being used by antiscience and anti-mask groups to further their agenda to eliminate masks in schools. By working in a collaboration with other science-based groups fighting misinformation, such as Unambiguous Science and SciMoms, a public comment titled "Our Children Deserve Better Science" (Bloomgarden et al. 2021) was registered with *JAMA Pediatrics* on why this was false. Then, to counter the already viral spread of this article, the team developed a series of infographics outlining the serious flaws in the methodology that put the validity of the conclusions of this article in question. Through a collaborative social media push among all the groups, these infographics were able to reach over 700,000 people. The study was retracted seventeen days later (Christakis and Fontanarosa 2021).

A Proactive Approach: IMPACT Model to Address Vaccine Hesitancy and Access

Once the COVID-19 vaccines were granted Emergency Use Authorization by the US Food and Drug Administration (FDA), IMPACT shifted its focus to targeting vaccine misinformation using a proactive coordinated approach. To address vaccine misinformation, IMPACT team members used social media to crowdsource the top myths health care professionals heard. This was done by probing closed Facebook groups, two national and one local, of health care professionals, which were largely physician women. One example of a question probe was, "What are the top reasons for vaccine hesitancy among health care workers in your area?" The two most prevalent reasons for hesitancy from this polling were fertility concerns and that the vaccine was "too rushed" or "too new" (see table 12.2). IMPACT identified additional reasons for hesitancy by reviewing common questions that team members encountered at work, from their communities, and across social networks. Using this targeted approach, IMPACT developed infographics to disseminate on social media that directly addressed vaccine hesitancy and misinformation and provided the public with accurate evidence-based information.

TABLE 12.2
Top Reasons for Vaccine Hesitancy from Health Care Workers

Themes	*Sample Sentiments*
Fertility concerns	Don't want to harm babies. Scared to impact chances of getting pregnant.
Too rushed or too new	Don't know the long term side effects.
Distrust of research or of government by minority community	Historic distrust due to racism.
Side effects/allergies	Concerned for an allergic reaction if I have an allergy.
Conspiracy theories	The vaccine changes DNA.
It's not serious for young people	I'm young and won't get sick.
Anti-vaccine sentiment	I never get vaccinated anyways.
Taking time off	I can't take off or work.

Note: Assembled from ~100 responses to a Facebook query in Health Care Worker closed Facebook groups of largely physician women.

Source: Vineet Arora, MD, MAPP. March 2021.

First, IMPACT created a core "infographics team" of volunteer student interns, a physician lead, and the IMPACT cofounders. Infographics were created following a stepwise process initially described by Mark Smiciklas (Kelly and Gaytan 2014). Infographics drafted by the core team were shared with the physician lead and one or more physician cofounders for initial review. Once approved, the infographic was then reviewed by the broader IMPACT team. The content for each infographic was gathered from federal agencies' sources, such as CDC or FDA, or peer-reviewed, evidence-based sources. Citations and dates of publication were included in each infographic. Key points were edited for lay audience with an eighth-grade literacy using the program Readable. Infographics were also translated into Spanish by bilingual team members.

IMPACT created two series of infographics to address vaccine misinformation: The Vaccine Series (see figure 12.1) and the Myth Debunkers Series (see figure 12.2). The Vaccine Series was designed to describe each US-authorized COVID-19 vaccine (Pfizer-BioNTech, Moderna, Janssen) as well as the technology behind each vaccine. Each infographic in this series began with a commonly asked question, added components to make the infographic visually appealing and simplify the data, and ended with reiterating the initial question and answering related follow-up questions. The Myth Debunkers Series utilized the "Fact, Myth, Fallacy, Fact" method from *The Debunking Handbook* (Lewandowsky et al. 2020) and incorporates the idea that combating misinformation is more effective when the audience is made to feel suspicious of the misinformation. Each infographic in this series follows the same pattern outlined in figure 12.3 leading with the fact, warning about the myth once, and then immediately explaining why the myth is false. The final step is restating the fact. The detailed refutation sandwiched between repetition of the fact is key to tackling misinformation without unintentionally perpetuating the myth.

Once finalized, these infographics were shared across the group's various social media platforms (see figure 12.4) and on the IMPACT website. In this way, IMPACT was able to rapidly disseminate information with an average turnaround time of five to ten days from idea to completion. Team members also shared the infographics individually, and many of the infographics were embedded into guidance for schools and hospital systems, displayed in physicians' offices, as well as shared by IMPACT partners nationally. While it is difficult

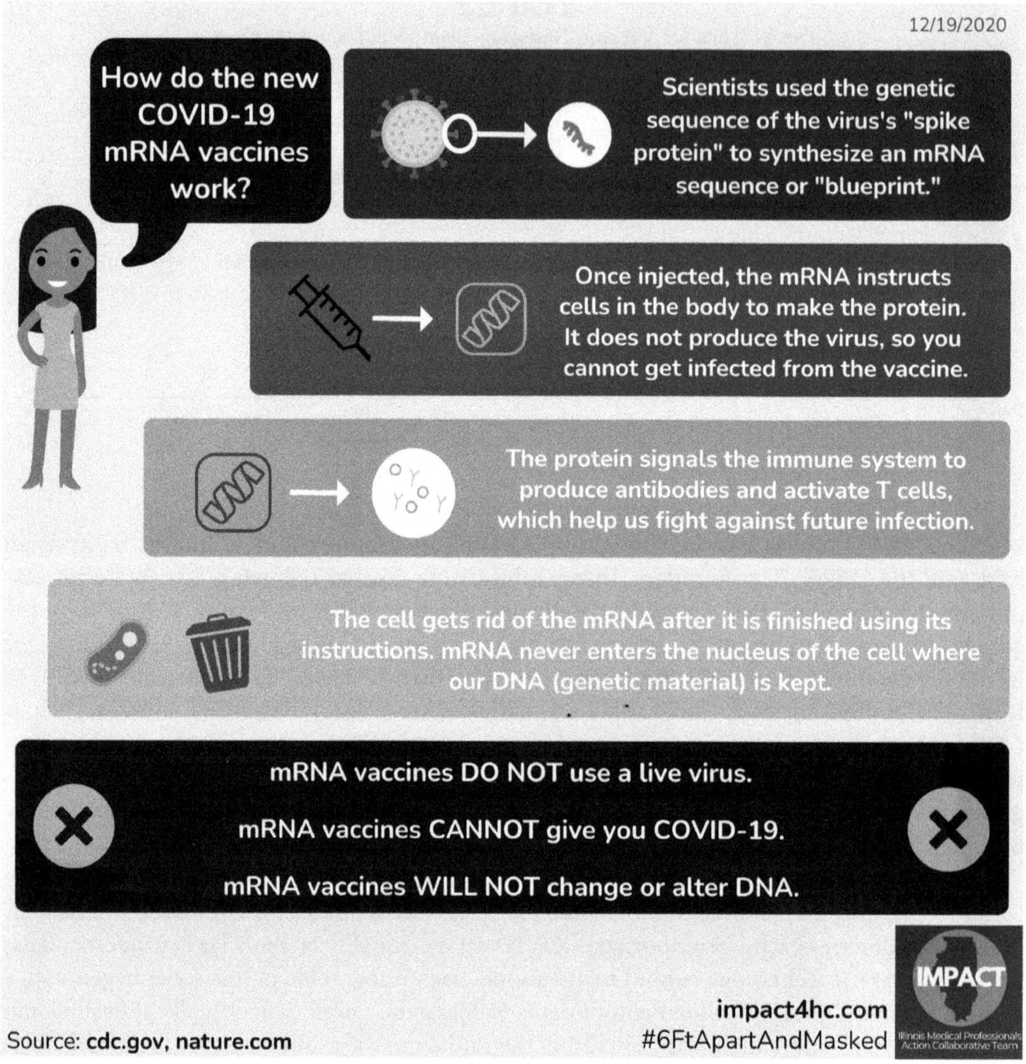

FIGURE 12.1
IMPACT4HC's Vaccine Series, How Do the New COVID-19 mRNA Vaccines Work?
Source: IMPACT4HC 2021.

to assess if these infographics impacted decision-making in every circumstance, numerous stories shared with the group speak to the impact that these infographics had to inform individuals and guide decision-making among those who had read or heard inaccurate information (Rotolo et al. 2021).

The rollout of the COVID-19 vaccines was immediately hindered by misinformation, confusion, and inequities in access in the city of Chicago as well. To expedite vaccine access, IMPACT mobilized and recruited over 1,500 medical and nonmedical volunteers through calls on social media to help staff over 300 vaccination events across Chicago's hardest-hit communities. When in the field, IMPACT volunteers were instructed to use copies of IMPACT infographics, vaccine Q&A sheets, and brochures to educate the community in person. Through these experiences, IMPACT members realized that there are many in the community who do

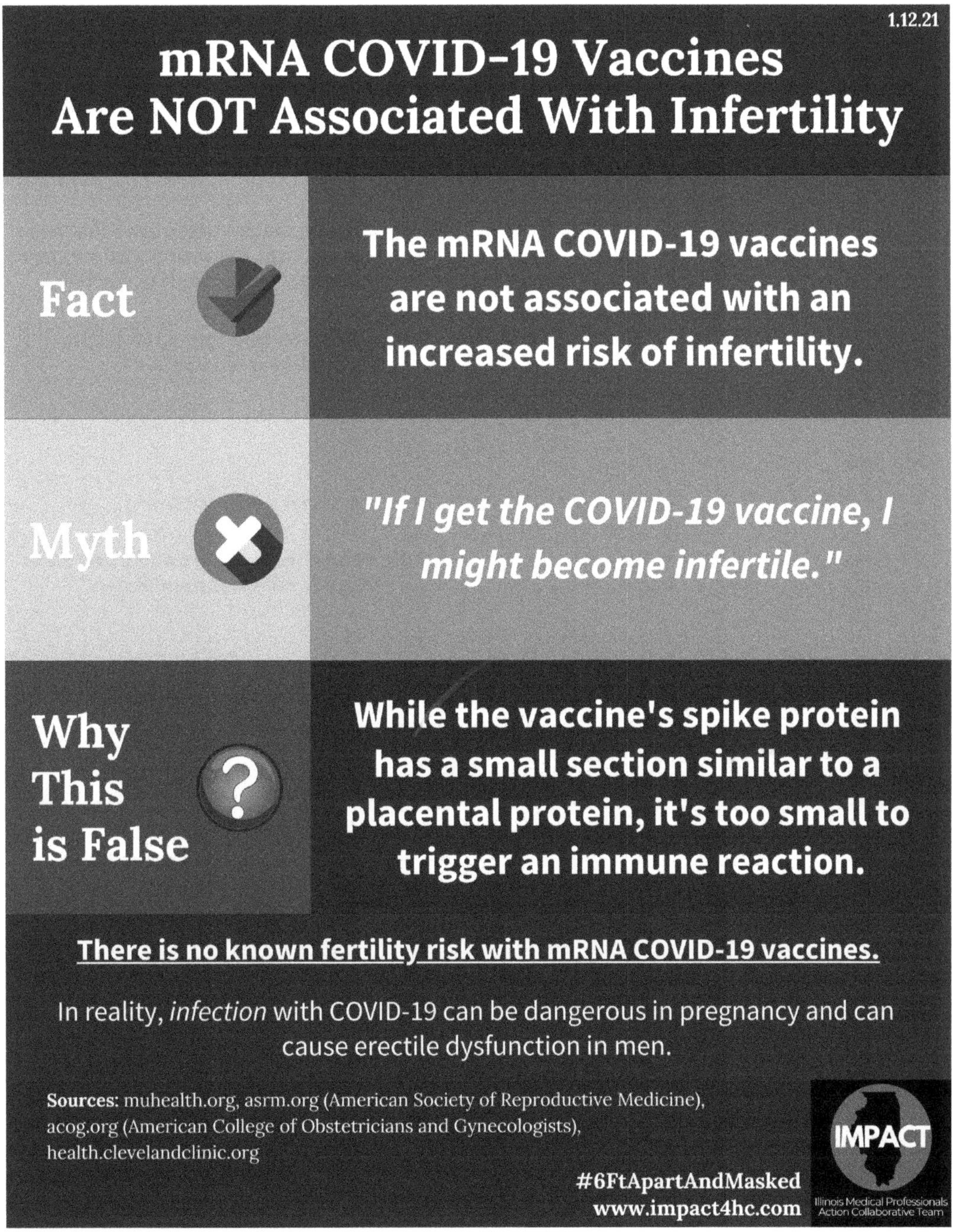

FIGURE 12.2
IMPACT4HC's Myth Debunkers Series, mRNA COVID-19 Vaccines Are NOT Associated with Infertility.
Source: IMPACT4HC 2020c.

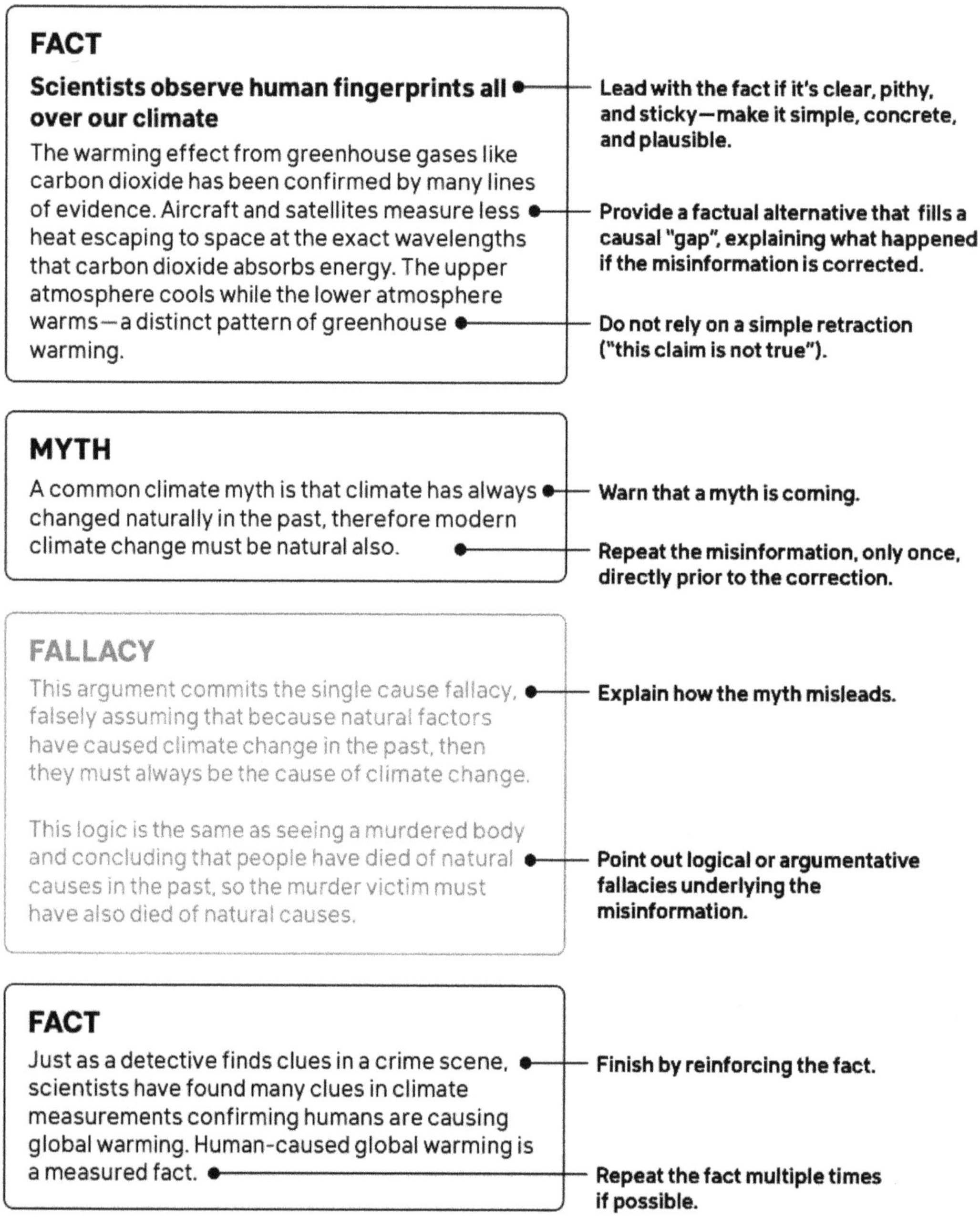

FIGURE 12.3
Example of a Refutation from *The Debunking Handbook 2020*.
Source: Lewandowsky et al. 2020.

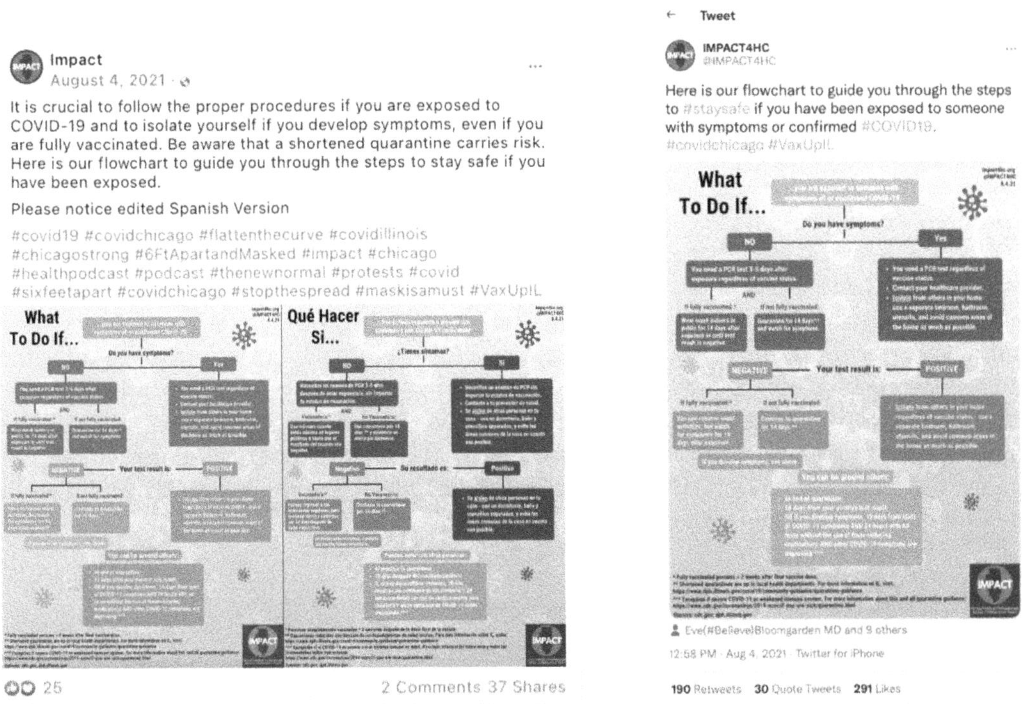

FIGURE 12.4
A sample *Facebook* (Left) and *Twitter* (Right) Post of an Original IMPACT4HC Infographic.

not have access to social media and technological resources. As a result, IMPACT created an IMPACT Speakers Bureau to help provide speakers for community events. Team members held "town hall Q&A sessions" upon request and reviewed accurate vaccine information and provided direct opportunities for community members to ask their questions. To expand the reach of IMPACT's information, IMPACT team members found it helpful to empower trusted messengers in local communities. One group of trusted messengers that specialize in community information are public librarians. Through a partnership with the Chicago Public Library, IMPACT speakers held online training for all public librarians in both English and Spanish.

Building on the success of the session with the public librarians, IMPACT representatives expanded their reach and have spoken at school events, vaccine events, and numerous other community engagement initiatives to answer questions and address concerns related to COVID-19 and the vaccines. In one school, only 50 percent of the staff was planning on initially receiving the vaccine and, after the Q&A session, this improved to 95 percent of those individuals either being vaccinated or scheduling a vaccine appointment.

Conclusion

The COVID-19 pandemic has underscored the influence that social media platforms hold when it comes to the rapid communication and dissemination of critical information. The pandemic has also highlighted the need for consistent messaging from health care professionals. Although health professionals are seen as trusted messengers with the credibility to effectively debunk misinformation, there are challenges to engaging in social media. Therefore, it is critical to create models that empower health care professionals to do this. The creation, evolution, and development of IMPACT provide a model for how medical professionals can effectively use social media to identify misinformation and reach a much larger audience. Specifically, having a presence on social media allows for intentional crowdsourcing and for the rapid dissemination of health information through visual aids (infographics). It also allows for rapid identification of health care inequities, such as vaccine access, and focusing of resources on areas that need them. The role of IMPACT in combating misinformation necessitated engaging the public on social media and reinforced the critical role of medical professionals in disseminating reliable and evidence-based information.

Acknowledgments

The authors would like to thank both past and present members as well as the partners of the Illinois Medical Professionals Action Collaborative Team. Additionally, the authors would like to thank the authors of *The Debunking Handbook* and the *Journal of the American Medical Association* for their permission for using figures in our chapter.

References

Agrawal, A. J. 2016. “What Do Social Media Algorithms Mean for You?” *Forbes*, April 20, 2016. https://www.forbes.com/sites/ajagrawal/2016/04/20/what-do-social-media-algorithms-mean-for-you/.

Allport, Gordon W., and Leo Postman. 1946. “An Analysis of Rumor.” The Public Opinion Quarterly 10 (4): 501–17.

Arora, Vineet M. (@FutureDocs). 2020. “Dear @GovPritzker, Over 300 IL Physicians Are Calling for Urgent Action to Enforce Social Distancing given Chicago Mass Gatherings (e.g. St. Patrick’s Day, O’hare). Help Us #FlattenTheCurve Now. #COVID19 https://Docs.Google.Com/Document/d/1uvDDiTm6DsIq_nT3aaQyPOYofR3YgO4VJP8yYopTnRo/Edit?Usp=sharing Cc @alikhan28 @ShikhaJainMD @LJoyZ @haroldpollack.” Twitter, March 15, 2020. https://twitter.com/FutureDocs/status/1239271918479474688.

Arora, Vineet M., Sonia Madison, and Lisa Simpson. 2020. “Addressing Medical Misinformation in the Patient-Clinician Relationship.” *JAMA* 324 (23): 2367. https://doi.org/10.1001/jama.2020.4263.

Arora, Vineet, and Shikha Jain. 2020. “The Messaging of Masks: Overcoming Disinformation.” Op-Med. August 19, 2020. https://opmed.doximity.com/articles/the-messaging-of-masks-overcoming-disinformation.

Arora, Vineet, Shikha Jain, Laura Zimmermann, Ali Khan, Amisha Wallia, and Eve Bloomgarden. 2020a. “Masks Are Not a Partisan Issue. They Are a Public Health Issue. #AmericaMaskUp.” KevinMD.Com, June 19, 2020. https://www.kevinmd.com/blog/2020/06/masks-are-not-a-partisan-issue-they-are-a-public-health-issue-americamaskup.html.

Arora, Vineet, Shikha Jain, Megan L. Ranney, and Helen Burstin. 2020b. “The Case for A National Universal Masking Mandate.” *Health Affairs*, August 5, 2020. https://www.healthaffairs.org/do/10.1377/hblog20200804.515241/full/.

Berry, Sarah D., Kimberly S. Johnson, Lonnita Myles, Laurie Herndon, Ana Montoya, Shekinah Fashaw, and David Gifford. 2021. "Lessons Learned from Frontline Skilled Nursing Facility Staff Regarding COVID-19 Vaccine Hesitancy." *Journal of the American Geriatrics Society* 69 (5): 1140–46. https://doi.org/10.1111/jgs.17136.

Bloomgarden, Eve, Elisabeth Marnik, Alison Bernstein, and Rebecca J. Heick. 2021. "Our Children Deserve Better Science." *JAMA Pediatrics Comments*, July 2, 2021. https://jamanetwork.com/journals/jamapediatrics/fullarticle/2781743.

Centers for Disease Control and Prevention. 2020. "Coronavirus Disease 2019 (COVID-19)." Accessed February 8, 2022. https://www.cdc.gov/coronavirus/2019-ncov/communication/vaccination-toolkit.html.

Centers for Disease Control and Prevention. 2021. "How to Address COVID-19 Vaccine Misinformation." Accessed February 8, 2022. https://www.cdc.gov/vaccines/covid-19/health-departments/addressing-vaccine-misinformation.html.

Christakis, Dimitri, and Phil B. Fontanarosa. 2021. "Notice of Retraction. Walach H, et al. Experimental Assessment of Carbon Dioxide Content in Inhaled Air With or Without Face Masks in Healthy Children: A Randomized Clinical Trial." *JAMA Pediatr.* Published Online June 30, 2021." *JAMA Pediatrics*, July, e213252. https://doi.org/10.1001/jamapediatrics.2021.3252.

Cinelli, Matteo, Gianmarco De Francisci Morales, Alessandro Galeazzi, Walter Quattrociocchi, and Michele Starnini. 2021. "The Echo Chamber Effect on Social Media." *Proceedings of the National Academy of Sciences* 118 (9): e2023301118. https://doi.org/10.1073/pnas.2023301118.

Clayman, Marla, Shikha Jain, and Vineet Arora. 2020. "Misinformation and Masking: Salvaging the Message." *Medium*, August 5, 2020. https://medium.com/@ShikhaJainMD/misinformation-and-masking-salvaging-the-message-339270f8d4f.

Conduct Science. 2019. "The Impact of Social Media on Knowledge Dissemination–Conduct Science." Accessed February 8, 2022. https://conductscience.com/the-impact-of-social-media-on-knowledge-dissemination/.

DataReportal. 2021. "Global Social Media Stats." Accessed February 8, 2022. https://datareportal.com/social-media-users.

Dockterman, Eliana. 2021. "These Moms Work as Doctors and Scientists. But They've Also Taken on Another Job: Fighting COVID-19 Misinformation Online." *TIME Magazine*, March 24, 2021. https://time.com/5947557/covid-19-vaccine-misinformation-moms/.

Fox32Chicago. 2020. "Chicago Doctors Come Together to Dispel Misinformation, Advise Officials on the Pandemic." Accessed February 8, 2022. https://www.fox32chicago.com/video/684221.

Goldstein, Carly M., Eleanor J. Murray, Jennifer Beard, Alexandra M. Schnoes, and Monica L. Wang. 2020. "Science Communication in the Age of Misinformation." *Annals of Behavioral Medicine* 54 (12): 985–90. https://doi.org/10.1093/abm/kaaa088.

Hopkins, Jared S., and Arian Campo-Flores. 2020. "As Pfizer's Covid-19 Vaccine Rolls Out, Next Step Is Getting People to Take It." *The Wall Street Journal*, December 13, 2020. https://www.wsj.com/articles/as-pfizers-covid-19-vaccine-rolls-out-next-step-is-getting-people-to-take-it-11607859001.

Hughes, Adam, and Stefan Wojcik. 2019. "10 Facts about Americans and Twitter." Pew Research Center, August 2, 2019. https://www.pewresearch.org/fact-tank/2019/08/02/10-facts-about-americans-and-twitter/.

Illinois Department of Public Health. 2020. "COVID-19 Ambassadors." Accessed February 8, 2022. https://www.dph.illinois.gov/ambassador.

IMPACT4HC. 2020a. "We Need a Federal Mask Mandate: #AmericaMaskUp." Change.Org, June 2020. https://www.change.org/p/nancy-pelosi-we-need-a-federal-mask-mandate-americamaskup.

IMPACT4HC. 2020b. "Universal Masking in Schools." Accessed February 8, 2022. https://static1.squarespace.com/static/5e80f9e9abd507573ed7f6c0/t/5f15ce02c17bc37b233776d1/1595264514635/UniversalMaskingInSchools_NoVaccineExemptions.pdf.

IMPACT4HC. 2020c. "How Do the New COVID-19 MRNA Vaccines Work?" Accessed July 13, 2022. https://www.impact4hc.com/impact-infographics.

IMPACT4HC. 2021. "IMPACT on BCB Live." Accessed February 8, 2022. https://www.impact4hc.com/impact-on-bcb-live.

Jain, Shikha (@ShikhaJainMD). 2020. "There Are Lines out the Door at Restaurants and the St. Patrick's Day Celebrations from Yesterday Were Absolutely Ridiculous. Please Move Quickly as We Are Already so Far behind the Curve and Our Hospitals Will Be Overrun Very Soon. Please Do Something ASAP." Twitter, March 15, 2020. https://twitter.com/ShikhaJainMD/status/1239234531586121730.

Johnson, Sarah. 2020. "NHS Staff Forbidden from Speaking out Publicly about Coronavirus." *The Guardian*, April 9, 2020. http://www.theguardian.com/society/2020/apr/09/nhs-staff-forbidden-speaking-out-publicly-about-coronavirus.

Kelly, Stephanie, and Jorge Gaytan. 2014. "Book Review: The Power of Infographics: Using Pictures to Communicate and Connect with Your Audience, by Smiciklas, M." *Business and Professional Communication Quarterly* 77 (2): 240–42. https://doi.org/10.1177/2329490614527821.

Kindelan, Katie, and Sarah Lang. 2020. "How to Talk to Kids about Race, Privilege amid George Floyd Protests | GMA." *Good Morning America*, June 1, 2020. https://www.goodmorningamerica.com/family/story/parents-talk-kids-racism-george-floyd-protests-70992137.

Letsas, George, and Virginia Mantouvalou. 2020. "COVID-19 and Free Speech: 'Gagging' NHS Staff Is Not Proportionate and Lawful." *British Politics and Policy at LSE*, April 17, 2020. https://blogs.lse.ac.uk/politicsandpolicy/covid-19-and-free-speech/.

Lewandowsky, Stephan, John Cook, Ullrich Ecker, Dolores Albarracín, Michelle A. Amazeen, Panayiota Kendeou, Doug Lombardi et al. 2020. *The Debunking Handbook 2020*. Databrary. https://doi.org/10.17910/B7.1182.

Lua, Alfred. 2019. "21 Top Social Media Sites to Consider for Your Brand." *Buffer Library*, January 24, 2019. https://buffer.com/library/social-media-sites/.

Murthy, Vivek H. 2021. "Confronting Health Misinformation: The U.S. Surgeon General's Advisory on Building a Healthy Information Environment." US Department of Health & Human Services. Accessed February 8, 2022. https://www.hhs.gov/sites/default/files/surgeon-general-misinformation-advisory.pdf.

Pan American Health Organization. 2020. "Understanding the Infodemic and Misinformation in the Fight Against COVID-19." Accessed February 8, 2022. https://www.paho.org/en/documents/understanding-infodemic-and-misinformation-fight-against-covid-19.

Pendergrast, Tricia R., Shikha Jain, N. Seth Trueger, Michael Gottlieb, Nicole C. Woitowich, and Vineet M. Arora. 2021. "Prevalence of Personal Attacks and Sexual Harassment of Physicians on Social Media." *JAMA Internal Medicine* 181 (4): 550. https://doi.org/10.1001/jamainternmed.2020.7235.

Reinhart, R. J. 2020. "Nurses Continue to Rate Highest in Honesty, Ethics." *Gallup*, January 6, 2020. https://news.gallup.com/poll/274673/nurses-continue-rate-highest-honesty-ethics.aspx.

Romo, Vanessa. 2021. "Poison Control Centers Are Fielding a Surge of Ivermectin Overdose Calls." NPR, September 4, 2021. https://www.npr.org/sections/coronavirus-live-updates/2021/09/04/1034217306/ivermectin-overdose-exposure-cases-poison-control-centers.

Rothkopf, David J. 2003. "When the Buzz Bites Back." *Washington Post*, May 11, 2003. https://www.washingtonpost.com/archive/opinions/2003/05/11/when-the-buzz-bites-back/bc8cd84f-cab6-4648-bf58-0277261af6cd/.

Rotolo, Shannon M., Shikha Jain, Serena Dhaon, Jack K. Dokhanchi, Elzbieta Kalata, Tejal Shah, Lisa J. Mordell et al. 2021. "A Coordinated Strategy to Develop and Distribute Infographics Addressing COVID-19 Vaccine Hesitancy and Misinformation." *Journal of the American Pharmacists Association*. 62(1):224-231. doi: 10.1016/j.japh.2021.08.016.

Saad, Lydia. 2020. "U.S. Ethics Ratings Rise for Medical Workers and Teachers." Gallup.com, December 22, 2020. https://news.gallup.com/poll/328136/ethics-ratings-rise-medical-workers-teachers.aspx.

Sayce, David. 2019. "The Number of Tweets per Day in 2020." David Sayce, December 3, 2019. https://www.dsayce.com/social-media/tweets-day/.

Sehl, Katie. 2020. "Everything Brands Need to Know About TikTok in 2020." *Social Media Marketing & Management Dashboard*, March 2, 2020. https://blog.hootsuite.com/what-is-tiktok/.

Solnick, Rachel E., Grace Chao, Ryan D. Ross, Gordon T. Kraft-Todd, and Keith E. Kocher. 2021. "Emergency Physicians and Personal Narratives Improve the Perceived Effectiveness of COVID-19 Public Health Recommendations on Social Media: A Randomized Experiment." *Academic Emergency Medicine: Official Journal of the Society for Academic Emergency Medicine* 28 (2): 172–83. https://doi.org/10.1111/acem.14188.

Statista. 2021. "Most Used Social Media 2021." Accessed February 8, 2022. https://www.statista.com/statistics/272014/global-social-networks-ranked-by-number-of-users/.

Staude-Müller, Frithjof, Britta Hansen, and Melanie Voss. 2012. "How Stressful Is Online Victimization? Effects of Victim's Personality and Properties of the Incident." *European Journal of Developmental Psychology* 9 (2): 260–74. https://doi.org/10.1080/17405629.2011.643170.

Thayer, Kate. 2020. "Chicago Doctors—Mostly Moms—Join Together to Advise Officials and the Public. 'We Can't Not Say Something.'" *Chicago Tribune*, May 7, 2020. https://www.chicagotribune.com/coronavirus/ct-life-coronavirus-mom-doctors-impact-group-tt-20200507-vyvtdwkpyzbytp2udja7ikpxyq-story.html.

Tsao, Shu-Feng, Helen Chen, Therese Tisseverasinghe, Yang Yang, Lianghua Li, and Zahid A. Butt. 2021. "What Social Media Told Us in the Time of COVID-19: A Scoping Review." *The Lancet Digital Health* 3 (3): e175–94. https://doi.org/10.1016/S2589-7500(20)30315-0.

Vosoughi, Soroush, Deb Roy, and Sinan Aral. 2018. "The Spread of True and False News Online." *Science* 359 (6380): 1146–51. https://doi.org/10.1126/science.aap9559.

Walker, Garth. 2020. "How Your Participation in the Census Could Lead to Greater Health Care Equity in Chicago." *Chicago Sun-Times*, October 1, 2020. https://chicago.suntimes.com/2020/10/1/21497236/chicago-healthcare-inequity-u-s-census-south-side-dr-garth-walker.

Wallia, Amisha, Ali Khan, Laura Zimmerman, Amish Desai, Julie Blankemeier, Eve Bloomgarden, Lisa Mordell, Alex Kenefake, Shikha Jain, and Vineet Arora. 2021. "Creation and Translation of IMPACT (Illinois Medical Professional Action Collaborative Team) to Amplify and Address Disparities in COVID-19: The Case of Vaccine Delivery." *Health Services Research* 56 (S2): 33–33. https://doi.org/10.1111/1475-6773.13764.

Wang, Yuxi, Martin McKee, Aleksandra Torbica, and David Stuckler. 2019. "Systematic Literature Review on the Spread of Health-Related Misinformation on Social Media." *Social Science & Medicine* 240 (November): 112552. https://doi.org/10.1016/j.socscimed.2019.112552.

Way, Katie. 2020. "Nurses Across the U.S. Are Getting Fired for Fighting PPE Shortages." *Vice*, April 21, 2020. https://www.vice.com/en/article/akwxze/nurses-across-united-states-fired-for-fighting-covid-19-ppe-shortages.

Wu, Katherine J. 2021. "Could a Smell Test Screen People for COVID-19?" *The New York Times*, January 19, 2021. https://www.nytimes.com/2021/01/19/health/smell-test-for-covid.html.

Zimmermann, Laura, Vineet Arora, Eve Bloomgarden, and Shikha Jain. 2020. "Letters: Is It Possible to Get Kids to Wear Masks in Schools? Yes, and It's Necessary." *Chicago Tribune*, July 20, 2020. https://www.chicagotribune.com/opinion/letters/ct-letters-vp-072120-20200720-rb2el7anenda3jgrgwoz4kxpry-story.html.

13

Participation, Empowerment, and Equity

Addressing eHealth Misinformation with Community Engagement in Libraries

Amanda J. Wilson and Laura Bartlett

Disclaimer: The opinions expressed by the authors are their own and this material should not be interpreted as representing the official viewpoint of the US Department of Health and Human Services, the National Institutes of Health, or the National Library of Medicine.

COMMUNITY ENGAGEMENT—"working collaboratively with and through groups of people . . . to address issues affecting [their] wellbeing" (Agency for Toxic Substances and Disease Registry 2011, 9)—is a powerful, localized, sustainable, and equitable practice from which libraries can build a suite of responses and programs for ehealth misinformation immunity. Eysenbach (2001) defines ehealth as "health services and information delivered or enhanced through the internet and related technologies" (para. 3), to which Eng (2001) adds that the outcome is enabled or improved health and health care. Communities and groups amplify ehealth information, misinformation, and disinformation through social media and other online platforms. Regardless of motivations, the prevalence of misinformation and disinformation erodes trust, increases the effort required to verify information, and reinforces barriers between groups online that translate into everyday behaviors offline (Lewandowsky 2012; Swire-Thompson and Lazer 2020). These impacts are social, in that they affect interpersonal relationships. Community engagement approaches provide specific, tailored solutions for these types of social impacts that complement the skills and tools libraries already used in equipping the public to accurately assess information and cope with information overload.

The problem of misinformation and disinformation in health is not new (Parmet and Rothstein 2018; Szymanski 1982). As with many aspects of public health and society overall, the COVID-19 pandemic is a singular, unique event that both exposed inequalities and provided new opportunities for innovation, collaboration, and engagement on a global scale (Callaway 2021; Mohammed et al. 2021; Peet 2021; Rathore and Farooq 2020; Walker 2021; Zarocostas 2020). In the context of library and information science, the World Health Organization (WHO) positioned the promise and challenges of information, misinformation, and information overload as pivotal with the establishment of the WHO Information Network for Epidemics that "seeks to give everyone access to timely, accurate, and easy-to-understand advice and information from trusted sources on public health events and outbreaks" after the COVID-19 disease outbreak (World Health Organization 2021, para. 1).

Two important factors are at the core of the WHO strategy to counter mis/disinformation. The first is managing information and promoting information access. While this is the core of the library and information science (LIS) professions, with libraries on the front lines helping the public manage information overload, a scoping review of health information overload for the public found only twenty-two articles from 2001 through 2018 that focused primarily on information overload in the health context (Khaleel et al. 2020). The second factor at the core of the WHO infodemic strategy is community voices—centering them to understand needs and challenges, inform actions, and identify influencers, as well as craft effective messages and dissemination mechanisms. Overall, infodemic management for the current crisis and similar future scenarios requires health information skill building (National Academies of Sciences, Engineering, and Medicine 2020), tailored messages from trusted managers (Chou et al. 2020; National Institutes of Health 2020), and responses at the same scale and frequency that misinformation spreads (Starbird 2019).

What does this mean for library-led community engagement to address misinformation? Focusing specifically on libraries that work with the general public, library workers have a long history and are experts at addressing factors identified by Klerings, Weinhandl, and Thaler (2015) as contributing to "filter failure" for information overload situations: inefficient systems to access information, the sheer volume and diversity of information, and low health literacy (286). Since library workers can serve as an access point to ehealth information, libraries are also uniquely situated to refute misinformation through information services and patron training. Through training, library workers can prepare to build resilience to misinformation, for example, by providing credible information or best scientific evidence available. For health information, the Medical Library Association (MLA) offers a Consumer Health Information Specialization to equip library workers with the skills to provide competent consumer health services, as well as an understanding of health literacy, ethical, legal, and social issues (ELSI), and other areas (Medical Library Association 2022). Library workers can enhance their skills in providing consumer health information, using specific examples of sources of mis/disinformation as an example for which ehealth information evaluation can be used. In the 2000s, the Bill and Melinda Gates Foundation (Becker et al. 2011), the National Library of Medicine (NLM), and other organizations funded computer labs and internet access in libraries across the United States to increase access to technology and online information for communities. With those tools came the need for libraries to teach computer and internet skills to the community, and those needs still exist. A 2016 Pew study revealed that 80 percent of respondents "definitely" wanted libraries to offer programs to teach patrons "how to use digital tools such as computers, smart phones, and apps" (Horrigan 2016, para. 2). As part of the social infrastructure of civic life (Hughes and LaPierre 2021; Klinenberg 2018), libraries that serve the general public are also effective community partners (Humphreys et al. 1999; Whitney et al. 2017). Library capacities and activities are already addressing many aspects of the WHO framework for infodemic management.

While libraries are already contributing to many aspects of the WHO infodemic management call to action, other opportunities exist for library-led community engagement. Specifically, those additional opportunities deepen the character of library community engagement efforts and expand their focus to more fully capture the spirit of the current infodemic management strategy and respond to any future ehealth misinformation challenges. Increasingly, public health professionals are looking to (and partnering with) libraries to address public health in local communities (National Institutes of Health 2017; Philbin et al. 2019; Whiteman et al. 2018). In work tracing the role of civic engagement through libraries, Kranich (2021) argues that community engagement in this era, particularly listening to communities, "necessitates the adoption of new competencies as well as a shift from a mission that informs citizens to one that also *engages* them" (12). This shift has already begun: the American Library Association's (ALA) Libraries Transforming Communities initiative and the Institute of Museum and Library Services (IMLS) Community Catalyst Initiative are increasing the capacity of library workers to listen for opportunities to better serve their community, facilitate community conversations, create shared visions and plans with community partners, and leverage user-centered design for tools and solutions. These are the exact skills and outcomes the WHO espoused for managing the COVID-19 infodemic and preventing the spread of misinformation.

Critical health literacy (CHL) provides a framework for engaging communities more equitably, inclusively, and collaboratively in order to build ehealth misinformation resilience over the long term. This is accomplished by building on functional (or basic) and interactive (or communication) literacies. CHL, which is "a process in which [community members] become aware of issues, participate in critical dialogue, and become involved in decision making for health" (Sykes et al. 2013, 2), puts communities at the center of the process, from needs assessment to conceptualizing solutions to implementation. To be most effective, CHL approaches used by libraries must engender and strengthen trust, by taking into account how inequalities are experienced by different groups and how their experiences affect trust or mistrust in ehealth misinformation (Jaiswal et al. 2020). Building this resilience is complex and multifaceted, as ehealth literacy involves traditional, health, scientific, media, digital, and information literacies (Norman and Skinner 2006). Using community-informed approaches through the lenses of inclusion and equity can provide libraries with the tools to work meaningfully with communities in active response to mis/disinformation and its resulting impact on health outcomes (Swire-Thompson and Lazer 2020; World Health Organization 2020b).

The remainder of this chapter will provide an overview of CHL, map how managing ehealth misinformation strategies can be addressed using CHL as a framework, discuss community-based participatory research (CBPR) as a source of evidence-based approaches for library-led community engagement, and conclude with recommended practical strategies for immediate implementation. This chapter draws primarily on public health literature, resources, and practices to inform many of the recommendations and strategies presented because both libraries and public health offer CHL and CBPR-informed work to their patron populations and communities and because partnerships between libraries and public health departments are increasing (DeGuzman et al. 2021).

Using CHL to Tackle eHealth Misinformation

Critical analysis of information, understanding of social determinants of health, and engagement in collective action are the three constituent domains of CHL, comprising the concepts of health knowledge, information skills, effective interaction, informed decision-making, and empowerment (Chinn 2011; Nutbeam 2000, 2008; Sykes et al. 2013). Dependencies for CHL include basic or functional health literacy and interactive or communications health literacy (Chinn 2011; Nutbeam 2000; Sykes et al. 2013). Functional health literacy focuses on basic understanding and personal health. Interactive health literacy builds on this foundation, with the focus at this level on the ability to communicate understandings about health information provided to and heard from others. Nutbeam et al. (2018) asserts that this

> categorisation also helps to distinguish between interventions that are task-based—designed to develop specific skills to manage prescribed activities (medication adherence, behaviour change), and interventions that are skills based—designed to develop generic, transferable skills that equip people to make a range of more autonomous decisions relating to their health, and to adapt to changing circumstances. (902)

From the foundation of functional and interactive health literacies, CHL can be achieved. When applied fully, the outcome of CHL is power-building that leads to community action(s) and, ultimately, advancing health equity at the population level.

A distinguishing factor of CHL from other literacies is the focus on building community empowerment for action, which makes equity and inclusion a primary focus. This is because CHL requires community participation at every stage of a project or initiative—from identifying needs to defining the problem to determining the next steps to driving (or pausing) the activity's timeline—which is the goal of the framework for individuals and communities: autonomy and greater control of health and health-related decisions (Nutbeam 2008). Enabling empowerment in communities through CHL also requires organizations to actively address structural equity, both internally and in working with communities.

A starting point for accomplishing CHL comes from the public health field of health promotion and focuses on three categories of activities: education, social mobilization, and advocacy. These categories map to the functional, interactive, and critical levels of health literacy. Nutbeam (2008) conceptualizes health literacy as an outcome of educational activities that both propels individual or collective social actions and also informs advocacy efforts to improve community health. In each of these areas, libraries are already offering programming and activities (e.g., ideas may be found on the WebJunction Health Happens in Libraries programming page). For example, an education activity in libraries could be a virtual misinformation Escape Room from the University of Washington; a community development activity could be engaging with the Keene Valley Library (Keene Valley, NY) OurStoryBridge project to create oral histories; and an activism activity could be libraries creating programs using the Human Library® model to challenge prejudice. Table 13.1 provides a more in-depth examination of how libraries and library workers can empower users through health literacy and better engagement with their community using Nutbeam's ten-step conceptual model of health literacy as a tool.

As libraries facilitate users' movement through Nutbeam's ten steps, the ability to use a wider range of empowerment, negotiation, and advocacy tools to influence others toward making health decisions also increases along with health literacy—this is CHL (National Academies of Sciences, Engineering, and Medicine 2021).

Depending on a library's context and mission, not all of these actions for CHL may be feasible. Moreover, the library's role as a place in communities may be an approach to meaningful support, but library workers might not actively engage in some higher-order CHL activities, or some may choose to remain neutral and not actively address community circumstances, social issues, and/or information phenomena such as misinformation. While the current debate on library neutrality and critical librarianship (Gibson et al. 2017; Critlib.org, n.d.) is ongoing, the imminent harm posed by ehealth misinformation and the COVID-19 pandemic may prompt libraries to take a more active stance in community engagement and ehealth literacy (i.e., educating for health and mobilizing collective energy, resource, and skills to improve and advocate for health [Nutbeam 2000]). Proposed strategies for managing the COVID-19 infodemic specifically and ehealth misinformation map to the CHL levels of literacy.

TABLE 13.1
Examples of the Potential Impact of Libraries on Users Aligned with Nutbeam's (2008) Conceptual Model of Health Literacy

Nutbeam's (2008) Steps to Critical Health Literacy	*Related Role(s) of Library Worker/Library*	*Potential Impact on Library Users*
1. Prior understanding of individual capacity—reading fluency, numeracy, existing knowledge	• Needs assessments—surveys, focus groups • Active use of community panels, user panels • Partnerships with health-supporting organizations—health departments, counseling centers, hospitals, individual health care providers, food banks, etc. • Community-level characteristics data such as from Census (caveat: individuals and communities are more than data and anecdotes. You can have a community with high literacy but low health literacy.) • Investigation and research into academic and nonacademic sources to discover what is "known" about your community segments—published papers, presentations at conferences, news reports, etc.	• By knowing users, libraries provide customized services, programming, and resources to meet their needs • Refer to the *Contexts* and *Partnership Process* domains of the CPBR Conceptual Model discussed later in this chapter for evidence-based approaches to establishing joint understanding and agreement between the library and their users and community on what they need
2. Tailored information, communication, education	• Using existing and established educational frameworks and tools in health literacy such as Shoemaker et al. (2013), CDC Clear Communication Index (2019), and child and adult education principles and practices • Use preferred communication methods of their community such as radio ads, social media challenges, gamification, and badges • Train library workers in the needed languages of their community including verbal, written/braille, and signed • Invite community co-leadership in the identification, design, testing, and implementation of new and redesigned services, programming, and resources	• Individual and community ownership of library services, programming, and resources • Agency of individuals and the community to participate in programming that is representative of their needs • Greatest benefit without wasted costs in library services, programming, and resources • Users recognize library "as a place" in their community

(*continued*)

TABLE 13.1 *Continued*

Nutbeam's (2008) Steps to Critical Health Literacy	*Related Role(s) of Library Worker/Library*	*Potential Impact on Library Users*
Steps 3–5 of Nutbeam's model are a result of the educational foundation. Each of these steps can happen independently, concurrently, or, in some cases, not applicable.		
3. Developed knowledge and capability	• Library workers have access to and use Continuing Education (CE) opportunities • Library workers use techniques for health comprehension such as the "Teach Back Method" when engaging with users • Libraries have at least one trained worker in health literacy and consumer health	• Users demonstrate knowledge and skills in health literacy and associated literacies such as digital health, data/numeracy, and research literacy • Users access resources and tools from the library to help with applying the literacies
4. Skills in social organization and advocacy	• Facilitating health-supporting organizations to be active and visible in libraries	• Users know how to access health support systems in their community
5. Skills in negotiation and self-management	• Libraries offer programing for users about advocating for their health and communicating with health care providers, and health support services and agencies	• Users help themselves, their social networks, and their community by being advocates for health • Users feel empowered and a critical part of their own health care management and treatment team
At this point Nutbeam states, "health literacy is the outcome of education and communication rather than a factor that may influence the outcome" (2075).		
6. Improved health literacy	• Library workers are trained, prepared, and confident in serving the health information needs of their communities • Libraries measure their knowledge and skills in health literacy • Libraries support the work of health-supporting organizations to advance community health needs and goals	• Users make informed decisions about their health such as understanding medication, treatment options, prevention, and maintenance of health • Users assess health information and identify misinformation
As a result of step 6, library users are better equipped to engage in a range of personal and community behaviors and practices. The authors would like to point out that even the actions that seem small (e.g., modeling a new healthy behavior) may have a large impact on the lives of the individuals and their community, e.g., that new behavior may ripple out through social networks.		
7. Changed health behaviors and practices	• Libraries recognize the importance of and improve library worker's health and well-being • Libraries remove physical and psychological hazards and barriers	• Users engage in library programming such as yoga classes • The community uses the library as a place for free blood pressure screenings • Users access library collections about health and wellness

Nutbeam's (2008) Steps to Critical Health Literacy	*Related Role(s) of Library Worker/Library*	*Potential Impact on Library Users*
8. Engagement in social action for health	• Libraries encourage and model community supporting health behaviors • Library workers demonstrate wellness practices such as taking a five-minute walk once an hour and encouraging healthy snack options for events	• Individuals and communities are active participants in civic engagement such as participating in health needs assessment, research studies, and decision-making of community health resource allocation. (the authors believe that when individuals are empowered to make a change, that is when change occurs in communities)
9. Participation in changing social norms and practices	• Libraries make space for and invite wellness and health by offering space to health-supporting organizations	• Users recognize opportunities for participation for themselves, for those in their social network, and for their community to engage in health improvement and maintenance practices such as screening, disease prevention, and modeling change behavior
In conclusion, the individual and community achieve CHL.		
10. Improved health outcomes, healthy choices, and opportunities	• Library workers and the library are key participants in advancing the health equity of their users and community through information	• Individual and community barriers to improved health outcomes and opportunities are removed • Health needs of the library community are realized • Individuals and the community move from health disparities to health equities

Managing Misinformation with the CHL Model

Strategies for addressing misinformation span all levels of the CHL model: the basic/functional health literacy level, the interactive/communication health literacy level, and the critical health literacy level. At the functional level of health literacy, ehealth misinformation management strategies include programming that strengthens capabilities that enable the public to know how to report misinformation on social networking sites, evaluating information sources, and double-checking facts (World Health Organization 2020a). At the interactive level, ehealth misinformation management strategies must actively address uncertainty, ideology, information source, messenger, trust, and predispositions to believe misinformation, as communication is at the core of this level. Successes and advancements at this interactive level of literacy enable CHL actions, such as collaborating with health care providers, engaging in counter-messaging campaigns with tailored messages for different communities/groups, nudging for behavior change, and engaging and collaborating with organizations trusted by underrepresented groups.

Trust and equity are imperative for both CHL and successful ehealth misinformation resilience. Libraries generally enjoy the benefits of the former with their communities and are positioned to significantly impact the latter for ehealth misinformation. Even with these, Sykes et al. (2013) admonish that to fully succeed, CHL "depends on the motivation and development of skills within the individual or community but also requires collaborative efforts at a structural level" (9). Libraries have and continue to do this, too. Libraries are places in the community that are trusted to provide space, resources, and expertise in information (Horrigan 2016; Klinenberg 2018). With materials and services created to satisfy the interests of persons across the lifespan, libraries enjoy a reputation that is often formed during childhood and continues through adulthood. A study by Pew Research Center (Geiger 2020) showed

> [a]bout eight-in-ten adults (78%) feel that public libraries help them find information that is trustworthy and reliable and 76% say libraries help them learn new things. Also, 56% believe libraries help them get information that aids with decisions they have to make. (para. 3)

Through this privileged status, libraries can effectively support their communities' battle with misinformation using CHL.

As ehealth misinformation continues to be "diffused significantly farther, faster, deeper, and more broadly" (Swire-Thompson and Lazer 2020, 437) than accurate information, libraries must maintain a bifurcated approach to also include people impacted by the digital divide and library nonusers in communities (Chou et al. 2020; DeGuzman et al. 2021; Wang et al. 2019). For example, Campos-Castillo and Laestadius (2020) discuss equity challenges through access; not all populations use social media equally. Strategies that leverage social networking and technology may not equally address or provide insight to all populations. For those already impacted by the digital divide, the absence of having access when information is critical can have grave health consequences. Like food stamps and subsidized housing benefits, libraries serve as a social safety net for access to the internet and computers (Klinenberg 2018). No access or limited access to online sources of information prevents individuals from having the tools needed to verify or challenge misinformation.

Community-Based and Community-Informed Approaches

As discussed previously, libraries are already involved in community engagement through specific outreach programs, community advisory panels, and participation in community and civic events. The degree to which libraries participate and develop programming with their community will differ. These differences—in available resources, knowledge, and trust with specific community populations or the library's prerogative in program and service design—impact their community engagement. This section introduces community-based participatory engagement and how it can be used to create programming that is inclusive of the community's needs.

Community-based participatory engagement borrows practice from community-based participatory research, which is a proven process for shared vision and responsibility in achieving community research. CBPR involves the community in all aspects of research—not just certain parts that are of convenience to the researcher or the community. CBPR aims to involve all partners to create the greatest outcome that each partner values and can use. The CBPR Conceptual Model developed by Wallerstein and Duran (2010) has evolved over the years, being influenced by what is taught and practiced in community engagement through public health and social sciences. NLM has been using CBPR-informed and CBPR-inspired practice for decades (Wallingford et al. 1996; Dutcher et al. 2007; Wood et al. 2005) as "outreach," which the Library's Office of Engagement and Training is now calling community-based participatory engagement. NLM's work in this area includes cocreating health information resources and elevating voices from communities to improve programs and resources. NLM has also provided technical assistance and funding awards to communities that are experiencing health inequities, underserved, or underrepresented. The awards are intended to help mitigate mis/disinformation issues and respond to information needs within communities.

The CBPR Conceptual Model developed by Wallerstein and Duran (2010) has four domains:

1. *Contexts*: This is preplanning work that typically precedes the development of research questions. This work can be done by the library before they engage with the community. Please refer to the CBPR Conceptual Model (https://engageforequity.org) to view videos and read examples of this important part of the process.
2. *Partnership Processes*: This domain is informed by the *Contexts* domain and examines how the partners interact with each other, including the power dynamics between them, and how communications and work are established. It is categorized into three areas:
   - Individual characters—the characteristics of individuals, their personalities, their cultural humilities, and other factors that relate to their ability to work with others.
   - Partnership structures—the values, goals, funding levels, and policies of each partner.
   - Relationships—how partners work together, develop trust, handle conflict, and so on.
3. *Intervention and Research:* This domain comprises the scientific processes and outputs that are influenced by *Contexts* and *Partnership Processes* to determine how research is carried out. This domain is not dominated by the researcher or by the research methods chosen by the researcher; this domain is a cocreation of the community and the researcher. The community may suggest research methods for which there is no "evidence-base," such as techniques or approaches that do not follow traditional Western-based science methods. Instead, the community may suggest methods that are informed by their values, beliefs, experiences, and community knowledge.
4. *Outcomes*: This domain not only covers the outcome of the research question/goal but also what the partners learn about how and with whom they want to partner with in the future, the sustainability of the intervention, and the community's ability to own and lead research in the future.

The Engage for Equity website (https://engageforequity.org/) on the CBPR Conceptual Model can be used by community-based organizations, such as libraries, to learn the CBPR process and utilize tools that can be used to envision community-based participatory engagement.

Libraries can work through the first two domains of the CBPR Conceptual Model to better understand their strengths and weaknesses in approaches to community-based engagement. It is not recommended that those libraries using the CBPR Conceptual Model move through the domains to envision a community-based engagement without the involvement of their community partners. Rather, libraries on their own can work through the first two domains, *Contexts* and *Partnership Processes*, to understand where the library is situated and interacts in community partnerships. After this work, libraries can then assess their role as a partner in the community and be better prepared to participate in CBPR-informed methods when engaging with their community.

In thinking about library programming and services to mitigate and respond to ehealth misinformation, the authors ask that you consider these questions in table 13.2, or develop your own, in the first domain of the CBPR Conceptual Model, *Contexts*.

TABLE 13.2
CBPR-Informed Questions that Libraries Can Ask that Align with Misinformation Categories Adapted from Wang et al.'s (2019) Systematic Review

Misinformation Category (adapted from Wang et al. 2019)	*Question*	*CBPR Contexts Domain*
Uncertainty in scientific process	What are your community members' experiences with health research and health care?	• How does health care access impact the feelings toward scientific processes? • Does your community have equal access to the highest level of health care? • Does the library understand the complexity of health care access in your community? • What can be the library's role in raising the health equity in the community?
Ideology	Does the library support intellectual freedom?	• What are the common ideologies that exist within the community? • Does the library support intellectual freedom of all viewpoints or behaviors that do not violate library policy?
Information sources	Does your community have the skills to evaluate health information online?	• What are the specific factors and barriers that limits the community's skills and how can the library address those gaps (such as access to internet)? • What has the library provided to communities to improve their evaluation and assessment skills? How were those services/programs conceived and evaluated? • What evidence-based health resources do library workers use within the library in assisting patrons?
Messenger and trust	Does your community have trusted health information and health care sources?	• Who are the trusted messengers for specific populations within your community? • Does the library invite and provide space for trusted messengers? • How does the library amplify trusted messengers through library information services, programming, and online?
Predisposition to believe misinformation	Does your library support critical thinking skills?	• What are the sources of misinformation in your community? • Does the library support members of the community with quick, condensed information sources, programs, and services? • How does the library teach or train the community to evaluate health information, in different modalities, and meeting different user needs?

TABLE 13.3
Libraries and Library Worker CBPR-Informed Self-Assessment Questions for Addressing Health Misinformation

CBPR Partnership Processes
Individual Characteristics
• Are library workers trained in health literacy, plain language, and interacting with lower health literacy patrons?
• Are library workers trained in "prescribing" evidence-based health information and not "diagnosing" health concerns?
• Are library workers trained and prepared to interact with patrons that may have different ideologies than their own?
• Are library workers able to interact objectively with patron questions about sources that may contain misinformation?
Partnership Structures
• What policies, procedures, and processes has the library developed to work with communities?
• How is funding for programs/services obtained?
• How does the library identify which populations within their community with whom to work?
• What are the shared goals between the library and the community?
• Do the library workers, volunteers, and advisory groups have members from all specific populations within the community?
Relationships
• What are the current partnerships the library has?
• How are partnerships started, maintained, and retired?
• What are the power dynamics in each partnership?

In thinking about library programming and services to mitigate and respond to health misinformation, consider these questions in the second domain of the CBPR Conceptual Model, *Partnership Processes* in table 13.3.

The CBPR Conceptual Model is approachable and easy to use for libraries and communities to adopt or strengthen a process for community-based participatory engagement. The evidence-informed processes and methods of community-driven research adapt well to planning, performing, and evaluating library-led engagement, and to the development of library programs and activities that are community-focused and community-driven.

How Libraries Are Positioned to Respond to Crises through Community Engagement

Considering our current health infodemic, libraries have successfully responded to support the work of public health departments and other response agencies to provide needed services to communities, which demonstrates—again—their crisis response capabilities. Libraries work with public health departments and other health organizations to respond in times of national crisis, emergencies, and disasters. During natural disasters, libraries have served as hubs for computer and internet access so patrons could sign up for disaster relief services and connect with the outside world (Bishop and Veil 2013). In response to Hurricane Katrina and Hurricane Sandy, libraries became lifelines to communities impacted by the storms. The MLA in conjunction with NLM support the training and competencies of library workers to become Disaster Information Specialists to "access, use, and manage information to support their institutions and communities in planning for, responding to, and recovering from disasters and emergencies" (Medical Library Association 2022). The Library Reserve Corps was formed in March 2020 to provide critical librarian skills to the WHO Global COVID-19 database to meet the need of timely and accurate information during the global pandemic (Library Reserve Corps 2022). In COVID-19, community leaders and governments have turned to libraries to distribute COVID-19 information and to open their virtual and physical doors to their impacted communities.

Partnerships with public health departments and health-serving organizations extend to libraries being a place for interactions between those agencies and communities that use libraries. Libraries are community hubs where nurses (Nursing News Highlights 2016), social workers (Lambert 2020), and health professionals along with library workers have partnered effectively in service of vulnerable, culturally diverse, and hard-to-reach communities. In times of crisis, libraries remain a trusted resource in the community. For example, following the 2014 Ferguson, Missouri, civil unrest, the Ferguson Municipal Public Library remained opened even when schools were closed (NBC News 2015). Other areas in which libraries align with public health goals include libraries providing access to health information through nutritional programs and exercise classes, access to language services, and safe spaces for community discussions (Philbin et al. 2019).

Libraries are also called on to bridge national initiatives to their local communities. During the 2013 roll-out of the Affordable Care Act (ACA) Health Insurance Marketplace, libraries were recognized as the place where many Americans use computers to access ehealth information and rely on librarians to assist in seeking information about health and health care (American Library Association 2013). Two federal government agencies, the Centers for Medicare and Medicaid Services (CMS) and the IMLS, provided funding and support to ensure libraries were prepared to assist patrons with their questions about the Health Insurance Marketplace. In 2021, libraries continue to provide support for patrons' enrollment (American Library Association 2021). Libraries have hosted and promoted virtual events with their communities in support of the National Institutes of Health (NIH) Community Engagement Alliance (CEAL) against COVID-19 Health Disparities. The initiative aims to address COVID-19 misinformation by using trusted partners as messengers to the communities they represent. The Network of the National Library of Medicine (NNLM) served as a cohost of two events with the Texas CEAL consortium in January 2021: "United to Debunk Misinformation in Our Communities: A Town Hall on COVID-19" and "Addressing Attitudes and Science Mistrust during the COVID-19 Pandemic." Many other libraries have partnered with trusted community research and health care providers to amplify their messages and to counteract misinformation.

Call to Action: Responding to eHealth Misinformation through Community Engagement

As trusted institutions within communities, libraries and library workers have the skills and resources to be responders in misinformation situations. Below are actions libraries can take.

Create a Health Equity Statement to Inform Your Health Information Policies

Create, implement, and evaluate the highest level of commitment to the health of your community by creating a health equity statement to inform your library's policies, values, and all partnerships, programs, and services. The health equity statement relates to the *Partnership*

Processes domain of the CBPR Conceptual Model, including the Individual Characteristics area and Partnership Structures area. The CBPR Conceptual Model can be used to create the statement collaboratively with your community.

Learn about CBPR Approaches and Models for Application in Your Library

LIS is interdisciplinary, and CBPR has methods that can be added to your skills toolbox. A considerable benefit of using the CBPR Conceptual Model and approaches is that it is well-defined, widely accepted, evidence-based, and evidence-informed. As discussed earlier, CBPR models and methods lend well to create a community-based participatory engagement plan for your community.

Learn about Health Literacy Approaches to Enhance Skills Working with Library Patrons

This chapter provides several examples of health literacy training programs from the NNLM, the MLA, and the ALA. Below are additional resources to learn about health literacy approaches, applications, and evaluation:

- Agency for Healthcare Research and Quality
  https://www.ahrq.gov/health-literacy/index.html
- Centers for Disease Control and Prevention
  https://www.cdc.gov/healthliteracy/index.html
- Boston University and CommunicateHealth: Health Literacy Toolshed
  https://healthliteracy.bu.edu/
- Rural Health Information Hub
  https://www.ruralhealthinfo.org/topics/social-determinants-of-health
- Health Resources and Services Administration
  https://www.hrsa.gov/about/organization/bureaus/ohe/health-literacy/index.html
- National Academies of Sciences, Engineering, and Medicine
  - National Academies of Sciences, Engineering, and Medicine Press: Press publication on health literacy
    https://www.nap.edu/topic/476/health-and-medicine/health-literacy
  - Roundtable on Health Literacy
    https://www.nationalacademies.org/our-work/roundtable-on-health-literacy

Go Local on the Internet

Locate where your community is on the internet to find "their corner of the internet":

- Ensure your library is an information provider listed on the websites and social media accounts of your health department, community centers and civic organizations, and educational institutions.
- Monitor community conversations through social media listening. This is a method often used for marketing purposes but is being adopted by public health and health care services to understand trends, sentiment, and map conversations to locations (Fung et al. 2015; Clemson University n.d.).

The Internet Is Your Community

Allow library workers to be a "virtual bookmobile"—going to spaces and places where misinformation happens to provide information remediation.

- Participate in or host a Wikipedia edit-a-thon to improve the quality of health information in Wikipedia articles (Network of the National Library of Medicine 2022; WebJunction, n.d.).
- Engage in community discussions, such as Reddit's "Ask Me Anything" (AMA), to provide links to evidence-based health and wellness resources. This popular Reddit discussion event allows users to ask experts any question within individual subreddits (Lai et al. 2020; Hara et al. 2019; Record et al. 2018).

Use Dual Formats of Programming to Translate In-Person Activities for Online Participation

To adapt to COVID-19, public libraries moved many in-person services online to accommodate their patrons when libraries were closed out of necessity. In "Public Libraries Respond to COVID-19" (2020), the Public Library Association captured how libraries were impacted by COVID-19: 61 percent of libraries planned to add virtual programming and 38 percent to expand phone reference services. When planning your programming and services, consider offering online options to accommodate many users who may have limited physical access to libraries. Also consider online programming that occurs through social media and new media channels to attract a broader audience.

Bring Health Care Providers, Health Professionals, and Researchers to Libraries to Speak Directly to Communities

Marc Morial (2021), president and CEO of the National Urban League, in a webinar about COVID-19 and vaccines information for Black Americans was asked the question "What do you see as the role of community-based organizations in the dissemination process?" Morial responded, "We can amplify messages from the right messengers. The right messengers are . . . African American physicians, doctors, and scientists. We've got to help people make the right decision with the right information."

Take Information Services Out into the Community

Dr Lisa Fitzpatrick, MD, MPH, MPA, is the trusted messenger for *Dr. Lisa on the Street* (Grapevine Health 2020), which is an outreach and engagement program that goes to the streets to video-interview community members about medical issues, get their responses, then provide accurate information about that medical issue to increase health literacy and equity. As has been discussed in this chapter, libraries and public health organizations have partnered to serve their communities both in and outside of the physical library. *Dr. Lisa on the Street* shows the public health interest in using popular digital formats for ehealth engagement. Libraries can expand their community-based participatory engagement using similar methods to expand services outside of the library and into the physical and digital communities.

Design Programs for Inclusion of All Members of Your Community; Do Not Limit to One Format

Due to COVID-19, libraries shifted their programming to virtual as an emergency means to keep offering services to their patrons. The NNLM's *All of Us* partnership library events, which seek to increase health literacy and knowledge of precision medicine and research (Network of the National Library of Medicine 2022), found that using this approach allowed a greater reach to patrons who could not come into libraries for in-person programming and expanded their partnership to provide opportunities with national minority health organizations.

Get Funding and Get Piloting!

Traditional library funding sources:

- Network of the National Library of Medicine, https://nnlm.gov/
- Institute for Museums and Libraries, https://imls.gov/
- American Library Association, http://www.ala.org/awardsgrants/

Pursue Nontraditional Funding Course through Partnering and Coalition-Building

This is part of the *Contexts* domain of the CBPR Conceptual Model. Libraries are not always eligible to apply for funding from government institutions and private foundations, but through partnerships in their communities, libraries can be collaborators in solving community issues. Sources of funding that have a focus on health communities and improving health equity, literacy, and communities include:

- Robert Wood Johnson Foundation, https://www.rwjf.org/en/how-we-work/grants-explorer/funding-opportunities.html
- Knight Foundation, https://knightfoundation.org
- Harwood Institute, https://theharwoodinstitute.org
- Centers for Disease Control and Prevention, https://www.cdc.gov/grants/index.html
- US Department of Health and Human Services Office of Minority Health, https://www.minorityhealth.hhs.gov/omh/
- Health Resources and Services Administration, https://www.hrsa.gov/grants/index.html

As libraries continue to develop deeper relationships and partnerships through community-led and community-driven engagement, public health and community-based organizations will seek out the libraries as a trusted institution in times of need. Libraries' role using CHL and CBPR to address ehealth misinformation also presents the opportunity to fill gaps in ehealth misinformation research (Chou and Gaysynsky 2020) and in the evidence base for CHL (Nutbeam, McGill, and Premkumar 2017). Libraries can continue deepening trusted relationships with communities by providing culturally informed training, services, and programs.

Acknowledgment

This work was carried out by staff of the National Library of Medicine (NLM), National Institutes of Health, with support from NLM.

References

Agency for Toxic Substances and Disease Registry. 2011. *Principles of Community Engagement.* Centers for Disease Control and Prevention. https://www.atsdr.cdc.gov/communityengagement/.

American Library Association. 2013. "Libraries and the Affordable Care Act." *American Libraries Magazine*, July 12, 2013. https://americanlibrariesmagazine.org/blogs/the-scoop/libraries-and-the-affordable-care-act/.

American Library Association. 2021. "Libraries Connecting You to Coverage: Affordable Care Act." Public Libraries Association, June 4, 2021. http://www.ala.org/pla/initiatives/connectingyoutocoverage.

Becker, Samantha, Michael D. Crandall, Karen E. Fisher, Rebecca Blakewood, Bo Kinney, and Cadi Russell-Sauvé. 2011. *Opportunity for All: How Library Policies and Practices Impact Public Internet Access.* Institute of Museum and Library Services. https://www.imls.gov/sites/default/files/publications/documents/oppforall2_0.pdf.

Bishop, Bradley Wade, and Shari R. Veil. 2013. "Public Libraries as POST-CRISIS Information Hubs." *Public Library Quarterly* 32, no. 1: 33–45. https://doi.org/10.1080/01616846.2013.760390.

Callaway, Jessica. 2021. "The Librarian RESERVE Corps: An Emergency Response." *Medical Reference Services Quarterly* 40, no. 1: 90–102. https://doi.org/10.1080/02763869.2021.1873627.

Campos-Castillo, Celeste, and Linnea I. Laestadius. 2020. "Racial and Ethnic Digital Divides in Posting COVID-19 Content on Social Media among US Adults: Secondary Survey Analysis." *Journal of Medical Internet Research* 22, no. 7. https://doi.org/10.2196/20472. https://www.jmir.org/2020/7/e20472/.

Centers for Disease Control and Prevention. 2019. *The CDC Clear Communications Index.* Last modified June 5, 2021. https://www.cdc.gov/ccindex/index.html.

Chinn, Deborah. 2011. "Critical Health Literacy: A Review and Critical Analysis." *Social Science &a Medicine* 73, no. 1: 60–67. https://doi.org/10.1016/j.socscimed.2011.04.004.

Chou, Wen-Ying Sylvia, and Anna Gaysynsky. 2020. "Where We Go from Here: Health Misinformation on Social Media." *AJPH Perspectives* Supplement 3, 110, no. S3. https://doi.org/10.2105/AJPH.2020.305905.

Chou, Wen-Ying Sylvia, Caitlin E. Burgdorf, Anna Gaysynsky, and Christine M. Hunger. 2020. "COVID-19 Vaccination Communication: Applying Behavioral and Social Science to Address Vaccine Hesitancy and Foster Vaccine Confidence." National Institutes of Health. https://obssr.od.nih.gov/sites/obssr/files/inline-files/OBSSR_VaccineWhitePaper_FINAL_508.pdf.

Clemson University. n.d. "Social Media Listening Center." College of Behavioral, Social and Health Sciences. Accessed February 11, 2022. https://www.clemson.edu/cbshs/centers-institutes/smlc/.

Critlib.org. n.d. "Recommended Resources." Accessed February 11, 2022. http://critlib.org/recommended-readings/.

DeGuzman, Pamela B., Neha Jain, and Christine G. Loureiro. 2021. "Public Libraries as Partners in Telemedicine Delivery: A Review and Research Agenda." *Public Library Quarterly*: 1–12. https://doi.org/10.1080/01616846.2021.1877080.

Dutcher, Gale A., Melvin Spann, and Cynthia Gaines. 2007. "Addressing Health Disparities and Environmental Justice: The National Library of Medicine's Environmental Health Information Outreach Program." *Journal of the Medical Library Association* 95 (3): 330–36. https://doi.org/10.3163/1536-5050.95.3.330.

Eng, Thomas R. 2001. *The e-Health Landscape: A Terrain Map of Emerging Information and Communication Technologies in Health and Health Care.* Princeton, NJ: The Robert Wood Johnson Foundation.

Engage for Equity. n.d. "Engage for Equity." Accessed March 23, 2021. https://engageforequity.org/.

Eysenbach, G. 2001. "What Is e-Health?" *Journal of Medical Internet Research* 3, no. 2. https://doi.org/10.2196/jmir.3.2.e20. https://www.jmir.org/2001/2/e20.

Fung, Isaac Chin-Hai, Zion Tsz Tse, and King-Wa Fu. 2015. "The Use of Social Media in Public Health Surveillance." *Western Pacific Surveillance and Response Journal* 6, no. 2: 3–6. https://doi.org/10.5365/wpsar.2015.6.1.019.

Geiger, Abigail W. "Most Americans Say Libraries Can Help Them Find Reliable, Trustworthy Information." *Pew Research Center*, May 30, 2020. https://www.pewresearch.org/fact-tank/2017/08/30/most-americans-especially-millennials-say-libraries-can-help-them-find-reliable-trustworthy-information/.

Gibson, Amelia N., Renate L. Chancellor, Nicole A. Cooke, Sarah Park Dahlen, Shari A. Lee, and Yasmeen L. Shorish. 2017. "Libraries on the Frontlines: Neutrality and Social Justice." *Equality, Diversity and Inclusion: An International Journal* 36, no. 8: 751–66. https://doi.org/10.1108/edi-11-2016-0100.

Grapevine Health. 2020. "Dr. Lisa on the Street" playlist of videos. https://www.youtube.com/watch?app=desktop&v=ONIgfnT7eLo&list=PLsCsggYFJT0B4DQ4.

Hara, Noriko, Jessica Abbazio, and Kathryn Perkins. 2019. "An Emerging Form of Public Engagement with Science: Ask Me Anything (AMA) Sessions on Reddit r/Science." *PLoS ONE* 14, no. 5. https://doi.org/10.1371/journal.pone.0216789.

Horrigan, John B. 2016. "Libraries 2016." *Pew Research Center: Internet, Science & Tech*, September 9, 2016. https://www.pewresearch.org/internet/2016/09/09/libraries-2016/.

Hughes, Kathleen, and Susan LaPierre, hosts. 2021. "Misinformation." FYI: The Public Libraries Podcast (podcast), March 24, 2021. http://publiclibrariesonline.org/2021/03/new-podcast-misinformation-disinformation-and-more.

Humphreys, Betsy L., Angela B. Ruffin, Majorie A. Cahn, and Neil Rambo. 1999. "Powerful Connections for Public Health: The National Library of Medicine and the National Network of Libraries of Medicine." *American Journal of Public Health* 89, no. 11: 1633–36. https://doi.org/10.2105/ajph.89.11.1633.

Jaiswal, J., C. LoSchiavo, and D. C. Perlman. 2020. "Disinformation, Misinformation and Inequality-Driven Mistrust in the Time of COVID-19: Lessons Unlearned from AIDS Denialism." *AIDS Behavior* 24 (10): 2776–2780. doi:10.1007/s10461-020-02925-y.

Khaleel, Israa, Barbara C. Wimmer, Gregory M. Peterson, Syed Tabish Zaidi, Erin Roehrer, Elizabeth Cummings, and Kenneth Lee. 2020. "Health Information Overload among Health Consumers: A Scoping Review." *Patient Education and Counseling* 103, no. 1: 15–32. https://doi.org/10.1016/j.pec.2019.08.008.

Klerings, Irma, Alexandra S. Weinhandl, and Kylie J. Thaler. 2015. "Information Overload in Healthcare: Too Much of a Good Thing?" *Zeitschrift für Evidenz, Fortbildung und Qualität im Gesundheitswesen* 109, no. 4–5: 285–90. https://doi.org/10.1016/j.zefq.2015.06.005.

Klinenberg, Eric. 2018. *Palaces for the People: How Social Infrastructure Can Help Fight Inequality, Polarization, and the Decline of Civic Life.* New York: Broadway Books.

Kranich, Nancy C. 2021. "Democracy, Community, and Libraries." In *Ask, Listen, Empower: Grounding Your Library Work in Community Engagement*, edited by M. D. Fournier and S. Ostman, 1–16. Chicago: ALA Editions.

Lai, Deborah, Daniel Wang, Joshua Calvano, Ali S. Raja, and Shuhan He. 2020. "Addressing Immediate Public Coronavirus (COVID-19) Concerns through Social Media: Utilizing Reddit's AMA as a Framework for Public Engagement with Science." *PLoS ONE* 15, no. 10. https://doi.org/10.1371/journal.pone.0240326.

Lambert, Christiane, P. 2020. "Libraries and Social Workers—Perfect Partners." *Social Work Today* 20, no. 2. https://www.socialworktoday.com/archive/MA20p20.shtml.

Library Reserve Corps. 2022. "Library Reserve Corps." Accessed February 11, 2022. https://librarianreservecorps.libguides.com/home.

Medical Library Association. 2022. "Professional Development: Specializations." Accessed February 11, 2022. https://www.mlanet.org/p/cm/ld/fid=42.

Mohammed, Mustapha, Abubakar Sha'aban, Abubakar Ibrahim Jatau, Ismaeel Yunusa, Abubakar Musa Isa, Abubakar Sadiq Wada, Kehinde Obamiro, Hadzliana Zainal, and Baharudin Ibrahim. 2021. "Assessment of COVID-19 Information Overload among the General Public." *Journal of Racial and Ethnic Health Disparities* 9: 184–92. https://doi.org/10.1007/s40615-020-00942-0.

Morial, Marc. "Making It Plain: What Black America Needs to Know About COVID-19 and Vaccines," streamed January 7, 2021, YouTube, 1:41:54. https://www.youtube.com/watch?app=desktop&v=fv2qR6xniq4.

National Academies of Sciences, Engineering, and Medicine. 2020. *Addressing Health Misinformation with Health Literacy Strategies: Proceedings of a Workshop in Brief.* Washington, DC: The National Academies Press. https://doi.org/10.17226/26021.

National Academies of Sciences, Engineering, and Medicine. 2021. *Exploring the Role of Critical Health Literacy in Addressing the Social Determinants of Health: Proceedings of A Workshop—In Brief.* Washington, DC: The National Academies Press. https://doi.org/10.17226/26214.

National Institutes of Health. 2017. "NIH's *All of Us* Research Program Partners with the National Library of Medicine to Reach Communities through Local Libraries." US Department of Health and Human Services, November 29, 2017. https://allofus.nih.gov/news-events-and-media/announcements/nihs-all-us-research-program-partners-national-library-medicine.

National Institutes of Health. 2020. "NIH Funds Community Engagement Research Efforts in Areas Hardest Hit by COVID-19." US Department of Health and Human Services, September 18, 2020. https://www.nih.gov/news-events/news-releases/nih-funds-community-engagement-research-efforts-areas-hardest-hit-covid-19.

NBC News. "'In This Together': Ferguson Library Stays Open Amid Violence." NBCUniversal News Group, June 11, 2015. https://www.nbcnews.com/storyline/michael-brown-shooting/together-ferguson-library-stays-open-amid-violence-n256346.

Network of the National Library of Medicine. "Virtual Health Programming." Accessed February 11, 2022. https://allofus.nnlm.gov/vhp.

Network of the National Library of Medicine. "Wikipedia Edit-a-thon." Accessed February 11, 2022. https://nnlm.gov/guides/wikipedia-edit-a-thon.

Norman, Cameron D., and Harvey A. Skinner. 2006. "EHealth Literacy: Essential Skills for Consumer Health in a Networked World." *Journal of Medical Internet Research* 8, no. 2. https://doi.org/10.2196/jmir.8.2.e9. https://www.jmir.org/2006/2/e9/.

Nursing News Highlights. 2016. "Does Your Community Have a Library Nurse?" Accessed February 11, 2022. https://nursing.jnj.com/nurses-leading-innovation/does-your-community-have-a-library-nurse.

Nutbeam, Don. 2000. "Health Literacy as a Public Health Goal: A Challenge for Contemporary Health Education and Communication Strategies into the 21st Century." *Health Promotion International* 15, no. 3: 259–67. https://doi.org/10.1093/heapro/15.3.259.

Nutbeam, Don. 2008. "The Evolving Concept of Health Literacy." *Social Science & Medicine* 67, no. 12: 2072–78. https://doi.org/10.1016/j.socscimed.2008.09.050.

Nutbeam, Don, Bronwyn McGill, and Pav Premkumar. 2018. "Improving Health Literacy in Community Populations: A Review of Progress." *Health Promotion International* 33, no. 5: 901–11. https://doi.org/10.1093/heapro/dax015.

Parmet, Wendy E., and Mark A. Rothstein. 2018. "The 1918 Influenza Pandemic: Lessons Learned and Not-Introduction to the Special Section." *American Journal of Public Health* 108, no. 11: 1435–36. https://doi.org/10.2105/AJPH.2018.304695.

Peet, Lisa. 2021. "Battling the Infodemic: LJ's 2021 Librarians of the Year." *Library Journal*, January 5, 2021. https://www.libraryjournal.com/?detailStory=Battling-the-Infodemic-LJs-2021-Librarians-of-the-Year-covid-19.

Philbin, Morgan M., Caroline M. Parker, Mary Grace Flaherty, and Jennifer S. Hirsch. 2019. "Public Libraries: A Community-Level Resource to Advance Population Health." *Journal of Community Health* 44, no. 1: 192–99. https://doi.org/10.1007/s10900-018-0547-4.

Public Library Association. 2020. "Public Libraries Respond to COVID-19." Accessed March 23, 2021. https://www.ala.org/pla/sites/ala.org.pla/files/content/advocacy/covid-19/PLA-Libraries-Respond-Survey_Aggregate-Results_FINAL2.pdf.

Rathore, Farooq, and Fareeha Farooq. 2020. "Information Overload and Infodemic in the COVID-19 Pandemic." *Journal of Pakistan Medical Association Peer-reviewed Journal* 70 (Suppl 3), no. 5: S162–S165.

Record, Rachel A., Will R. Silberman, Joshua E. Santiago, and Taewook Ham. 2018. "I Sought It, I Reddit: Examining Health Information Engagement Behaviors among Reddit Users." *Journal of Health Communication* 23, no. 5: 470–76. https://doi.org/10.1080/10810730.2018.1465493.

Shoemaker, Sarah J., Michael S. Wolf, and Cindy Brach. 2013. *The Patient Education Materials Assessment Tool (PEMAT) and User's Guide*. Agency for Healthcare Research and Quality. https://www.ahrq.gov/health-literacy/patient-education/pemat.html.

Starbird, Kate. 2019. "Disinformation's Spread: Bots, Trolls and All of Us." *Nature* 571, no. 7766: 449–49. https://doi.org/10.1038/d41586-019-02235-x.

Swire-Thompson, Briony, and David Lazer. 2020. "Public Health and Online Misinformation: Challenges and Recommendations." *Annual Review of Public Health* 41, no. 1: 433–51. https://doi.org/10.1146/annurev-publhealth-040119-094127.

Sykes, Susie, Jane Wills, Gillian Rowlands, and Keith Popple. 2013. "Understanding Critical Health Literacy: A Concept Analysis." *BMC Public Health* 13, no. 1. https://doi.org/10.1186/1471-2458-13-150. https://bmcpublichealth.biomedcentral.com/articles/10.1186/1471-2458-13-150.

Szymanski, Albert. 1982. "On the Uses of Disinformation to Legitimize the Revival of the Cold War: Health in the U.S.S.R." *International Journal of Health Services* 12, no. 3: 481–96.

Walker, Philip. 2021. "The Library's Role in Countering Infodemics." *Journal of the Medical Library Association* 109, no. 1. https://doi.org/10.5195/jmla.2021.1044.

Wallerstein, Nina, and Bonnie Duran. 2010. "Community-Based Participatory Research Contribution to Intervention Research: The Intersection of Science and Practice to Improve Health Equity." *American Journal of Public Health* 100, no. S1. https://doi.org/10.2105/ajph.2009.184036. https://www.ncbi.nlm.nih.gov/pmc/articles/PMC2837458/.

Wallingford, K. T., A. B. Ruffin, K. A. Ginter, M. L. Spann, F. E. Johnson, G. A. Dutcher, R. Mehnert et al. 1996. "Outreach Activities of the National Library of Medicine: A Five-Year Review." *Journal of the Medical Library Association* 84 (2 Suppl): 1–60. https://www.ncbi.nlm.nih.gov/pmc/articles/PMC226815/.

Wang, Yuxi, Martin McKee, Aleksandra Torbica, and David Stuckler. 2019. "Systematic Literature Review on the Spread of Health-Related Misinformation on Social Media." *Social Science & Medicine* 240: 112552. https://doi.org/10.1016/j.socscimed.2019.112552.

WebJunction. n.d. "Wikipedia + Libraries: Better Together." Accessed March 23, 2021. https://www.webjunction.org/explore-topics/wikipedia-libraries.html.

Whiteman, Elizia D., Roxanne Dupuis, Anna U. Morgan, Bernadette D'Alonzo, Caleb Epstein, Heather Klusaritz, and Carolyn C. Cannuscio. 2018. "Public Libraries as Partners for Health." *Preventing Chronic Disease* 15. https://doi.org/10.5888/pcd15.170392.

Whitney, Wanda, Alla Keselman, and Betsy Humphreys. 2017. "Libraries and Librarians: Key Partners for Progress in Health Literacy Research and Practice." *Information Services & Use* 37, no. 1: 85–100. https://doi.org/10.3233/isu-170821.

Wood, Frederick B., Elliot R. Siegel, Gale A. Dutcher, Angela Ruffin, Robert A. Logan, and John C. Scott. 2005. "The National Library of Medicine's Native American Outreach Portfolio: A Descriptive Overview." *Journal of the Medical Library Association* 93 (4 Suppl): S21–S34. https://www.ncbi.nlm.nih.gov/pmc/articles/PMC1255750/.

World Health Organization. 2020a. "7 Steps to Flatten the Infodemic Curve." October 2, 2020. https://www.who.int/news-room/spotlight/let-s-flatten-the-infodemic-curve.

World Health Organization. 2020b. "Managing the COVID-19 Infodemic: Promoting Healthy Behaviours and Mitigating the Harm from Misinformation and Disinformation." September 23, 2020. https://www.who.int/news/item/23-09-2020-managing-the-covid-19-infodemic-promoting-healthy-behaviours-and-mitigating-the-harm-from-misinformation-and-disinformation.

World Health Organization. 2021."EPI-WIN: WHO Information Network for Epidemics." Accessed February 11, 2022. https://www.who.int/teams/risk-communication.

Zarocostas, John. 2020. "How to Fight an Infodemic." *Lancet* 395, no. 10225: 676.

14

Addressing Health Misinformation in the Infodemic Era

The Alaska Public Health Information Response Team

Jennifer Meyer, Joy Chavez Mapaye, Alexandra Edwards, Thomas Hennessy, Tim Hinterberger, and Mary Ryan

THIS CHAPTER DISCUSSES the Alaska Public Health Information Response Team, a community-engaged public health intervention designed to monitor and rapidly respond online to health misinformation on Facebook. Launched in October 2020, we developed a cross-disciplinary system to provide fact-based information that supports Alaskans in making health decisions. This collaboration between the University of Alaska Anchorage and the Alaska Public Health Association is the first known effort to address online misinformation in Alaska.

This effort combines the scientific expertise of public health, strategic communications theory, and computer science. Our team has worked to assess the significance of the misinformation problem and evaluate our efforts to mitigate the impact of misinformation on the local media landscape, potentially influencing community norms and individual health behaviors.

Alongside climate change, infectious diseases, and air pollution, vaccine hesitancy was named one of the top ten threats to global health by the World Health Organization (2019). Online misinformation undermines adherence to public health mitigation guidance and vaccine uptake locally, nationally, and globally (Hoffman et al. 2019; Larson 2018). The spread of health misinformation through social media has been identified as one of the most significant global health risks (Larson 2018; Vogel 2017). The COVID-19 pandemic has intensified these concerns, leading the World Health Organization to warn of an "infodemic" spreading misinformation about vaccine safety, downplaying the potential severity of disease, discrediting protective behaviors, and promoting unsafe or ineffective treatments that can directly harm people's health and well-being ("The COVID-19 Infodemic" 2020).

Efforts to describe and determine key characteristics of misinformation and its virality, along with effective interventions for reaching vaccine-hesitant groups, will be necessary to overcome the COVID-19 epidemic globally. Until we can meet this need, vaccine uptake will lag, and hesitancy among at-risk populations will persist, placing families and communities at risk for future outbreaks (MacDonald 2015). Health misinformation in general and COVID-19 misinformation specifically have led to dramatic gaps in the application of COVID-19 mitigation strategies and vaccine uptake. These disparities disproportionately impact historically marginalized racial and ethnic groups, as well as groups with limited access to health care information and services. An equity-informed strategy to combat misinformation has the potential to reduce health disparities and improve population health outcomes by generating increased public support for science-based public health policies.

History

Misinformation in the public sphere has existed for centuries, and in the last seventy years, it has been expertly exploited by those aiming to further their interests (Oreskes and Conway 2010). Recall the now-famous 1969 tobacco industry memo, noted by Milberger et al. (2006), from public relations firm Brown & Williamson, which stated, "Doubt is our product since it is the best means of competing with the body of fact that exists in the mind of the general public. It is also a means of establishing a controversy."

Selling doubt is a far easier task than explaining the nuances of scientific findings, which always have limitations. The anti-vaccine disinformation apparatus manufactures doubt by leveraging scientific uncertainty and elements of human psychology to help their claims penetrate the global media landscape (Oreskes and Conway 2010; Romer and Jamieson 2021). Filling gaps in human understanding with conspiracies or false claims brings both comfort to and commitment from the consumer. Not only has the internet allowed false claims to travel quickly, but technology now allows those claims to sit in people's pockets, constantly ready to support confirmation bias, and acts as an easily accessible dispensary of fake cures and supplements (Howard 2019). Scientists and physicians have sounded the alarm against anti-vaccine misinformation for decades (Hotez 2020). Others have sought to build the public's media and science literacy skills (Caulfield 2020), while still more voices have urged scientists to become better communicators (Offit 2011; Sagan and Druyan 1997).

At the beginning of the COVID-19 pandemic, leaders of the World Health Organization and the United Nations warned of an "infodemic" of misinformation ("Managing the COVID-19 Infodemic: Promoting Healthy Behaviours and Mitigating the Harm from Misinformation and Disinformation," n.d.). To prevent the global public health response from being undermined by misinformation, they urged solidarity, information surveillance, collaboration with communications specialists, and myth-busting to blunt its impact. The Alaska Public Health Information Response Team aimed to answer this call to action.

Alaska

Demographer Chad Ferrell notes that Anchorage, Alaska, is home to one of the most diverse census tracts in the United States (Farrell and Lee 2018). Alaska is also home to large populations of those deeply impacted by past and present pandemics, such as Indigenous peoples and others whose historical oppression places them at higher risk of negative health outcomes (Fortuine 1989; Hatcher 2020).

Racial/ethnic minorities in Alaska are vulnerable to disparate COVID-19 outcomes. People who were identified as Native Hawaiian or Pacific Islander, Alaska Native/American Indian, Asian, or Black had higher COVID-19 death rates than the general population (McLaughlin and Castrodale 2021a; Shiels et al. 2021). As of April 2021, more than half (52 percent) of non-white Alaskans had not received a COVID-19 vaccine (Alaska Department of Health and Social Services Coronavirus Response Hub, n.d.). In a March 2021 statewide survey, among non-white respondents who had not received a COVID-19 vaccine, more than 70 percent were hesitant to be vaccinated compared to 35 percent of the general population (McLaughlin and Castrodale 2021b). Most vaccine-hesitant survey respondents reported that their primary reasons for not being vaccinated were safety concerns, belief that COVID-19 was not serious, or that they were at low risk for illness, mistrust of the vaccine, or endorsing misconceptions/conspiracy theories regarding the vaccine (McLaughlin and Castrodale 2021b). These findings suggest that misinformation may support vaccine hesitancy.

While literature describing the depth, breadth, and spread of health misinformation on social media has expanded over the last decade, few articles have examined strategies for responding to and correcting misinformation, and even fewer have examined how medical and public health professionals might confront health misinformation (Caulfield 2020). Recent studies that have explored this question have found that there is substantial potential for medical and health professionals to successfully address and correct health misinformation, especially if they are provided with proper training and resources (Office of the Surgeon General 2021). The search for solutions to the COVID-19 misinformation problem can be informed by the experiences of colleagues who have addressed very similar communication challenges around climate change (Cook, Lewandowsky, and Ecker 2017).

Response

The Office of the US Surgeon General's July 2021 advisory report called health misinformation an "urgent threat" and offered a comprehensive set of recommendations for health professionals and health organizations to partner with local organizations to prevent and address it. The report called on doctors, nurses, and other clinicians to be proactive about health misinformation and to engage with patients and the public in meaningful ways. The surgeon general also encouraged the use of media platforms and other technology to share accurate health information. The Alaska Public Health Information Response Team offers one example of how public health and health care practitioners partnered with communications experts and technical applications to respond to online health misinformation. This project may provide a case study and inform best practices going forward.

Organizing for Success

The inspiration for the Alaska Public Health Information Response Team came from two earlier public health response projects. The first was the University of Alaska Anchorage's smoke- and tobacco-free campaign, which led to a systemwide smoke- and tobacco-free policy for the University of Alaska Anchorage (2015). Students who were enrolled in a strategic communications campaigns class, along with public health practitioners from tobacco-free coalitions, mobilized online to combat misinformation regarding the proposed policy. The second inspiration was the work of Dr. Todd Wolynn, whose medical practice was attacked on social media by anti-vaccine activists. In response, Dr. Wolynn developed defense strategies and organized a volunteer group of health professionals ("Shots Heard Round the World") to rapidly respond to similar attacks on other health care providers (Wolynn and Hermann 2021). Both examples demonstrate the need for real-time responses to online misinformation from subject matter experts.

The United Nations Children's Fund (2020), along with partners at Yale University and the Public Good Projects, also offers a useful Misinformation Management Field Guide, which contains a broad, four-step approach to managing misinformation. These four steps are: prepare a team, perform media listening, analyze the types of misinformation and develop responses, and then engage strategically through coordinated campaigns while monitoring for impact. Based on the recommendations of the US surgeon general, UNICEF, and these earlier inspirational efforts, the team has now developed a set of best practices to mitigate the spread of misinformation and the resulting health and social harms it may cause. Overall, strategies to address health misinformation and the infodemic can be summarized as follows: (1) build health and news media literacy; (2) monitor social media for misinformation patterns and trends; (3) respond to and correct identified misinformation with credible and accurate messages that do not inadvertently increase the spread of misinformation; (4) amplify trusted voices; (5) implement algorithms and other mechanisms for identifying and slowing the spread of online misinformation by technology companies; and (6) build coalitions among government agencies, news media, community organizations, and the scientific community to share resources, information, and consistent messaging. These principles have influenced the Alaska team's approach.

Developing Response Skills

In consideration of these principles, our team also applies three core elements to counter misinformation: real-time surveillance, accurate diagnosis, and a rapid response that is modeled after basic applied field epidemiology concepts. Typically, for infectious disease surveillance, epidemiologists define the characteristics of the "case" by analyzing descriptive statistics, such as frequency among different demographics, and by identifying factors that enhance or reduce an individual's susceptibility to infection (Rassmusen and Goodman 2018). We assess similar factors in misinformation identified through regular social media listening and daily media surveillance of Facebook—the most heavily used social media platform. The second step includes accurate diagnosis of the types of misinformation that appear to have high spread; in other words, prioritize the most serious cases for response. Third, we rapidly develop and deliver counter-messaging that could mitigate the impact of the misinformation.

The Alaska Public Health Information Response Team has two primary goals:

1. Reduce the spread of misinformation related to COVID-19 by responding with science-based messages on key Alaska public-facing Facebook pages.
2. Increase public trust in public health prevention and intervention strategies.

In addition to these goals, the team hopes that its presence on Facebook threads helps "break through the silence." The spiral of silence mass communication theory describes how individuals fear isolation and stay silent if their views are in the minority (Noelle-Neumann 1974). The spiral begins when individuals perceived to be in the minority stop speaking out, leaving the opinion of the perceived majority to be incorrectly recognized as dominant. In one analysis, just twelve people drove most vaccine misinformation on social media (Bond 2021). An internal Facebook study divided US users, groups, and pages into 638 population segments. Research found that just 10 of the 638 segments contained 50 percent of vaccine-hesitant content (Dwoskin 2021). This vocal minority can appear dominant in some individuals' social media news feeds. Figure 14.1 illustrates an example of breaking this spiral of silence to allow space for another voice to enter the conversation.

The volunteers were taught to respond using the "Triple E" approach developed by the team: empathy, education, and engagement. The volunteers also received training on using a "truth sandwich," a communication technique described in the guidance from *The Debunking Handbook 2020* (Lewandowsky et al. 2020) to help frame responses. The volunteers were taught to simply correct misinformation using facts from credible sources. We sought to avoid distracting, back-and-forth arguments with the person who posted the misinformation by refraining from using their name, as well as not using personal attacks or derogatory comments. The team aimed to write for the readers of the comment thread, not the person posting the misinformation. The volunteers were asked to either respond directly to the misinformation comment (see figure 14.2) with a referenced source (Vraga and Bode 2018) or place a new general comment at the top of the thread expressing either an overall observation and/or correction (see figure 14.1) or a positive public health message that includes graphics and other visuals to help engage readers (see figure 14.3).

Process

Since the inception of the project, the team has received requests from communities across Alaska to monitor popular public pages. Students now conduct media listening and monitoring for misinformation on more than twenty-five public-facing Facebook pages. The process was cyclical and included social media monitoring, identifying misinformation, notifying course instructors, vetting, alerting volunteer responders, and responding. For monitoring, the students looked for relevant health misinformation on selected public Facebook pages, particularly on topics related to COVID-19, such as false claims regarding remedies, vaccines, and case numbers; personal opinions were excluded. The student monitors used the World Health Organization and Centers for Disease Control and Prevention websites as factual references. Once misinformation was found, the students copied the unique URL link to the Facebook comment, noted the nature of the comment, and took a screenshot. The students then notified the course instructor via a free two-way communications application on smartphones for classroom announcements (Remind). The course instructor confirmed that the posts contained factually incorrect information regarding COVID-19 mitigation strategies, policies, or vaccines and sent them on to the volunteer responders via both email and Remind. These alerts also included direct links to the Facebook misinformation posts. Misinformation comments flagged by student monitors, as well as responses from the team, were collected and organized in Microsoft Excel for later analysis. A computer science student assisting with the project later developed an application specifically for data capture and analysis for the project. Figures 14.4 and 14.5 illustrate sample periodic surveillance figures created to help team members visualize the frequency and topic themes of misinformation in near real time, as well as document the volume of debunking and prebunking responses from volunteer responders.

Evaluating the Impact

A process evaluation was conducted for the project to assist us with organizational management and help us identify areas of strengths, weaknesses, and opportunities to remedy problems. The process evaluation focused on describing team organization, monitoring team members' responses to misinformation comments during a specific time period, and the col-

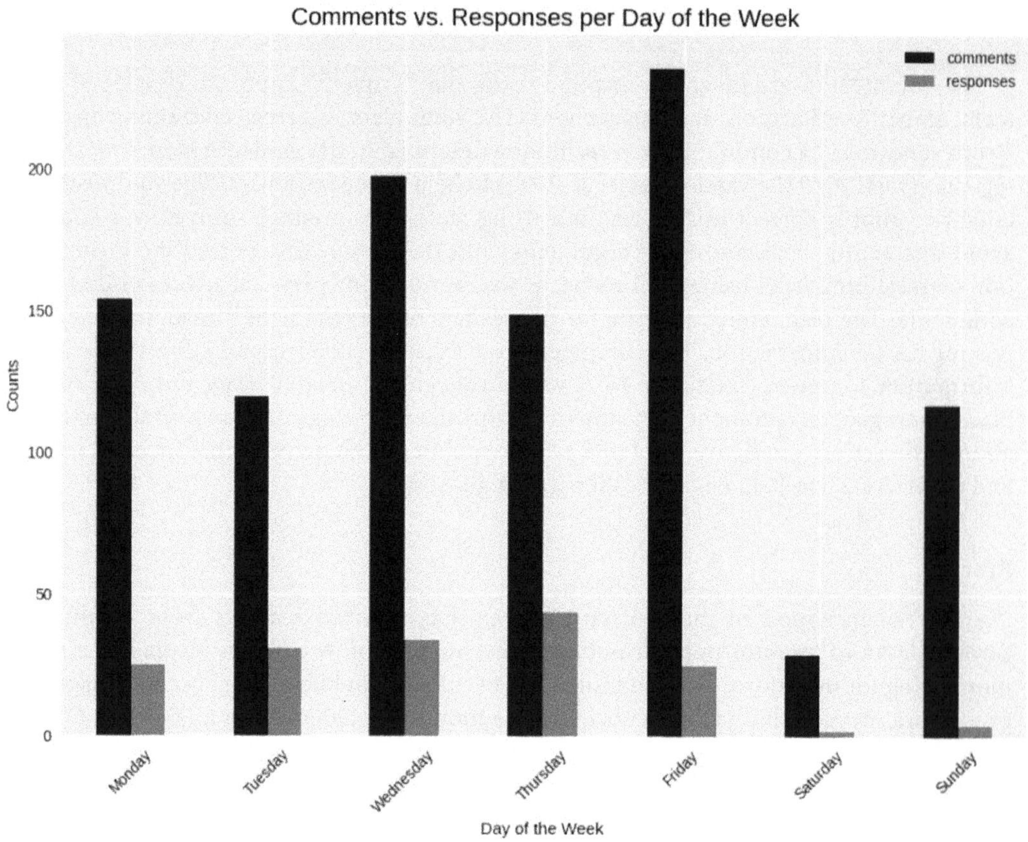

FIGURE 14.4
Weekly Display of Misinformation Comment Flags/Alerts and Team Responses.

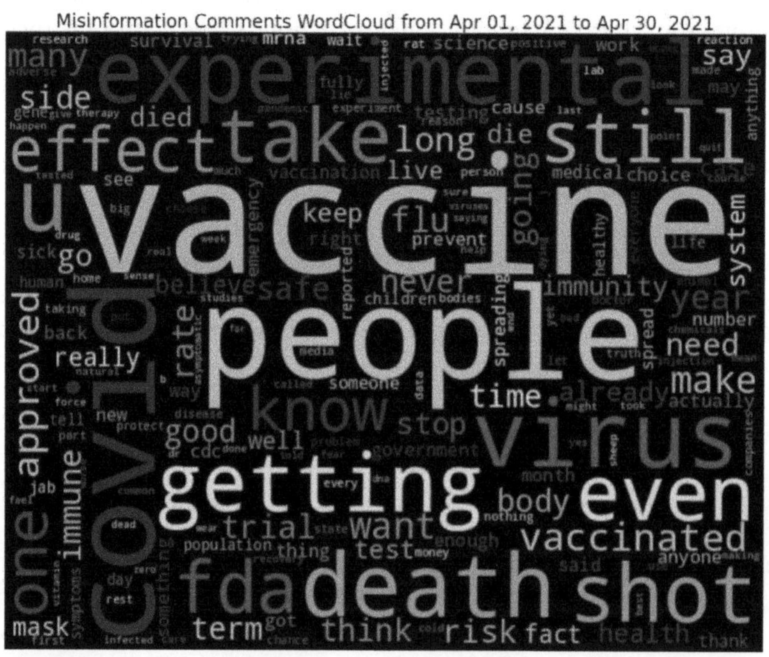

FIGURE 14.5
Wordcloud Illustrating Misinformation Topic Frequency during April 2021.

lection of feedback from team members on their involvement and training needs. The goals the process evaluation intended to help are focused on team organization, monitoring team members' responses to misinformation comments during a specific time period, and the collection of feedback from team members on their involvement and training needs. Using this process evaluation, we were ultimately able to identify data needs more accurately for measuring impact going forward as the project expands. Four key questions have provided a framework for evaluation activities thus far:

1. How is the team organized?
2. How are Facebook comments monitored?
3. How does the team respond to comments?
4. Do team responses to misinformation result in a change in public engagement with comments with misinformation?

Research on the effectiveness of correcting misinformation has largely focused on the identification and correction of misinformation in experimental settings (Bode and Vraga 2018) or been performed through surveys documenting health professionals' experiences correcting misinformation on social media (Bautista, Zhang, and Gwizdka 2021). As such, there does not yet seem to be a model framework for monitoring and evaluating the effectiveness of our real-world project. Adding to this challenge, Facebook no longer allows the automated collection of posts and comment data. Even newer methods of data collection, such as the Facebook-owned CrowdTangle ("What Data Is CrowdTangle Tracking?" n.d.), do not allow for the gathering of engagement information at the comment level. Furthermore, data are only available for public-facing Facebook pages with more than fifty thousand likes, which would eliminate all but three of the Alaska Facebook pages being monitored by the project.

These challenges necessitated the development of ad hoc data collection tools, including an online form to record each misinformation alert distributed through the Remind app and a cloud-based app developed specifically for the Alaska Public Health Information Response Team that used machine learning to analyze flagged misinformation comments. Both methods required the manual review and logging of each link to identify such comments, and the cloud-based app also required manual copying and pasting of the comments. Data collected through the online form included the Facebook post date, time, and topic (e.g., vaccines); the Remind alert date and time; public engagement with the post (i.e., the number of comments on the post; the number and type of reaction emojis such as likes, hearts, and angry faces; and the number of shares); the link to the misinformation comment; the misinformation topic (e.g., vaccines cause autism); whether and how many team members provided a correction and the types of public engagement with the correction(s); and whether and how many team members commented elsewhere under the post. In addition, graphic memes posted as comments by misinformation commenters were archived for later analysis.

From January 1 to April 30, 2021, monitors flagged 338 posts with 443 misinformation comments on Alaska-based Facebook pages. Almost three-quarters (73 percent) of the identified comments were made on one of three pages—two popular local news pages and the page of the Alaska Department of Health and Social Services. Once triaged, 82 percent of the misinformation comments were sent as alerts to volunteers within forty-eight hours of the comment being made (minimum thirty-five minutes, maximum thirty-four days). Posts with misinformation comments had an average of 118 comments, 68 shares, and 216 reactions in the full thread. Approximately, 46 percent of the misinformation posts were related to COVID-19 vaccines,

17 percent were related to COVID-19 mitigation strategies (not vaccines), and 4 percent were about emergency orders such as masking and capacity restrictions. Additional topics fell below the 4 percent threshold and made up the remainder.

Each identified misinformation post had an average of two team members providing countering comments, either directly to the misinformation comment or elsewhere in the comment threads. Approximately, 80 percent of all the identified misinformation comments had a team member respond in some way, either directly or generally at the top of the thread, while 41 percent had a team member provide a direct countering response. Between January 1 and April 30, 2021, team members collectively made 1,212 comments correcting misinformation. Positive public engagement (positive reactions or supportive comments) outweighed negative engagement: there were 2,948 comments and reactions to team corrections and only 28 percent were negative.

Challenges and Next Steps

While thirty volunteer responders were recruited between January and April 2021, only approximately one-third of the volunteers consistently provided corrections on Facebook. In one brief team member survey conducted in April 2021, volunteer responders cited time as a barrier to participation, and some noted that they feared harassment or that they found participation mentally and emotionally taxing. They also felt that they needed more training on how to respond or preferred to use already-developed template responses to ensure that they were providing accurate counter-information. We recommended changes to the dissemination of alerts, added resources, and made training adjustments. Additional team processes were needed to reduce the barriers to participation and increase team members' sense of team support.

Although the team has gained clarity of purpose through practice and received positive feedback from readers, community members, public information officers, and Alaska-based media coverage, challenges remain. For example, data monitoring indicates that the volume of misinformation outnumbers the team members' capacity to correct it. Maintaining and growing the number of volunteer responders are challenges yet to be addressed. As with any volunteer effort, it can be difficult to balance the demands of work and family, and the unpleasant nature of social media can be a deterrent to participation. To meet the goal of responding in force to each post of misinformation, it will be necessary to encourage a higher level of participation and engage in frequent recruitment efforts.

The next phase of the project will use a more comprehensive approach to addressing online misinformation, building on the monitoring and response efforts already established. In public health, successful interventions aim simultaneously at multiple levels. At the individual level, we plan to continue prebunking and debunking misinformation online and to study the effects of different types of responses. At the community level, we plan to work with educators and students to develop media literacy skills to identify and respond effectively to misinformation. At the systems level, the team has developed relationships with marketing and public relations agencies and social media professionals to discuss methods for reducing the spread of misinformation at the source. We also intend to improve our own process and evaluation efforts by increasingly automating the tracking and monitoring of sources and the spread of misinformation in Alaska. The team is also working on machine learning technologies that could potentially assist and automate online misinformation monitoring and response.

We will build on the efforts of the Alaska Public Health Information Response Team to strengthen trust and mitigate the threat of vaccine misinformation among vulnerable populations. The objectives of the next phase are:

1. Identify factors that influence individual-, family- and community-level COVID-19 vaccine acceptance among vulnerable populations by the end of the first quarter of the project.
2. Neutralize 5 percent or more of identified COVID-19 misinformation on selected Facebook pages every week throughout the span of the project.
3. Develop and disseminate targeted and culturally appropriate COVID-19 vaccine messages to increase vaccine acceptability among vulnerable populations by the end of the second quarter of the project.

The project team has experience accomplishing similar objectives through previous work on COVID-19 behavioral health surveys, misinformation response, and the development and dissemination of targeted COVID-19 vaccine messaging to vulnerable groups. Given this background, the team knows that the internet is just one component of the larger picture of misinformation in the infodemic era. This next phase calls for addressing misinformation using a holistic approach that incorporates online platforms and in-person spaces and communities. This comprehensive public health approach to misinformation is advocated by the US surgeon general as part of a "whole-of-society" effort to address misinformation. The Alaska Public Health Information Response Team is well positioned to answer this call to action.

Acknowledgments

Special acknowledgment to Katie Cueva, ScD MAT MPH, and Rebecca Van Wyke for editorial and formatting support.

References

Alaska Department of Health and Social Services Coronavirus Response Hub. n.d. "Alaska COVID-19 Information Hub." Accessed January 23, 2022. https://alaska-coronavirus-vaccine-outreach-alaska-dhss.hub.arcgis.com/.

Bautista, John R., Yan Zhang, and Jacek Gwizdka. 2021. "Healthcare Professionals' Acts of Correcting Health Misinformation on Social Media." *International Journal of Medical Informatics* 148 (April): 104375. https://doi.org/10.1016/j.ijmedinf.2021.104375.

Bode, Leticia, and Emily K. Vraga. 2018. "See Something, Say Something: Correction of Global Health Misinformation on Social Media." *Health Communication* 33, no. 9: 1131–40. https://doi.org/10.1080/10410236.2017.1331312.

Bond, Shannon. 2021. "Just 12 People Are Behind Most Vaccine Hoaxes On Social Media, Research Shows." NPR, May 14, 2021. https://www.npr.org/2021/05/13/996570855/disinformation-dozen-test-facebooks-twitters-ability-to-curb-vaccine-hoaxes.

Caulfield, Timothy. 2020. "Pseudoscience and COVID-19—We've Had Enough Already." *Nature*, April 27, 2020. https://doi.org/10.1038/d41586-020-01266-z.

Cook, John, Stephan Lewandowsky, and Ullrich K. H. Ecker. 2017. "Neutralizing Misinformation through Inoculation: Exposing Misleading Argumentation Techniques Reduces Their Influence." *PLoS ONE* 12, no. 5: e0175799. https://doi.org/10.1371/journal.pone.0175799.

Dwoskin, Elizabeth. 2021. "Massive Facebook Study on Users' Doubt in Vaccines Finds a Small Group Appears to Play a Big Role in Pushing the Skepticism." *Washington Post*, March 14, 2021. https://www.washingtonpost.com/technology/2021/03/14/facebook-vaccine-hesistancy-qanon/.

Farrell, Chad R., and Barrett A. Lee. 2018. "No-Majority Communities: Racial Diversity and Change at the Local Level." *Urban Affairs Review* 54, no. 5: 866–97. https://doi.org/10.1177/1078087416682320.

Fortuine, Robert. 1989. *Chills and Fever: Health and Disease in the Early History of Alaska*. Fairbanks, AK: University of Alaska Press.

Hatcher, Sarah M. 2020. "COVID-19 Among American Indian and Alaska Native Persons—23 States, January 31–July 3, 2020." *MMWR. Morbidity and Mortality Weekly Report* 69. https://doi.org/10.15585/mmwr.mm6934e1.

Hoffman, Beth L., Elizabeth M. Felter, Kar-Hai Chu, Ariel Shensa, Chad Hermann, Todd Wolynn, Daria Williams, and Brian A. Primack. 2019. "It's Not All about Autism: The Emerging Landscape of Anti-Vaccination Sentiment on Facebook." *Vaccine* 37, no. 16: 2216–23. https://doi.org/10.1016/j.vaccine.2019.03.003.

Hotez, Peter J. 2020. "Combating Antiscience: Are We Preparing for the 2020s?" *PLoS Biology* 18 (3): e3000683. https://doi.org/10.1371/journal.pbio.3000683.

Howard, Jonathan. 2019. *Cognitive Errors and Diagnostic Mistakes: A Case-Based Guide to Critical Thinking in Medicine*. Cham, Switzerland: Springer.

Larson, Heidi J. 2018. "The Biggest Pandemic Risk? Viral Misinformation." *Nature* 562 (7727): 309. https://doi.org/10.1038/d41586-018-07034-4.

Lewandowsky, S., J. Cook, U. K. H. Ecker, D. Albarracín, M. A. Amazeen, P. Kendeou, et al. 2020. *The Debunking Handbook 2020*. Databrary. https://doi.org/10.17910/b7.1182.

MacDonald, Noni E. 2015. "Vaccine Hesitancy: Definition, Scope and Determinants." *Vaccine*, WHO Recommendations Regarding Vaccine Hesitancy 33 (34): 4161–64. https://doi.org/10.1016/j.vaccine.2015.04.036.

"Managing the COVID-19 Infodemic: Promoting Healthy Behaviours and Mitigating the Harm from Misinformation and Disinformation." n.d. Accessed February 11, 2022. https://www.who.int/news/item/23-09-2020-managing-the-covid-19-infodemic-promoting-healthy-behaviours-and-mitigating-the-harm-from-misinformation-and-disinformation.

McLaughlin, Joe, and Louisa Castrodale. 2021a. "Summary of COVID-19 Deaths—Alaska, January 1 through October 15, 2020." Accessed January 10, 2022. http://www.epi.alaska.gov/bulletins/docs/b2020_13.pdf.

McLaughlin, Joe, and Louisa Castrodale. 2021b. "Statewide COVID-19 Survey Results." Accessed January 23, 2022. http://www.epi.alaska.gov/bulletins/docs/rr2021_02.pdf.

Milberger, Sharon, Ronald M. Davis, Clifford E. Douglas, John K. Beasley, David Burns, Thomas Houston, and Donald Shopland. 2006. "Tobacco Manufacturers' Defence against Plaintiffs' Claims of Cancer Causation: Throwing Mud at the Wall and Hoping Some of It Will Stick." *Tobacco Control* 15 (Suppl 4), no. Suppl 4: iv17–26. https://doi.org/10.1136/tc.2006.016956.

Noelle-Neumann, Elisabeth. 1974. "The Spiral of Silence A Theory of Public Opinion." *Journal of Communication* 24, no. 2: 43–51. https://doi.org/10.1111/j.1460-2466.1974.tb00367.x.

Office of the Surgeon General. 2021. *Confronting Health Misinformation: The U.S. Surgeon General's Advisory on Building a Healthy Information Environment*. Washington, DC: US Department of Health and Human Services.

Offit, Paul A. 2011. *Deadly Choices: How the Anti-Vaccine Movement Threatens Us All*. New York, NY: Basic Books.

Oreskes, Naomi, and Erik M. Conway. 2010. *Merchants of Doubt: How a Handful of Scientists Obscured the Truth on Issues from Tobacco Smoke to Global Warming*. New York, NY: Bloomsbury Press.

Rassmusen, Sonja, and Richard Goodman. 2018. *The CDC Field Epidemiology Manual*. Oxford, New York: Oxford University Press.

Romer, Daniel, and Kathleen H. Jamieson. 2021. "Patterns of Media Use, Strength of Belief in COVID-19 Conspiracy Theories, and the Prevention of COVID-19 from March to July 2020 in the United States: Survey Study." *Journal of Medical Internet Research* 23, no. 4: e25215. https://doi.org/10.2196/25215.

Sagan, Carl, and Ann Druyan. 1997. *The Demon-Haunted World: Science as a Candle in the Dark*. New York, NY: Random House.

Shiels, Meredith S., Anika T. Haque, Emily A. Haozous, Paul S. Albert, Jonas S. Almeida, Montserrat García-Closas, Anna M. Nápoles, Eliseo J. Pérez-Stable, Neal D. Freedman, and Amy Berrington de González. 2021. "Racial and Ethnic Disparities in Excess Deaths During the COVID-19 Pandemic, March to December 2020." *Annals of Internal Medicine*, October. https://doi.org/10.7326/M21-2134.

"The COVID-19 Infodemic." 2020. *The Lancet Infectious Diseases* 20, no. 8: 875. https://doi.org/10.1016/s1473-3099(20)30565-x.

United Nations Children's Fund. 2020. "Vaccine Misinformation Management Field Guide." Accessed January 15, 2022. https://www.unicef.org/mena/reports/vaccine-misinformation-management-field-guide.

University of AlaskaAnchorage. 2015. "UAA to Go Tobacco-Free Nov. 19, 2015." Accessed January 23, 2022. https://www.uaa.alaska.edu/news/archive/2015/03/uaa-to-go-tobacco-free-nov-19-2015.cshtml.

Vogel, Lauren. 2017. "Viral Misinformation Threatens Public Health." *CMAJ* 189, no. 50: E1567. https://doi.org/10.1503/cmaj.109-5536.

Vraga, Emily K., and Leticia Bode. 2018. "I Do Not Believe You: How Providing a Source Corrects Health Misperceptions across Social Media Platforms." *Information, Communication & Society* 21, no. 10: 1337–53. https://doi.org/10.1080/1369118X.2017.1313883.

"What Data Is CrowdTangle Tracking?" n.d. Accessed February 11, 2022. http://help.crowdtangle.com/en/articles/1140930-what-data-is-crowdtangle-tracking.

Wolynn, Todd, and Chad Hermann. 2021. "Shots Heard Round the World: Better Communication Holds the Key to Increasing Vaccine Acceptance." *Nature Immunology* 22, no. 9: 1068–70. https://doi.org/10.1038/s41590-021-00998-y.

World Health Organization. 2019. "Ten Threats to Global Health in 2019." Accessed January 22, 2022. https://www.who.int/news-room/spotlight/ten-threats-to-global-health-in-2019.

Index

AAPI. *See* Asian Americans and Pacific Islanders
Abadie, Roberto, 115
absolute differences, 81
ACA. *See* Affordable Care Act
accuracy, of health information, 71–72
Achterberg, P., 106, 107
Adams, Samantha, 73
advertising, misleading, 7
Affordable Care Act (ACA), 198
Agley, J., 111, 115–16
Aguillo, Isidro, 69
AIDS: conspiracy theories about, 20, 109; COVID-19 pandemic parallels with, 19–20; denialism, 19–20; disinformation and, 19–20; misinformation and, 19–20; racism and, 19. *See also* HIV
ALA. *See* American Library Association
Alaska: COVID-19 in, 208–9, 217; demographics of, 208–9; heath misinformation in, 209; racism in, 208–9
Alaska Department of Health and Social Services, 215
Alaska Public Health Information Response Team, 207; challenges to, 216–17; establishment, 209–10; goals of, 210–11; impact of, 213–16; process of, 213; response skills of, 210–11
algorithms, on social media, 31–32
AlKhaja, Alwaleed K., 10
Al Khaja, Khalid A. J., 10
Allam, Ahmed, 69
alternative facts, 17
alternative medicine. *See* complementary and alternative medicine
Alvarez-Galvez, Javier, 34, 36
AMA. *See* American Medical Association
American Association for the Advancement of Science, 98
American College of Physicians, 101
American Library Association (ALA), 63; Libraries Transforming Communities initiative, 189
American Medical Association (AMA), 67, 68
American Public Health Association, 211
analytical thinking, 24, 34–35
Annona muricata, 7
antibiotics, 141–42
anti-vaccine movement, 45; on Facebook, 35; on social media, 23–24, 25–26
anxiety, OHI and, 62–63
Aral, Sinan, 32
Ashgedom, Ermias Joseph, 121
Asian Americans and Pacific Islanders (AAPI), 125; discrimination against, 127–28
AstraZeneca, 7
autism, vaccines and, 9, 92
automated bots. *See* bots
axis scaling, 82, *82*

bar charts, 82
Barrett, Stephen, 66
Beauchamp, A. L., 111
belief narratives, 47
Bell, Chris, 106

benchmarks, for misinformation, 9
Best, Alicia L., 113
best available evidence, 9
Bhatti, Rubina, 22
bias, 8, 23–24
Biden, Joe, 126
Biermann, J., 66
Bill and Melinda Gates Foundation, 188
biomedicine, 99–100
Black, Indigenous, and People of Color (BIPOC), 121–22, 127–29; disinformation effects on, 124–25; health outcomes of, 123–24; misinformation effects on, 124–25
Black Americans, 19–20, 200
Blaming Others (Sabatier & Tinker), 20
de Bont, Antoinette, 73
Book Selection Policies for Baltimore's Enoch Pratt Free Library, 64
bots: defining, 21–22; misinformation spread by, 32; proliferation of, on social media, 21–22
Boudewyns, Vanessa, 141
Bowman, Alfredo, 121
Boyer, Pascal, 55
Braden, Gregg, 92
Brainard, Julii, 53
Brashier, Nadia, 150
Bump Club & Beyond, 175
Burkell, Jacquelyn, 72

calculations, 81
Calories Don't Count (Davis), 63–64
Campos-Castillo, Celeste, 194
Canaries in the Coal Min (Collins-Dexter), 128
Caveant Lector et Viewor (article), 65
CBPR. *See* community-based participatory research
CDC. *See* Centers for Disease Control and Prevention
C. difficile, 145
CEAL. *See* Community Engagement Alliance
Centers for Countering Digital Hate, 23, 35
Centers for Disease Control and Prevention (CDC), 9, 93, 97, 105, 170, 213
Centers for Medicare and Medicaid Services (CMS), 198
Chen, Liang, 8
cherry-picking, 7
Chicago Vaccine Hunters, 173
Childs, Sue, 68
China Uncensored, 126
Chinese Americans, 126
Chinese Communist Party, 20
CHL. *See* critical health literacy
Chou, Wen-Ying Sylvia, 4, 10
Christensen, Helen, 69
Churchill, Winston, 93
Circumcision Resource Center, 98
CLAIM Evaluation Tool, 156, 159–60
climate change, 207
CMS. *See* Centers for Medicare and Medicaid Services
Code of Administrative Offenses, 56n1
Cognitive Reflection Test (CRT), 24
Collins-Dexter, Brandi, 128
colloidal silver, 22; for COVID-19, 10
community-based participatory research (CBPR), ix, 189; coalition-building in, 201; Conceptual Model, 195; defining, 194–95; formats, 200; Internet in, 199–200; libraries in, 199; on misinformation categories, *196*, *197*; online participation in, 200; outreach, 194–95; partnership processes, 197
community engagement: CHL for, 189; defining, 187; in eHealth, 198–201; Kranich on, 188–89; libraries in, 197–98
Community Engagement Alliance (CEAL), 198
community-informed approaches, 194–98
complementary and alternative medicine, 34, 51
conservatism, 110–11
conspiracy beliefs, defining, 6
conspiracy theories: about AIDS, 20, 109; COVID-19, 20, 45–46; about COVID-19 vaccines, 22, 95; during crises, 7; defining, 6, 7, 20; echo chambers and, 23–24; psychological predispositions to, 23–24; about vaccines, 25–26; verifiability of, 7
Consumer Health Information Specialization Group, 188
Continuing Medical Education, 143
Cooke, Nicole A., 123, 127
core standards, 66
Corriher, Sarah, 72
Corriher, Thomas, 72
counts, 77
COVID-19, vii, 105, 144, 207; AIDS pandemic parallels with, 19–20; in Alaska, 208–9, 217; case counts, 85; colloidal silver for, 10; conspiracy theories, 20, 45–46; denialism, 19–20; disinformation about, 22–23; Facebook posts on, 22–23; fake news about, 22; false claims about, 22; health literacy and, 62; health misinformation, 168; infodemic in,

17, 25, 50–51; information seeking during, *18*; isolation in, 23; Marathon Webinar, 21; misinformation, 18–19; mortality from, 25, 85; numeracy skills and, 85–86; OHI and disinformation about, 22–23; pseudoscientific health therapies for, 22; racism and, 19; in Russia, 46–47; science evolution in, 168; scientific uncertainty surrounding, 108; SDoH in, 25; social and cognitive disruptions in, 23; in Sub-Saharan Africa, 128; Twitter posts on, 22–23; vaping and, 7, 9. *See also* vaccines, COVID-19
critical cultural literacy, 122; in action, 128–29; defining, 127
critical health literacy (CHL), ix; for community engagement, 189; eHealth and, 189–90; health misinformation and, 193–94; Nutbeam on, *191–93*; trust and, 194
CrowdTangle, 215
CRT. *See* Cognitive Reflection Test
cyber troops, 21
Cynefin framework, 98

Da, Jingwei, 24
DAERI database, 67
Daraz, Lubna, 68
data: access to, 38; collection of, on social media, 31–32, 215; on Facebook, 215; graphics, 82; metadata, 68
Davis, Adele, 63–64
decision-making, 189; of HCPs, 140–41
Delamothe, Tony, 70
democracy, science and, 93
demographics, on social media, 31
denialism, vii; AIDS, 19–20; COVID-19, 19–20; scientific, 108
denominators, 81
Derakhshan, Hossein, 123
Deshpande, Aniruddha K., 8
Deshpande, Shruti Balvalli, 8
Dhaliwal, D., 92
Dhanani, L. Y., 114
diabetes, 97
Diepgen, Thomas L., 69
digital health, 116
directionality, 84
disbelief narratives, 47
DISCERN instrument, 68, 71–72
disinformation: AIDS and, 19–20; BIPOC impacted by, 124–25; about COVID-19, 22–23; defining, vii, 6, 17; misinformation distinguished from, 8, 92; psychological predispositions to, 23–24
DNA, COVID-19 vaccines and, 95, 97
Dow, Benjamin J., 23
Down Syndrome, 94
drug advertising, 7
Drummond, C., 112
Duesberg, Peter, 19
Duesberg hypothesis, 19
Duke Program on Medical Misinformation, 138
Duke University, 143
Dunn, Dana S., 162
Duran, Bonnie, 194–95

eating disorders, 32
EBM. *See* evidence-based medicine
echo chambers: conspiracy theories and, 23–24; social media, 31–32
Ecker, Ullrich K. H., 10
Eckert, Erin, 142
ecological model, of information seeking, 18
education, trust in science and, 112
eHealth: CHL and, 189–90; community engagement in, 198–201; defining, 187; Eysenbach on, 187; misinformation, 189–90
Einstein, Albert, 81
Engage for Equity, 195
engagement. *See* community engagement
Environmental Protection Agency (EPA), 110
epistemic vigilance, 55
Epoch Times, 126
Escape Room, 190
evaluative categories, 84
Evans, Kiameesha R., 113
evidence-based medicine (EBM), 140; defining, 91; misinformation and, 101–2
evidence-based practices, 9; of HCPs, 140
Eysenbach, G., 68, 72; on eHealth, 187

Facebook, 36, 207, 210; anti-vaccine movement on, 35; COVID-19 posts on, 22–23; data on, 215; IMPACT on, 172–73
face-to-face settings, 7
fact-checking, 9
fake news: about COVID-19, 22; defining, 6, 7; IPC and receptivity towards, 24–25
fake news laws, 46
Fallis, Don, 8
false claims, 8; about COVID-19, 22; defining, 9–10
Family Doctor, 63

FDA. *See* Food and Drug Administration
Federal Trade Commission, 39
Feinstein, N. W., 100
Fensham, Peter, 98
Ferguson Municipal Public Library, 198
Ferrell, Chad, 208
filter failure, 188
First Amendment, 33
Fischhoff, B., 112
Fitzpatrick, Lisa, 200
Fletcher, Jim, 95
Fletcher, Rita, 95
Food and Drug Administration (FDA), 7, 105, 176
food stamps, 194
Franz, B., 114
fraud, 91–92; victimization from, 66
freedom of expression, 33
freedom of speech, on social media, 33
Freelon, Deen, 125–26
Freimuth, Vicki S., 109

Gab, 37
Gagliardi, Anna, 70–71
Galinsky, Adam, 49
Gauchat, G., 110
Geeng, Christine, 35
generally recognized as safe (GRAS), 7
General Social Survey (GSS), 106, 110
Ghebreyesus, Tedros Adhanom, 168
Ghenai, Amira, 38
Ghosh, Isha, 37
Google Machine, 69
Google Trends, 69
government, trust in, 108–9
GRAS. *See* generally recognized as safe
Greenhill, Kelly, 49
Greenwald, Anthony G., 122
Griffiths, Kathleen, 69
GroupSense, 126
GSS. *See* General Social Survey
Guidry, Jeanine, 35
Gusmano, Michael K., 113
Guyatt, Gordon, 91

H1N1, 109
Haines, Helen, 63
Halpern, Diane F., 162
Hanif, Faisal, 63
Harb, Jenna, 126
harmful behavior, social media reinforcing, 32
HCPs. *See* health care professionals
Healthcare 4.0, 116
health care professionals (HCPs), 137; challenges for, 138; decision-making of, 140–41; EBPs of, 140; health information combated by, 171–81; mitigation strategies of, 142–44; on social media, 170–71; time constraints of, 138–39; training for, 139–42; trust in, 170–71
health equity statements, 198–99
health information: accuracy of, 71–72; challenges in, 69–71; evaluation of, 69–71; HCPs combating, 171–81; proxies and, 71–73; public access to, 62–65; quality of, 71; reliability of, 150; solutions to problems, 67–69
health interventions: defining, 149; in low-income settings, 149–50
health literacy, 61; books and, 63–64; COVID-19 and, 62; information selection and, 63–64; public libraries and, 63; selection criteria, 64–65
health misinformation: automated detection of, 37; case studies on combating, 174–81; challenges in, 7–10; CHL and, 193–94; consistency of terminology in, 7–8; corrections for, 35–36; COVID-19, 168; defining, 3–5, *4*, *5*, 9, 10, 167–68; future research on, 36–39; IMPACT combating, 173–81; in patient-clinician relationship, *169*; prevalence of, 122–24; proposed solutions for, 67–69; public health and, 139; research gaps on, 36–39; science mistrust and, 105–7; on social media, 34–36, 122–24, 169–70
health number communications, 77–78
Health of the Net (HON) Foundation, 67, 72
HealthWyze.com, 72
Heath, Chip, 83
heath misinformation, in Alaska, 209
Henne, Kathryn, 126
heuristics and biases program, 23–24
HIV, vii, 19–20; myths about, 94
Hmielowski, J. D., 114
Holder, Eric Ronald, Jr., 121
HONCode, 71, 72; certification, 68; Toolbar, 73
HON Foundation. *See* Health of the Net Foundation
Hooper, Monica Webb, 113
human papillomavirus (HPV), 35, 113
Hunter, Paul, 53
Hurricane Katrina, 197–98
Hurricane Sandy, 197–98
hydroxychloroquine, 168

identity protective cognition (IPC), fake news receptivity and, 24–25
ideology, *196*; political, 109–11
IHC. *See* Informed Health Choices
Illinois Department of Public Health, 170
Illinois Medical Professionals Action Collaborative Team (IMPACT): case studies, 174–81; on COVID-19 vaccines, 176–78; on Facebook, 172–73; health misinformation combated by, 173–81; infographics, 177, *178*, *179*, *180*, *181*; on Instagram, YouTube, and TikTok, 173; on masking, 175–76; messaging of, 175–76; partnerships, 175; rapid response team, 174–75; on Twitter, 171–72
IMLS. *See* Institute Museum and Library Services
immigrant communities, 36–37
IMPACT. *See* Illinois Medical Professionals Action Collaborative Team
Imperva Cyber Security, 21–22
Impicciatore, Pietro, 71
inaccurate claims: defining, 9–10; in misleading advertising, 7
inappropriately applied science, *169*
Indigenous Americans, 126
infodemic, 3, 45, 91–92, 167–68; causes of, 55–56; coalition building in, 55–56; in COVID-19, 17, 25, 50–51; defining, *6*; dynamics of, *48*; motifs, 46–52; origins of, 52–55; in Russia, 48–56; spread of, *49*; timing of, 48–49; vaccine, *54*; WHO on, 188–89
information evaluability, 83
information seeking: during COVID-19, *18*; ecological model of, 18
information vacuums, 35
Informed Health Choices (IHC), 151; child experience in, 160; context constraints, 154; curricula, 161–62; end-of-term trial, 157; evaluations, 156–58; Key Concepts, *152*, 152–53, *153*; learning resources in, 160–61; measurements of, 156–57; one-year follow-up study, 157–58; primary school learning resources, 153–58; process evaluation, 158–59; teacher experience in, 160; teacher training in, 161; translation, 158–62; use of, in other settings, 158–59; user needs, 154
Instagram, 36, 37; IMPACT on, 173
Institute Museum and Library Services (IMLS), 189
institutional review board (IRB), 113
intent, misinformation and, 8
Internet Book of Critical Care, 21
IPC. *See* identity protective cognition
IRB. *See* institutional review board
von Isenburg, Megan, 142
isolation, in COVID-19, 23
ivermectin, 168

Jackson, Joseph, 138, 142
Jackson, Michael, 121
Jadad, Alejandro R., 70–71
Jaiswal, Jessica, 115
Johnson, B. B., 99, 108
Jones, Alex, 17
Journal of the American Medical Association, 65, 168
junk science, *169*

Kahan, Dan, 24
Kahneman, Daniel, 24
Kashani, Beeta M., 125
Kaufman, D. R., 94
Keene Valley Library, 190
Kennedy, Shirley Duglin, 68
Keselman, A., 94, 97, 101
Kessler, Fondazione Bruno, 22
Khan, Aqsa, 22
Kinkead, Laura, 69
Kitta, Andrea, 53, 55
Klein, William M. P., 4, 10
Klerings, Irma, 188
Klimov, Yura, 50–51
Kouzy, Ramez, 34
Kranich, Nancy C., 188–89
Krauthammer, Michael, 69
Kreps, S. E., 108
Kriner, D. L., 108
Krishna, Arunima, 8

Laestadius, Linnea I., 194
Lambert, F. B., 92
Lancet, 170
Lau, Kimberly, 51
Layton, D. E., 94
Lazer, David, 4, 9
lead, 83
Lee, Jung Jae, 22
levels, 77–78
Lewis, Daniel, 95
library and information science (LIS), 188
Library Reserve Corps, 197–98
Liddell, Jessica, 125
van der Linden, 36

linear scaling, 82
LIS. *See* library and information science
Loomba, Sahil, 22
Lopes, Lisa, 121
low-credibility information, on social media, 22–23
low-income settings, health interventions in, 149–50
Luganda, 154, 159

machine learning, 71
Madraki, Golshan, 37
Making Numbers Count (Heath & Starr), 83
malicious content, 33
malinformation, 123
Mann, Jonathan M., 19, 111, 115
Mannion, C., 92
Marsh, Elizabeth J., 150
masking, IMPACT on, 175–76
Mayo Clinic, 20, 144
Mbeki, Tabo, 19–20
MEDCERTAIN, 67, 68
Medem, 68
media: mistrust in mainstream, 17; science attitudes and, 114. *See also* social media
media literacy, defining, 127
Medialogia, 47
medical folk wisdom (MFW), *6*
Medical Library Association (MLA), 188
medical misinformation. *See* health misinformation
medical mistrust, 112–13
Medscape, 138
Mejova, Yelena, 38
Mesch, G. S., 109
messengers, 196
metadata, 68
MFW. *See* medical folk wisdom
microbiome, 145
Miller, Vicky, 125
miscalibration, 112
misinformation: AIDS and, 19–20; benchmarks for, 9; BIPOC impacted by, 124–25; bots spreading, 32; CBPR on categories of, 196; COVID-19, 18–19; defining, vii, 8–10, 17; disinformation distinguished from, 8, 92; eHealth, 189-90; evidence-based medicine and, 101–2; harm from, 66; history of, 208; intent and, 8; lack of agreement on features of, 8–10; movement of, 37; perceptions and, 8; predisposition for believing, *196*; research on, 33–34; on social media, 17, 32; social media policies for, 38; speed of spread of, 32; susceptibility to, 38; tracking, 34; understandings of, shifting, 33; wordcloud, *214. See also specific topics*
misleading advertising, 7
misleading information, defining, *6*
misperception, defining, *6*
mistrust: in mainstream media, 17; medical, 112–13
MLA. *See* Medical Library Association
MMR, 126, 137
mobile social networking apps (MSNs), 18
Molina, Theda, vii
Morial, Marc, 200
Morton, Deborah J., 113
MRI, 98
MSNs. *See* mobile social networking apps
multimodal approaches, 37–38
multisector efforts, 38–39
Muret, Marc, 69
Murphy, Eddie, 121

Naeem, Salman Bin, 22
Nagler, R. H., 114
NARCH. *See* Native American Research Center for Health
National Academies of Sciences, Engineering, and Medicine, 96
National Health Service, 170
National Institutes of Health (NIH), 109, 198
National Library of Medicine (NLM), 63, 188, 194
National Research Council, 98
Native American Research Center for Health (NARCH), 113
Native Americans, 123
nature of science (NOS), 98
Navar, Ann Marie, 143
Network of the National Library of Medicine, 61
New Tang Dynasty TV, 126
New York Online Access to Health (NOAH), 68
New York Times, 95
Next Generation Science Standards, 98
NIH. *See* National Institutes of Health
NLM. *See* National Library of Medicine
NOAH. *See* New York Online Access to Health
Norway, 154
Norwegian Research Council, 151
NOS. *See* nature of science
numeracy: ambiguity navigation, 80–83; clear communication of health numbers, *87*;

COVID-19 and, 85–86; difficulty of, 80–83; number confusion, avoiding, 86–87; universal precautions approaches to, 79–80; use-relevant context in, 83–85
nurses, 198
Nutbeam, Don, 190; on CHL, *191–93*

O'Brien, Colleen, 8
OECD. *See* Organisation for Economic Cooperation and Development
Oh, April, 4, 10
OHI. *See* online health information
online harassment, 170–71
online health information (OHI): anxiety and, 62–63; COVID-19 disinformation and, 22–23; ecology of, 20–21; quality criteria for, 65–67; social media and, 17–18
online participation, 200
Onondaga County Public Library, 64
Oppenheim, Ben, 49
Organisation for Economic Cooperation and Development (OECD), 97
OurStoryBridge, 190
outdated science, *169*
Oxford University, 72–73

partisanship, 114
partnership structures, *197*
Patel, Vimla L., 94
patient-clinician relationship, health misinformation in, *169*
PCPs. *See* primary care providers
Pearl Harbor, 127–28
peer-review, 3–4, 9
Peng, Tai-Quan, 8
Pennycook, Gordon, 24
perceptions: defining, 8; misinformation and, 8. *See also* misperception
Pew Internet Project, 20
Pew Research Center, 31, 110
Pew surveys, 17
Physician Mommies Chicago, 172
pie charts, 82
Pinchuk, Lindsay, 175
Pinterest, 35, 36
PISA. *See* Program for International Student Assessment
Plambeck, Benjamin, 123
political ideology, in scientific trust, 109–11
popular orientalism, 51
prebunking, 35
presidential election, ,2016, vii
primary care providers (PCPs), 141
Program for International Student Assessment (PISA), 97
progress, narratives of, 46
protection advice, 56n5
proxies, health information and, 71–73
PRSSA. *See* Public Relations Student Society of America
pseudoscience, 23, *169*
pseudoscientific health therapies, for COVID-19, 22
psychological predispositions: to conspiracy theories, 23–24; to disinformation, 23–24
public health, 32; health misinformation and, 139
public libraries, health literacy and, 63
Public Relations Student Society of America (PRSSA), 211
PubMed, 93
Purcell, Gretchen P., 70
Putin, Vladimir, 46

quacks, 121
Quackwatch, 66
quality criteria: for OHI, 65–67; public access of, 62–65; Six Senses, 68
Quinn, S. C., 109, 114

racism: AIDS pandemic and, 19; in Alaska, 208–9; COVID-19 pandemic and, 19
Rand, David G., 24
randomized controlled trials (RCTs), 9
Reddit, 36, 37
reference class, 81
relief thresholds, 84
religion, trust in science and, 111
replication crisis, 99–100
research databases, 3–4
Rios, K., 111
Rissler, L. J., 111
Roozenbeek, Jon, 36
Roy, Deb, 32
rumors: defining, 6, 7; on Twitter, 23
Russia: COVID-19 in, 46–47; infodemic in, 48–56; medical attitudes in, 52–53; vaccines in, 52–54

Sabatier, Renée, 20
Sabin, Janice A., 122
Sandy Hook massacre, 17
Scherer, Laura D., 34
Schleifer, Cyrus, 111, 115

Schwirian, K. P., 109
science: attitudes about, 106–7; conflicting interpretations of, *169*; consensus in, 107; in COVID-19 pandemic, 168; democracy and, 93; education and trust in, 112; inappropriately applied, *169*; interventions for public trust in, 114–16; junk, *169*; knowledge of, 96–99; layperson use of, 93–95; legitimacy of, 99; literacy, 95–101; media and attitudes toward, 114; methodological imperfects of, 99–100; mistrust of and health misinformation, 105–7; nature of, 98; outdated, *169*; political ideology in, 109–11; process of, 107; public understanding of, 107; religion and trust in, 111; social contextual factors and trust in, 112–13; trust in government and, 108–9; uncertainty in, 107–8, *196*
science confidence gap, 107
scientific denialism, 108
SDoH. *See* social determinants of health
search engines, 57n7
Searcher (magazine), 66
self-care management, 20
self-citations, 69
Sequiera, Reginald P., 10
Sheble, Laura, 143
Silberg, William M., 66, 67, 70–71
Sims, James Marion, 124
Singh, Vivek K., 37
Sivaramakrishnan, M., 94
Six Senses, 69; quality criteria, 68
Slovic, P., 99, 108
SLS. *See* social live streaming services
snake oil, 66, 91–92
social contextual factors, trust in science and, 112–13
social determinants of health (SDoH), 113; in COVID-19, 25
social live streaming services (SLS), 18
social media: algorithms on, 31–32; anti-vaccine movement on, 23–24, 25–26; bots proliferating on, 21–22; data collection on, 31–32, 215; decentralization of, 37; demographics on, 31; echo chambers, 31–32; freedom of speech on, 33; harmful behaviors reinforced by, 32; HCP on, 170–71; health care advocates for, 21; health misinformation on, 34–36, 122–24, 169–70; information disseminated on, 21; infrastructure of, 21–22; low-credibility posts on, 22–23; misinformation on, 17, 32; misinformation policies of, 38; news on, 17; OHI and, 17–18; shift to, 20–21
social safety net, 194
social workers, 198
Solomon, M., 108
Sonagara, Darshan, 37
Southwell, Brian G., 139, 142–43
spiral of silence, *211*
Sputnik-V program, 54
Stanford Center for Continuing Medical Education, 144
Stanley, Clark, 91–92
Starr, Karla, 83
Suarez-Lledo, Victor, 34, 36
Sub-Saharan Africans, 124, 151; COVID-19 impact on, 128
Sugerydoor, 65
Swahili, 154
Swire-Thompson, Briony, 4, 9
syndemics, 25
System-1 thinking, 24
System-2 thinking, 24

Taiwan, 51–52
Taiwanese Americans, 125
Tangherlini, Timothy, 47
Testing Treatments, 152
Thaler, Kylie J., 188
Thompson, Teresa L., 8
Thorson, 143
TikTok, 34; IMPACT on, 173
time interval, 81
Tinari, Paul D., 98
Tinker, John, 20
Tomeny, T. S., 92
Towne, Jordan, 123
traditional Chinese medicine, 51
transparency, 38
Triple E approach, *212*, 213
troll-farms, 21, 125–26
Trump, Donald, 20, 125–26
trust: CHL and, 194; education and scientific, 112; in government, 108–9; in HCPs, 170–71; health misinformation and, 105–7; increasing, 116; interventions for, in science, 114–16; mainstream media distrust, 17; of messengers, 196; political ideology and scientific, 109–11; religion and scientific, 111; social contextual factors, 112–13; urban communities and levels of, 113

Tumblr, 36
Tuskegee experiment, 124
Tversky, Amos, 24
Twitter, 36, 37; COVID-19 posts on, 22–23; IMPACT on, 171–72; rumors on, 23; vaccine discourse on, 35

Uganda, 151, 154, 158
uncertainty, scientific, *196*; of COVID-19, 108; in science, 107–8
United Nations International Children's Emergency Fund, 209–10
units, 81
universal precautions, for numeracy skills, 79–80
urban legends, 48–49

vaccines: autism and, 9, 92; conspiracy theories about, 25–26; hesitancy about, 52, 207; infodemic, *54*; in Russia, 52–54; Twitter discourse on, 35; WHO on, 207
vaccines, COVID-19, 139; availability of, 168; conspiracy theories about, 22, 95; DNA and, 95, 97; efficacy of, 86; Emergency Use Authorization, 168; hesitancy about, 176–78; IMPACT on, 176–78; risks, 85–86
VanEvery, Rachel, 125
vaping, COVID-19 and, 7, 9
Vardavas, C., 109
Velasquez, Nicolas, 37
verifiability, of conspiracy theories, 7
Vietnam War, 10, 127
Vincent, 143
Vosoughi, Soroush, 32

Wallerstein, Nina, 194–95
Wang, Xiahohui, 8
Wardle, Claire, 123
Watergate, 10
WebMD, 20
WeChat, 126
Weinhandl, Alexandra S., 188
WhatsApp, 124
Whetten, K., 109
Whitson, Jennifer, 49
WHO. *See* World Health Organization
WHO Information Network for Epidemics, 187
Wikipedia, 200
Wilson, Petra, 70
Wisconsin Health Literacy, 61–62
Wolynn, Todd, 209
Wood, Jamie L., 139, 142, 143
World Health Organization (WHO), 3, 9, 17, 45, 187, 213; on infodemic, 188–89; on vaccines, 207
Wright, Amy L., 125
Wuhan lab, 20
Wyatt, Jeremy C., 71

Yan, Jiaqi, 24
Yang, Ching, 22, 24
yellow journalism, vii
YouTube, 36, 37, 92; IMPACT on, 173

Zhao, Yuehua, 24
Zhukivska, S., 92
Zika, 32
Zikmund-Fisher, Brian J., 83
Zoom, 142

About the Editors

Alla Keselman, PhD, MA, is a senior social science analyst in the Office of Engagement and Training (OET), National Library of Medicine (NLM). She holds a PhD in Human Cognition and Learning and an MA in Biomedical Informatics from Columbia University. Dr. Keselman coordinates NLM efforts in evaluating the impact of its health information outreach and community engagement programs and serves as the NLM lead in the NLM collaboration with the Network of the National Library of Medicine (NNLM) Evaluation Center. Her research interests include the public's understanding of complex health concepts, scientific literacy, and the provision of health information outside clinical settings. She has done work on bringing health and environment-related topics to the science classroom and conducted research into the role of libraries in providing health information to the public.

Catherine Arnott Smith, PhD, is a professor in the Information School at the University of Wisconsin-Madison. She is a former medical librarian who moved into biomedical informatics for her PhD through the Center (now Department) of Biomedical Informatics at the University of Pittsburgh (2002), where she was a National Library of Medicine medical informatics predoctoral trainee. She holds an AMLS (Library and Information Science), MA (American History/Administration of Archives), MSIS (Information Science/Medical Informatics), and PhD (Library and Information Science/Medical Informatics). Her research centers on consumer interactions with clinical information systems, mediated through text, in settings that range from patient portals, to public libraries, to disabilities support centers.

Jointly, **Dr. Catherine Arnott Smith** and **Dr. Alla Keselman** coedited *Meeting Health Information Needs Outside Of Healthcare: Opportunities and Challenges* (2015, Elsevier) and cowrote *Consumer Health Informatics: Enabling Digital Health for Everyone* (2020, Chapman & Hall).

Amanda J. Wilson, MSLS, is chief, Office of Engagement and Training (OET) at the National Library of Medicine (NLM). She holds an MS in Library Science from the University of North Carolina at Chapel Hill and a BA in Music and Psychology from Emory University.

Her leadership of OET focuses on delivering effective, equitable engagement programs that facilitate access to and dissemination of NLM's trusted biomedical and health information resources. Major programs in OET's domestic and international portfolio include the Network of the National Library of Medicine (NNLM), the Environmental Health Information Partnership, and the National Library of Medicine Associate Fellowship program. Ms. Wilson is also an adjunct professor at The Catholic University of America Department of Library and Information Science.

About the Contributors

Chapter 1

Yuan Wang, MPhil, is a doctoral candidate in the Department of Communication at the University of Maryland.

Kathryn Thier, MS, is a doctoral candidate in the Department of Communication at the University of Maryland.

Xiaoli Nan, PhD, is a distinguished scholar-teacher and professor of Communication at the University of Maryland.

Chapter 2

David R. Kaufman, PhD, FACMI, is a clinical associate professor of Medical Informatics in the School of Health Professions at SUNY Downstate Health Sciences University.

Adiebonye E. Jumbo, PhD, ITIL, is an assistant professor of Medical Informatics in the School of Health Professions at SUNY Downstate Health Sciences University.

Tonya N. Taylor, PhD, MS, is an assistant professor in the Department of Medicine, Division of Infectious Disease and STAR Program at SUNY Downstate Health Sciences University.

Chapter 3

Wen-Ying Sylvia Chou, PhD, MPH, is a program director in the Health Communication and Informatics Research Branch at the National Cancer Institute.

Anna Gaysynsky, MPH, is a senior associate at ICF Next, providing programmatic support to the Health Communication and Informatics Research Branch at the National Cancer Institute.

Yuki Lama, PhD, MPH, is a Cancer Research Training Award Fellow in the Health Communication and Informatics Research Branch at the National Cancer Institute.

Chapter 4

Alexandra Arkhipova, PhD, is a senior research fellow at the School of Advanced Studies in Humanities, Presidential Academy for National Economics and Public Administration, Moscow, and a Visiting Research Fellow in Laboratoire d'Anthropologie Sociale, École des hautes études en sciences sociales, Paris, France.

Ian Brodie, PhD, is the professor of Folklore at Cape Breton University, Nova Scotia, Canada.

Chapter 5

Catherine Arnott Smith, PhD, is the professor at the Information School, University of Wisconsin-Madison.

Chapter 6

Brian J. Zikmund-Fisher, PhD, is a professor of Health Behavior and Health Education, a research professor of Internal Medicine, and associate director of the Center for Bioethics and Social Sciences in Medicine at the University of Michigan in Ann Arbor.

Jessica S. Ancker, MPH, PhD, is professor and vice chair for Educational Affairs in the Department of Biomedical Informatics at Vanderbilt University Medical Center.

Chapter 7

Alla Keselman, PhD, MA, is a senior social science analyst in the Office of Engagement and Training, National Library of Medicine, US National Institutes of Health.

Chapter 8

Alla Keselman, PhD, MA, is a senior social science analyst in the Office of Engagement and Training, National Library of Medicine, US National Institutes of Health.

Amanda J. Wilson, MSLS, is chief, Office of Engagement and Training, National Library of Medicine, US National Institutes of Health.

Chapter 9

Jason Alston, PhD, is assistant teaching professor, School of Information Science & Learning Technologies, University of Missouri.

Nicole A. Cooke, PhD, is Augusta Baker Endowed Chair and associate professor, School of Information Science, University of South Carolina.

Chapter 10

Jamie L. Wood, PhD, is assistant professor of the Practice of Medical Education, Duke University School of Medicine.

Erin Eckert, MPA, CPPS, is education coordinator, Duke Center for Healthcare Safety and Quality, Duke University Health System.

Megan von Isenburg, MSLS, is associate dean, Medical Center Library, Duke University.

Joseph Jackson, MD, is associate professor of Pediatrics, General Pediatrics & Adolescent Health, Duke University School of Medicine.

Brian G. Southwell, PhD, is senior director, Science in the Public Sphere Program, RTI International, and adjunct professor, Internal Medicine, Duke University.

Chapter 11

Sarah Rosenbaum, PhD, is a design researcher at the Centre for Epidemic Interventions Research, Norwegian Institute of Public Health.

Allen Nsangi, PhD, is a research fellow at the College of Health Sciences, Makerere University, Uganda.

Daniel Semakula, PhD, is a research fellow at the College of Health Sciences, Makerere University, Uganda.

Chapter 12

Lisa Mordell, MS, is a medical student at the Loyola University Chicago Stritch School of Medicine.

Eve Bloomgarden, MD, is the director of Thyroid and director of Endocrine Innovation and Education Division of Endocrinology at NorthShore University Health Systems.

Shikha Jain, MD, FACP, is an assistant professor of Medicine and the director of Communication Strategies in Medicine at the University of Illinois Chicago.

Vineet Arora, MD, MAPP, is the Herbert T. Abelson Professor of Medicine and the dean for Medical Education at the University of Chicago Pritzker School of Medicine.

Chapter 13

Amanda J. Wilson, MSLS, is chief, Office of Engagement and Training, National Library of Medicine, US National Institutes of Health.

Laura Bartlett, MLS, is a technical information specialist in the Office of Engagement and Training, National Library of Medicine, US National Institutes of Health.

Chapter 14

Jennifer Meyer, PhD, MPH, CPH, RN, is an assistant professor of Public Health at the University of Alaska Anchorage.

Joy Chavez Mapaye, PhD, is a professor of Journalism and Public Communications at the University of Alaska Anchorage.

Alexandra Edwards, MA, MPH, is a research professional III with the Institute of Social and Economic Research at the University of Alaska Anchorage.

Thomas Hennessy, MD, MPH, is an affiliate faculty with the College of Health at the University of Alaska Anchorage.

Tim Hinterberger, PhD, is a professor of Biology with the Alaska WWAMI School of Medical Education.

Mary Ryan, BA, is a University of Alaska Anchorage Alumna and past president of the UAA Public Relations Student Society of America.

www.ingramcontent.com/pod-product-compliance
Ingram Content Group UK Ltd.
Pitfield, Milton Keynes, MK11 3LW, UK
UKHW051932150926
475560UK00005B/361

9 781538 162194